Mickey C. Smith
Editor

Studies
in Pharmaceutical
Economics

Pre-publication
REVIEWS,
COMMENTARIES,
EVALUATIONS . . .

"**S**tudies in Pharmaceutical Economics is a superb and indispensable collection. Sections in the book cover public policy, intervention studies, economics and marketing, economics of noncompliance, and effects on pharmacy services. Each section includes several important chapters that cover topics such as paying for medical technology, Medicaid cost containment, the Iowa capitation experiment, physicians' perceptions of drug prices, economics of drug advertising, worldwide marketing, impacts of noncompliance, managed care, and prescription plans.

Pharmaceutical economics is an evolving research area and an understanding of these papers is critical for survival in the dynamic health care marketplace. This book will be a valuable resource for students, practitioners, and researchers. This is a significant collection of studies and anyone interested in pharmaceuticals and economics should have this book in their personal library."

William F. McGhan, PharmD
Professor, Philadelphia College of Pharmacy and Science

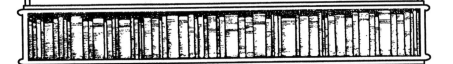

More pre-publication
REVIEWS, COMMENTARIES, EVALUATIONS . . .

"**S**tudies in Pharmaceutical Economics, edited by Mickey C. Smith, provides the academic researcher, student, and practitioner with a valuable pharmacoeconomic resource. This compilation of significant articles, case studies, and research reports covers a wide spectrum of pharmacoeconomic issues relevant to today's rapidly evolving healthcare environment. This timely book assists the reader in achieving a basic understanding of the myriad of factors that impact the cost of pharmaceutical care at the level of the patient, pharmacist, prescriber, manufacturer, and health system. Further, public policy issues discussed create a practical framework for the successful incorporation of the more technical aspects of understanding and controlling pharmaceutical utilization and cost. Most importantly, Dr. Smith presents strategies for improving the utilization of medication by changing prescribing behaviors, dispensing patterns, and consumer medication-taking habits. The value of any book of this type is in its utility in solving 'real-world' pharmacoeconomic problems. *Studies in Pharmaceutical Economics* succeeds in the role of a pharmacoeconomic problem-solving tool for practitioners and educators at many levels."

E. Paul Larrat, PhD
Assistant Professor of Epidemiology,
University of Rhode Island

"**A**n excellent summary of where we've been in pharmaceutical marketing with an 'eye to the future.' The marketing research discussion provides an excellent perspective on the current state of the art and customers' needs. The section on pricing gets to the heart of the matter–defining the value of the pharmaceutical product in the context of the macro environment."

J. Martin Jernigan, PhD
Manager, U.S. Commercial Development, Hoechs Marion Roussel, Inc.

"**A**gain, Mickey Smith has done an outstanding job in selecting the key issues and then providing the perspectives of recognized researchers in the discipline on those topics.

The book is must reading for anyone interested in the area of health economics and would be a valuable addition to every researcher's library. The book allows the reader to explore the philosophical aspects of the field of pharmacoeconomics, past and present, and provides concrete research examples across a variety of research questions."

Andreas M. Pleil, PhD
Senior Health Economist,
Pharmacia & Upjohn, Inc.

Studies in Pharmaceutical Economics

PHARMACEUTICAL PRODUCTS PRESS
Pharmaceutical Sciences
Mickey C. Smith, PhD
Executive Editor

Studies
in Pharmaceutical
Economics

Mickey C. Smith
Editor

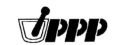

Pharmaceutical Products Press
An Imprint of The Haworth Press, Inc.
New York • London

Published by

Pharmaceutical Products Press, an imprint of The Haworth Press, Inc., 10 Alice Street, Binghamton, NY 13904-1580

The development, preparation, and publication of this work has been undertaken with great care. However, the publisher, employees, editors, and agents of The Haworth Press are not responsible for any errors contained herein or for consequences that may ensue from use of materials or information contained in this work. The opinions expressed by the author(s) are not necessarily those of The Haworth Press, Inc.

Library of Congress Cataloging-in-Publication Data

Studies in pharmaceutical economics / Mickey C. Smith, editor.
    p. cm.
Includes bibliographical references and index.
ISBN 0-7890-0062-8 (hard : alk. paper)
    1. Pharmaceutical industry. 2. Pharmaceutical industry–United States. 3 Drugs–Prices.
I. Smith, Mickey C.
HD9665.5.S776 1996
338.4'76151'0973–dc20
96-4736
CIP

CONTENTS

ABOUT THE EDITOR

Mickey C. Smith, RPh, PhD, is F.A.P. Barnard Distinguished Professor at the University of Mississippi School of Pharmacy. He has published more than 300 research and professional articles in more than 100 different journals. He has published eight books and presented more than 150 papers at professional meetings. Smith is editor of the *Journal of Pharmaceutical Marketing & Management* and the *Journal of Research in Pharmaceutical Economics* and Executive Editor of Pharmaceutical Products Press. His research interests include the determinants of medication use, medication compliance, and medication use in the elderly.

Contributors

Steven R. Arikian, MD, Professor, University of Toronto

Benjamin F. Banahan III, PhD, Professor, University of Mississippi

Kristina Baum, MBA, Independent Consultant

J. Lyle Bootman PhD, Dean, College of Pharmacy, University of Arizona

Norman V. Carroll, PhD, Professor, Virginia Commonwealth University

Frederic R. Curtiss, PhD, Reimbursement Consultant

Thomas R. Einarson, PhD, Professor, University of Toronto

Anne Elixhauser, PhD, Battelle

Anita L. Foster, MA, Georgia Department of Medical Assistance

Carol Brignoli Gable, PhD, State and Federal Associates, Inc.

Robert A. Freeman, PhD, Consultant, New York

Rhonda B. Friedman, ScD, The Medstat Group

Donnell L. Harris, BS, University of Maryland

Thomas K. Hazlet, PharmD, California Department of Health Services

Susan Sedory Holzer, MA, The Medstat Group

Cheryl Huey (now Kendrick), PharmD, Pru-Care Hospital, Atlanta

Christine Huttin, PhD, Associate Professor, University of Paris X Nanterre

Joseph D. Jackson, PhD, Bristol-Myers Squibb

Richard A. Jackson, PhD, Professor, Mercer University

Charlotte A. Jankel (now McMillan), PhD, Janssen
Pharmaceutical

John P. Juergens, PhD, Associate Professor, University
of Mississippi

Alison Keith, PhD, Pfizer Inc.

E. M. Kolassa, PhD, Research Associate, University
of Mississippi

Jeffrey A. Kotzan, PhD, Professor, Pharmacy Care Administration,
University of Georgia

Christopher M. Kozma, PhD, Associate Professor,
University of South Carolina

David H. Kreling, PhD, Professor, University of Wisconsin

Lon N. Larson, PhD, Associate Professor, Drake University

Earle W. Lingle, PhD, Associate Professor, University
of South Carolina

Ming-haw Liu, MS, University of Maryland

Brian Lovatt, Health Economist, ICI Pharmaceuticals

Bryan R. Luce, PhD, MEDTAP

David J. McCaffrey III, PhD, Assistant Professor,
University of Mississippi

Judy S. McKay, BS, University of Maryland

John A. McMillan, PhD, McNeil Laboratories

David W. Miller, BS, Glaxo

Lisa Muggeo, BA, Formerly Survey Statistician,
Bureau of the Census

C. Daniel Mullins, PhD, Assistant Professor, University
of Maryland

Dev S. Pathak, PhD, Professor, The Ohio State University

Matthew Perri III, PhD, Associate Professor, University
of Georgia

Margaret A. Pirl, MS, formerly Assistant Professor,
Mercer University

Sylvie Poirier, PhD, Assistant Professor, University of Georgia

Dennis W. Raisch, PhD, V.A. Hospital, Albuquerque, New Mexico

Gregory Reardon, PhD, Consultant, Columbus, Ohio

C. Eugene Reeder, PhD, Professor, University of South Carolina

Paul H. Rubin, PhD, Professor, Emory University

T. Donald Rucker, Consultant, Health Insurance
and Prescription Drug Policy

David Alexander Sclar, PhD, Associate Professor, Washington
State University

Neil H. Shear, MD, Professor, University of Toronto

Tracy L. Skaer, PharmD, Assistant Professor, Washington State
University

Mickey C. Smith, PhD, Professor, University of Mississippi

Stuart S. Speedie, PhD, Professor, University of Minnesota

Bruce Stuart, PhD, Professor, Pennsylvania State University

Sean D. Sullivan, PhD, Assistant Professor, University
of Washington

Sheryl L. Szeinbach, PhD, Associate Professor, University
of Mississippi

Rachel F. Tasch, MBA, Technology Assessment Group

James A. Visconti, PhD, Professor, The Ohio State University

Alan P. Wolfgang, PhD, Associate Professor, Purdue University

Charles Yesalis, ScD, Professor of Health Policy and Administration,
Pennsylvania State University

Foreword

When the *Journal of Research in Pharmaceutical Economics* (JRPE) was founded, there existed no other peer-reviewed, academic-based journal devoted to the field. As this is being written (in 1996), that is still the case.

In the inaugural issue we solicited and received comments from a variety of professional, trade, and government organization leaders on future research needs in the field of pharmaceutical economics. Examples of thought-provoking ideas presented follow:

- "What would be the effects of extending Medicare coverage to outpatient prescription drugs, especially on the market shares of leading brands and generics?" Daniel Oliver, Federal Trade Commission
- "Studies examining the impact of different methods for controlling costs on patient compliance and therapeutic outcomes . . . are needed so that those who are responsible for managing pharmacy benefits in private and government-sponsored health programs can base their decisions on hard data." John Schlegel, (then) American Pharmaceutical Association
- "What value do pharmacists add to the medical care process beyond the act of drug product dispensing? . . . What is the economic effect of clinical pharmacy services on length of stay, on hospital admissions, on patient compliance, on adverse reactions, and on physician prescribing habits?" Joseph Oddis, American Society of Hospital Pharmacists
- "What is the impact of multi-tier pricing on both pharmacists and consumers?" Donald W. Arthur, National Association of Retail Druggists
- "The application of cost-benefit and cost-effectiveness analysis to community pharmacy services will go a long way toward documenting the value-added component of care that pharmacists provide." Ronald L. Ziegler, National Association of Chain Drug Stores
- "What effects do restrictions on the use of prescription drugs have on the use and cost of other health care services?" Gerald Mossinghoff, Pharmaceutical Manufacturers Association (now PHRMA)

The answers to questions posed and issues raised by these and other contributors to the *Journal* remain elusive, but not necessarily beyond capture. The chapters in this collection are evidence of the intense and expert efforts to bring economic research to bear on the health problems of the world, especially as they relate to pharmaceuticals. Most of the papers appeared in *Journal of Research in Pharmaceutical Economics*, but a few, because of their relevance, have been added from our companion publication, *Journal of Pharmaceutical Marketing and Management.*

PART I:
PUBLIC POLICY ISSUES

This section begins with a look backward nearly 30 years to the HEW (Department of Health, Education, and Welfare) Task Force on Prescription Drugs and establishes very well that some problems just do not go away. Freeman follows with an argument for the need for and value of economic research in forming health policy. He then combines with Tasch in a conceptual financing scheme for new technology. McMillan and Jankel focus on a specific policy issue, Medicaid cost containment, and Rucker closes with a pragmatic critique of product prices and public policy.

Chapter 1

The HEW Task Force on Prescription Drugs: An Insider's Perspective

T. Donald Rucker

INTRODUCTION

In May of 1967, upon a directive from President Lyndon B. Johnson, the Secretary of Health and Human Services (then the U.S. Department of Health, Education, and Welfare) established the Task Force on Prescription Drugs. This body was charged with undertaking "a comprehensive study of the problems of including the cost of prescription drugs under Medicare." The Task Force (TF) consisted of nine top officials in the department, including its chairman, Philip R. Lee, MD, Assistant Secretary for Health, and Staff Director, Milton Silverman, PhD. Field work was supported by a professional staff of ten, although effective manpower was probably closer to six full-time equivalents.

During the subsequent months, the TF met periodically to review the work of its staff and to approve the release of the final report and the five background papers that are enumerated in Table 1.1. These volumes, prepared by Dr. Silverman, total 667 pages and represent a singular achievement both as a conceptual effort and as an accomplishment within the federal bureaucracy.

In addition to developing unique data and extensive surveys of the literature, the staff consulted with various federal agencies and more than 160 representatives from industry, the health professions, academia, consumer groups, and foreign governments. Although the project was sched-

Previously published in *Journal of Research in Pharmaceutical Economics*, Vol. 1(1), 1989.

TABLE 1.1. Publications[†] of the HEW[††] Task Force on Prescription Drugs, 1968-1969.

Final Report: Task Force on Prescription Drugs. Washington: GPO, (1969).
    86 pages.

Approaches to Drug Insurance Design. Washington: GPO, (1969).
    95 pages.

Current American and Foreign Programs. Washington: GPO, (1968).
    205 pages.

The Drug Makers and The Drug Distributors. Washington: GPO, (1968).
    86 pages.

The Drug Prescribers. Washington: GPO, (1968). 50 pages.

The Drug Users. Washington: GPO: (1968). 145 pages.

[†]Five interim reports were also issued between March 7, 1968, and January 10, 1969, and served, in part, as the basis for the *Final Report.* In light of the substantial documentation furnished in the five background papers, the reason for publication of these reports is unclear.
[††]Since 1980, the U.S. Department of Health and Human Services.

uled for completion in six months, these factors helped to extend the duration to 20.

In 1968, government (federal and state) outlays for drug benefits under Medicaid (Title 19) amounted to $208 million but had jumped to nearly $3 billion by 1987. With the passage and signing of the Catastrophic Health Insurance Amendments of 1988, which include a prescription drug benefit for aged and disabled individuals protected by Part B of Title 18, these expenditures seem destined to double by 1993 when the law would become fully operative.* Thus, basic public policy questions regarding prescription coverage for ambulatory patients have become economically important. This occasion provides, therefore, an opportunity not only to

---

*Editor's Note: Readers should note that these amendments were quickly repealed and thus these predictions could not be tested.

review a pioneering work 20 years later, but also to contemplate its value in light of the current legislative reality for which the TF was created. This critique has been prepared by a health economist who, in 1966, had begun to examine the question of drug insurance for the Social Security Administration and was detailed to aid in the formal investigation; hence, the economist was given the appellation "insider."

RESEARCH, FINDINGS, AND RECOMMENDATIONS

As Table 1.2 indicates, the call for a comprehensive study of the problems associated with prescription drug benefits led the TF to examine many related issues as well. Consequently, a total of 48 findings and 25 recommendations was put forward. These pertained to drug coverage, the quality of care associated with prescribed medications, the economic use of resources, professional education and proficiency, regulatory considerations at the federal and state level, and federal policy pertaining to pharmaceuticals in general. In short, the TF recognized that optimal drug benefit design could not be realized within the context of the insurance model and that analysis of the complex infrastructure underlying the role of prescribed medications in our society was also necessary.[1]

Drug Benefits for the Aged

The TF reported that many persons 65 years of age and older lacked financial resources to pay for prescribed medicines. Therefore, a need existed for an out-of-hospital insurance program under Medicare.[2] Moreover, such a program "has been shown to be economically feasible in many countries," although "no single method will by itself guarantee program efficiency, but without at least two features–reasonable formulary restrictions and effective data processing procedures–program controls will be ineffective."

In order to ensure reasonable program cost, the TF noted a positive relationship associated with additional features such as copayment or coinsurance (which was preferred over a deductible), use of low-cost chemical equivalents where possible, broad population coverage (to minimize adverse selection), vendor payment based on actual acquisition cost, and drug utilization review (to minimize irrational prescribing). Because of the nascent status of the latter, the TF reported that "there is an urgent need for further research to develop and test various approaches to effec-

TABLE 1.2. Statistical Summary of Task Force Findings and Recommendations According to Primary Area of Inquiry

Area*	Findings*	Recommendations**
Drug Insurance Benefits for the Aged	1, 2, 6, 9, 10, 12, 17, 20, 21, 22, 24, 26, 27, 28, 29, 30 31, 32, 33, 34, 35, 36, 37, 38, 39, 40, 41, 42	2(d); 17
Quality of Care: Drug Use Process	8, 11, 14, 18, 19 21, 28	4, 10, 12, 18(a), (b), (c); 20
Economic Issues	3, 4, 5, 7, 17, 22, 23	1, 2(a), (c), (d); 3(a), (b), (c); 5, 6, 12
Professional Education and Proficiency	8	7(a), (b), (c); 9, 11
HEW/State Government Regulatory Implications	14, 15, 16, 25	2(b); 8, 14, 15, 16, 21, 23, 24, 25
Federal Policy–Pharmaceuticals	13, 16, 43, 44, 45 46, 47, 48	3(a), (b), (c); 13, 19, 22

*   The TF utilized 17 categories for summarizing its work but the six-part framework here provides a more meaningful focus for this critique.

** As appropriate, several items have been assigned dual classifications.

Source: Task Force on Prescription Drugs. *Final Report.* Washington: GPO, (1969).

tive utilization review" as well as a universal coding and classification scheme covering all drug products. For administrative (and probably cost) reasons, the TF stressed that the program provide partial benefits initially, such as those deemed essential in the treatment of serious long-term illness (i.e., "maintenance drugs"). Finally, physician ownership of repackaging companies was cited as a conflict-of-interest situation that should be prohibited, and the need to study physician dispensing, for the same reason, was noted.

Although some 28 findings pertaining to a drug benefit for ambulatory patients under Medicare were put forward, the TF failed to make a formal recommendation to this effect. Only the transmittal letter from Dr. Lee to the Secretary specified "that such a program be instituted." However, the TF did recommend that more effective methods be found to determine the actual acquisition cost of pharmaceutical products (AWP [average wholesale price] was recognized as inconsistent with the fiduciary responsibility of a government program), and furthermore, that several departments test the proposed drug classification system.

Quality of Care: Drug Use Process

The TF found that prescriber decisions were often suboptimal and believed that cooperation among health professionals, suppliers, and government could contribute to more rational prescribing. In addition, it clarified the distinctions between chemical, biological, and clinical equivalents and reported that "lack of clinical equivalency among chemical equivalents meeting all official standards has been grossly exaggerated. . . ." Moreover, the TF enumerated certain criteria for implementing a sound formulary while noting that the exclusion of "certain combination products, duplicative drugs, and noncritical products from federal reimbursement would contribute significantly" to both rational prescribing and reduced program cost.

Economic Issues

The TF observed that much of the drug industry's research and development activities appeared "to provide only minor contributions to medical progress." The economic sequelae associated with this result include a waste of skilled resources and a confusing proliferation of drug products that combine to produce a burden on patients or taxpayers who ultimately must pay the costs. Further, the exceptionally high rate of profits attained by large manufacturers was not accompanied by excessive risk or the inability to attract capital.

While the TF was unable to document the efficiency of vendor (pharmacy) operations, it contended that significant program savings must be realized at this level as well. It also contended that payments should be limited to expenses that are directly related to dispensing, and "no portion of program payments should be made for unrelated functions or grossly inefficient vendor services."

Use of low-cost chemical equivalents, when of high quality, could yield savings of approximately 5% percent at the retail level. Finally, cooperative efforts on the part of professional associations and consumer groups were needed to help patients obtain better information on local prescription prices.

In order to confront these economic issues, the TF recommended that HEW conduct continuing surveys of product costs, prescription prices, and drug use. With respect to the manufacturing industry, it advocated study of incentives to stimulate the discovery and production of significant therapeutic agents and to discourage the output of marginal items. The TF also noted the need to limit the supply of free samples for physicians and to develop more effective methods for ascertaining the actual acquisition costs of prescription products. It called for an interagency investigation to consider discriminatory product pricing practices, discrepancy between foreign and domestic prices for the same product offered by a given firm, and possible revision of patent and trademark laws.

The TF also recommended wider use of prepackaging at the dispensing level, support for research to improve the efficiency and effectiveness of community and hospital pharmacy operations, and publication and distribution of a compendium covering all marketed products, including their respective prices.

Professional Education/Proficiency

The inability of most physicians to question their competency in making therapeutic judgments was lamented by the TF. It recommended development of curricula in medical and pharmacy schools to train pharmacists as drug information specialists on the health team. It stressed the desirability of strengthening pharmacy education along with preparation of pharmacy aides to provide their professional superiors with more time to engage in clinical functions. The TF also asserted that HEW should strengthen the teaching of clinical pharmacology in medical schools and support continuing education for physicians regarding rational prescribing.

Government Regulatory Duties

In reviewing the role of government as a regulator of pharmaceutical products, the TF found that the lack of clinical equivalency among chemical equivalents had been grossly exaggerated. Since uniform standards of product quality and efficacy should apply to all federally supported drug programs, the committee held that cost differentials due simply to the use of brand or generic terms could not be justified under reimbursement policy. The TF anticipated that the drug efficacy studies of products marketed between 1938 and 1962 would be completed by 1971. It noted that any increase in financial resources required to strengthen controls on product quality should not be attributed to the expense of federally assisted drug programs because these activities benefit the public in general.

The TF recommended that all products licensed for distribution in interstate commerce be subject to the quality control standards established by the FDA (Food and Drug Administration) and that this agency be provided with adequate financial resources to command internal and external expertise to exercise its scientific and regulatory responsibilities. In addition, it recommended that the FDA establish intramural clinical and laboratory research capabilities to help attract and retain the best scientific personnel. It also specified the need to study whether three classifications–new drugs and "not new" drugs, certifiable products, and biologics–were appropriate to ensure uniform quality. Finally, the TF recommended that HEW support studies on pharmacist licensure and reciprocity to facilitate expanded functions for these professionals and to ensure, rather than impede, fair competition.

Federal Policy

The TF found that a permanent mechanism was needed at the federal level to collect, analyze, and exchange information and to provide effective coordination of drug-related activities, such as uniform standards of quality, among the agencies involved. However, it found no need to centralize all drug-related functions within the department. As a result, the regulatory, discovery, manpower, and scientific information divisions of HEW would remain largely as organized.

As reported under the heading "Economic Issues" above, the TF recommended a joint study by the Departments of HEW, Commerce, Justice, and other agencies, including the Federal Trade Commission, to consider (1) drug product price differentials that persist between community and hospital pharmacies as well as foreign and domestic suppliers, and (2) the possible revision of patent and trademark laws governing pharmaceutical preparations. One of the major reasons for convening an industry conference was to permit drug firms to specify various marketing practices that could be defined as "unfair trade." These activities would be outlawed and hence place no firm at a competitive disadvantage.

The TF recommended establishment of a Federal Interdepartmental Health Policy Council to coordinate all federal prescription drug purchase and reimbursement programs. It also recommended adoption of a standardized drug code (to facilitate efficiency in processing prescription drug claims) and surveillance of drug costs, prescription prices, and drug use by the SSA (Social Security Administration).[3]

AN INDEPENDENT ASSESSMENT

As the *Final Report* of the TF was being issued, a new administration took office in Washington. On March 24, 1969, Secretary Robert H. Finch asked a diverse group of 17 leaders from outside the government to assist him in determining the course of action regarding selected aspects of the Task Force's work.

Within a period of four months, and without staff support, Dr. John T. Dunlop, Professor of Political Economy at Harvard, had elicited a response from each of his Review Committee members covering four basic issues: (1) the feasibility of adding prescription drug coverage to Medicare; (2) federal policy pertaining to chemical/biological/clinical equivalency; (3) economic matters related to drug manufacturing and distribution; and (4) methods for improving the flow of information regarding drugs to practicing physicians.

With only one dissent, the Review Committee concluded that the Medicare program should be expanded to include drug benefits and that HEW should develop more detailed plans concerning program regulations, data processing procedures, and cost computations necessary for legislative consideration. However, the Committee noted that (1) limitation of benefits to chronic disease treatments was neither advisable nor administrable; (2) an age limitation above 65 was undesirable; (3) a deductible should be avoided because of the record-keeping burden it placed on patients; (4) co-payment was preferable to coinsurance; and (5) only a "purely advisory national formulary . . . might possibly be appropriate." The drug program should be built around co-payment (with perhaps an annual ceiling beyond which the patient could be reimbursed), vendor payment based on a flat dispensing fee, coverage under Part A of Medicare, and utilization review.

In discussing the pharmacologic issues, the Committee recommended that the FDA continue developing reference standards for generic drugs to assure biologic equivalency, that advisory committees be established to assist in evaluating compliance with such standards, and that improved quality control in drug manufacturing through registration/licensure, as called for by the TF, be supported.

When the Review Committee confronted the major economic questions, there was general agreement that (1) pharmaceutical manufacturers' profits were high, relative to other industries; (2) a study should be made of price differentials that exist when products were sold to various types of buyers; and (3) patients needed better information about prescription prices. The Committee recommended that the department support research to improve the efficiency of community and hospital pharmacy operations and generally prohibit reimbursement of physician-owned repackaging companies. However, there was less agreement among Committee members regarding the TF discovery of duplicate and wasteful research by drug manufacturers.

With respect to TF recommendations pertaining to better information for prescribers, the Review Committee supported guidelines concerned with rational drug therapy and publication of a comprehensive compendium. In both cases though, it contended that the scientific basis for these compilations should emanate from nongovernment sources although major funding would be supplied by the public purse.

Given the fact that eight of the Committee members were provider-oriented, the extent of consensus regarding government policy on prescription drugs seems nothing less than remarkable.

IMPACT OF THE TASK FORCE'S WORK

The impact of the Task Force on Prescription Drugs is difficult to assess because results are a function of different criteria that may be employed and of evaluator interpretation. With respect to legislative efforts to extend drug coverage for aged persons, numerous bills were introduced in Congress for many years after the *Final Report* was issued in February 1969. However, during the three to four years prior to that date, more than 50 bills were introduced. While comparison of legislative components might be attempted via content analysis, the TF never recommended a model law as such. In fact, no administration–Republican or Democratic–has ever sponsored a bill to add prescription benefits to Medicare or even included them in a national health insurance plan. If the drug benefit under the 1988 amendments is used for analysis, the major staff paper [4] shaping this legislation incorporated only one reference (out of 71) that might be traced to the TF effort.

The impact of the TF may also be inferred from the literature dealing with drug insurance and related issues as outlined in Table 1.2. In this connection, the selected references presented in the Appendix reflect a major extension of the drug policy and drug insurance activities initiated by the TF. The prolific output of Dr. Silverman and associates represents a significant achievement in delineating major policy issues on the domestic scene and effecting changes in promotional and information practices conducted by large multinational pharmaceutical firms within many developing nations. A uniform cost accounting system for community pharmacy, developed by Dr. Bruce R. Siecker, stands as a beacon that illuminates how economic data should serve as the cornerstone for determining vendor reimbursement.

Studies such as those by Avorn and Soumerai;[5] Ray, Schaffner, and Federspiel;[6] Richards;[7] and Soumerai, Avorn, Ross-Degnan, and Gortmayer[8] coupled with important publications by USP[9,10,11] and AMA,[12] treat various aspects of the central questions addressed by the TF. However, neither of the compendia published by USP (United States Pharmacopoeia) and AMA (American Medical Association) incorporates the product price information so strongly advocated by the TF. While methods of introducing price information into clinical decision making represents a complex topic beyond the focus of this overview, adding price data to compendia raises questions about relative effectiveness of alternative models: (1) should not the physician give first consideration to selecting the drug of choice; (2) should not physicians have access to all prices per therapeutic category via computer terminal, rather than a published document, when they are originating a prescription order; and (3) should not reimbursement policy constitute the primary foundation for adjudicating product prices rather than trying to transform a busy clinician into a haphazard drug economist?[13]

If one moves from the legislative and literature models to the impact that the TF had on bureaucratic function, one can claim that its work stimulated the FDA to establish external advisory panels of outside experts to review New Drug Applications and develop the National Drug Code Directory. Unfortunately, the efficiency of this universal coding system was vitiated when the Pharmaceutical Manufacturers Association (PMA) insisted that each multiple source product be identified by both a manufacturer's prefix and a unique four-digit code.

The TF was also instrumental in inducing the FDA (via NAS/NRI) to review the efficacy of drugs approved between 1938 and 1962 (DESI project). In 1987, though, the Health Care Financing Administration was still listing 107 drug products identified by the DESI program as ineligible for reimbursement under Medicaid.[14] The TF recommendation for transferring the Division of Biologic Standards from the NIH (National Institutes of Health) to the FDA was carried out. Finally, the TF facilitated the agency's role "in dealing with the complex problems of drug quality, chemical equivalents, bioavailability, and clinical equivalency."[15]

DISCUSSION

The work of the TF represented the first systematic attempt by the administrative branch of the federal government to define and evaluate major public policy issues associated with drug use and insurance beyond the traditional regulatory matters pertaining to product purity, safety, and efficacy. In this endeavor, the TF made available the first national profile of drug use among the elderly; defined rational prescribing; documented the prevalence of irrational prescribing; and stressed the contribution that drug utilization review[16] could make, first in reducing inappropriate prescribing, and secondly in controlling program cost. The TF also put forward a number of innovative proposals, such as the ideas that exclusive rights to a product's trademark should last no longer than the patent, that drug program design should be simple enough that patients do not become unduly burdened in obtaining benefits, and that drug programs under Medicare and Medicaid should be coordinated.

The TF disclosed the nature of drug industry profits and resources dissipated in the marketing of products. It also demonstrated the waste associated with most "me-too" products and fixed combination preparations. It emphasized the potential value of clinical pharmacists' contributions to program goals and patient health status.

While many of these issues have subsequently entered the public domain, some were sufficiently radical to induce the President of the PMA to make a personal trip to the HEW in the spring of 1972 to help derail the research of the Drug Studies Branch in the Department[17] that focused on his clients. While the TF contributions to social welfare were numerous, the Committee also waffled by calling for more study of the role of physician-owned pharmacies, dispensing physicians, and, understandably, methods an insurance program should follow to reimburse providers for product cost. In addition, the *Final Report* was so preoccupied with identifying competing formula for reimbursing vendors for product cost and professional overhead that it neglected to mention what type of data was required for closely approximating the true economic cost of an efficient provider, regardless of methodology.

The TF pointed out the financial reasons for adding drug benefits to Part A of Medicare, but it never recognized the value of merging physician and drug claims under Part B as a means of making the DUR (Drug Utilization Review) function more effectively. Further, while stressing the patient burden of records keeping associated with a high deductible, the *Final Report* did not point out that this means of patient cost sharing is also likely to decimate quality assurance activities designed to raise beneficiary health status.

Although the TF provided a clear statement regarding the contribution of a drug formulary to program administration, it probably distorted our understanding of this mechanism by failing to differentiate between limitations in the scope of benefits (deletion of an entire therapeutic category) and formulary restrictions within an approved category. It also failed to clarify that administrative controls on drug quantity and product price can be promulgated in the absence of a formulary, and hence, such measures should not be ascribed to formulary performance for either positive or negative attribution.

The TF confused the reason for providing drug benefits only to patients who had reached age 70 or 72 (all retirement and medicare benefits commence when an individual reaches age 65). Because cost, both initially and subsequently, is always a consideration with any federal program, the argument was advanced that a higher age limit was one means of dealing with the financial constraint. However, this proposal was suggested by staff to confront the claim volume problem with the understanding that the age limit would be temporary and dropped to 65 just as soon as claim-processing capabilities permitted rapid handling of the larger administrative load.

The department never tested the drug classification system discussed above, but the Veterans Administration has utilized this source in preparing its own system.[18] Finally, the problem of inappropriate prescribing and inadequate education for prescribers remains[19] despite the heroic efforts of the TF to confront this social malady. It was hoped that the 1988 addition of drug benefits to the Medicare program would help resurrect this and other public policy matters initiated by the HEW Task Force on Prescription Drugs two decades ago, but of course that did not happen.

POSTSCRIPT

Two incidents related to the work of the TF illustrate a basic social problem concerning the relationship of the pharmaceutical manufacturing industry to efforts to develop prudent public policy.

During the latter part of 1968, an attorney employed by one of the largest drug firms approached the author for an advance copy of the *Third* or *Fourth Interim Report*. When he perceived after several minutes of discussion that I was unwilling to provide this document (it was sitting in a filing cabinet less than a foot from his head), he snorted, "Oh, the hell with it; we will steal it," and stomped out of the room.

The second incident occurred a decade later when the author was a professor in Columbus, Ohio. A representative from another large firm stopped for an unannounced visit as had often been his practice during my seven-year tenure in Washington. It was now a rare event, however, for him, or any other industry official, to make the trek to the Midwest for business or social purposes.

"Well, Alan, what are you doing in town?" I asked. "Oh," he remarked, "headquarters wants to know what our pricing policy is, and I am doing a field survey among our customers to find out what they paid for our products!" A decade later, another official of the same firm appeared in my office in Chicago. When I related this incident about his employer, he responded, "I can understand that."

These two examples illustrate how arrogance and obfuscation often stand as impediments to the development of a reimbursement policy that attempts to encompass the legitimate claims of both providers and society.

APPENDIX

Selected References Prompted by the Work of the Task Force on Prescription Drugs

American Pharmaceutical Association. *White paper on the pharmacist's role in product selection*. Washington: APhA, (1971).

Berger, B.A. Coverage of non-drug items under a major drug insurance program. *Pharmacy Management*, 152 (May-June 1980): 110-112;117.

Brodie, R.C. *Drug utilization and drug utilization review and control*. Health Services and Mental Health Administration. DHEW Pub. No. (HSM) 72-3002, (1970).

Campbell, W.H., Johnson, R.E. and Christensen, D.B. A procedural and conceptual analysis of drug use review. *Drugs in Health Care*, 2 (Fall 1975): 211-230.

Christensen, D.B. Guiding principles for pharmacy services under national health insurance. *Pharmacy Management*, 152 (September-October 1980): 205-209.

Cotton, H.A. and Rucker, T.D. Prescription cost determination in Kansas. *Journal of the American Pharmaceutical Association*, NS12 (August 1972): 412-415.

Fink, J.L. Some legal aspects of the hospital formulary system. *American Journal of Hospital Pharmacy*, 31 (January 1974): 86-90.

Fink, J.L. Coverage of prescription drugs for non-hospitalized medicare patients. *Clearinghouse Law Review*, 8 (February 1975): 712-720.

Fink, J.L. *Manager's guide to third-party programs*. Washington: American Pharmaceutical Association, (1982): 90 pages.

Fulda, T.R. Drug cost control: the road to maximum allowable cost regulations. In: *Toward a national health policy, public policy in the control of health care cost*, Friedman, K. and Raxoff, S. (eds.). Lexington, MA: Lexington Books, (1977); 55-67.

Gagnon, J.P., Nelson, A.A., and Rodowskas, C.A., Jr. A comparison of maintenance and nonmaintenance outpatient prescription directions, duration of coverage and costs per day. *Medical Care*, 13 (January 1975): 47-58.

Gagnon, J.P. and Rodowskas, C.A. Two controversial problems in third-party outpatient prescription plans. *Journal of Risk and Insurance*, 39 (December 1972): 603-611.

Gardner, V. Maximum allowable cost: estimated acquisition cost. *California Pharmacist*, 24 (July 1976): 36-39.

Health Care Financing Administration. *Guide to prescription drug costs*. Baltimore: HCFA–02104, (April 1980).

Jacoby, E.M. and Hefner, D.L. Domestic and foreign prescription drug prices. *Social Security Bulletin*, 34 (May 1971): 15-22.

Johnson, R.C. Overview and objectives of drug program management. *California Pharmacist*, 25 (January 1978): 19-24.

Knapp, D.A. and Palumbo, F.B. *Containing costs in third-party programs*. Hamilton, IL: Drug Intelligence Publications, Inc., (1978).

Knapp, D.A. Review article: paying for outpatient prescription drugs and related services in third-party programs. *Medical Care Review*, 28 (August 1971): 826-859.

Knapp, D.A. The restrictive formulary and drug use review in a medicare out-of-hospital prescription drug program. *NARD Journal*, 95 (October 15, 1973): 14-16.

Lee, P.R. The task force on prescription drugs: a review of problems, progress and possibilities. *Drug Information Journal*, 11 (March 1977): 7-10.

Lipton, H.L. and Lee, P.R. *Drugs and the elderly*. Stanford, CA: Stanford Univ. Press, (1988).

Maronde, R.F., Lee, P.V., McCarron, M.M., and Seibert, S. A study of prescribing patterns. *Medical Care*, 9 (September/October 1971); 383-395.

Maronde, R.F., Seibert, S., Katzoff, J., and Silverman, M. Drug data processing: its role in the control of drug abuse. *California Medicine*, 117 (September 1972): 22-28.

Maronde, R.F. and Silverman, M. Prescribing hypnotic and anti-anxiety drugs. *Annals Internal Medicine*, 79 (September 1973): 452.

Maronde, R.F. *Drug utilization review with on-line computer capability*. ORS/SSA, staff paper #13, DHEW Pub. No. (SSA) 73-11853, (1972); 81 pages.

Maronde, R.F. Drug utilization review. In: *Perspectives on medicines in society*, Wertheimer, A.I. and Bush, P.J. (eds.). Hamilton, IL: Drug Intelligence Publications, (1977): 169-191.

Massachusetts Department of Public Health. The Massachusetts drug formulary. *New England Journal Medicine*, 285 (July 22, 1971): 232-233.

Morse, M.L., Leroy, A., Gaylord, T.A., and Kellenberger, T. Reducing drug therapy-induced hospitalization: impact of drug utilization review. *Drug Information Journal*, 16 (October/December 1982): 199-202.

Muller, C. Drug benefits in health insurance. *International Journal of Health Services*, 4 (Winter 1974): 157-170.

Muller, C. Payment mechanisms. In: *Perspectives on medicines in society*, Wertheimer, A.I. and Bush, P.J. (eds.). Hamilton, IL: Drug Intelligence Publications, (1977): 429-449.

Olejar, P.D. (ed.). *Proceedings: computer-based information system in the practice of pharmacy*. Chapel Hill, NC: School of Pharmacy, University of North Carolina, (1971): 199 pages.

Pan American Health Organization. *Development and implementation of drug formularies*. Washington: PAHO Scientific Publication 474, (1984).

Report of the secretary's review committee of the task force on prescription drugs, (T. Dunlop, chairman). Washington: Office of the Secretary, U.S. Dept. HEW, (July 23, 1969): 164 pages.

Rucker, T.D. Pharmacy and third parties in the 1970's. *Michigan Pharmacist*, 7 (July 1970): 829-834.

Rucker, T.D. The need for drug utilization review. *American Journal of Hospital Pharmacy*, 27 (August 1970): 654-658.

Rucker, T.D. Drug insurance and vendor compensation. *California Pharmacist*, 18 (October 1970): 20-27.

Rucker, T.D. Possible impact of a government drug program on community pharmacies. *Journal of the American Pharmaceutical Association*, NS11 (June 1971): 334-337.

Rucker, T.D. Problems in measuring overhead costs for prescription services. *Texas Pharmacy*, 90 (October 1971): 24-37.

Rucker, T.D. Drug insurance, formularies and pharmacy. *Medical Marketing and Media*, 6 (October 1971): 11-18.

Rucker, T.D. The role of computers in drug utilization review. *American Journal of Hospital Pharmacy*, 29 (February 1972): 128-133.

Rucker, T.D. The pharmacist and national health insurance–potentials and problems. *California Pharmacist*, 19 (April 1972): 24-29.

Rucker, T.D. Economic problems in drug distribution. *Inquiry*, 9 (September 1972): 43-50.

Rucker, T.D. A model information system for prescription drug services. *The Wisconsin Pharmacist*, 41 (December 1972): 411-415.

Rucker, T.D. National health insurance—prerequisites and principles. *The Wisconsin Pharmacist*, 42 (January 1973): 33-38.

Rucker, T.D. Theory and practice in drug insurance design. *Illinois Pharmacist*, 37 (January 1973): 25-29.

Rucker, T.D. Economic aspects of drug overuse. *Medical Annals of the District of Columbia*, 42 (December 1973): 609-614.

Rucker, T.D. and Krautheim, D. A computer-oriented pharmacy information system: macro considerations. *Journal of Clinical Computing*, 3 (January 1974): 317-328.

Rucker, T.D. Public policy considerations in the use of psychoactive drugs. *Drugs in Health Care*, 1 (Summer 1974): 5-15.

Rucker, T.D. Public policy considerations in the pricing of prescription drugs. *International Journal of Health Services*, 4 (Winter 1974): 171-179.

Rucker, T.D. The pharmaceutical manufacturing industry's role in a dynamic health care system. *Drugs in Health Care*, 2 (Spring 1975): 86-95.

Rucker, T.D. Drug information for prescribers and dispensers: toward a model system. *Medical Care*, 14 (February 1976): 156-165.

Rucker, T.D. Commentary on: A.M. Lee, Constraining costs on pharmaceutical programs: lessons from abroad. In: *Impact of public policy on drug innovation and pricing*, Mitchell, S.A. and Link, E.A. (eds.). Washington: The American University, (1976): 177-189.

Rucker, T.D. Commentary on: Gordon Trapnell, Medicaid drug insurance progress: a comparison of the effect of contrasting approaches. In: *Impact of public policy on drug innovation and pricing*, Mitchell, S.A. and Link, E.A. (eds.). Washington: The American University, (1976): 230-233.

Rucker, T.D. National health insurance and prescription benefits. *Drug Intelligence and Clinical Pharmacy*, 10 (September 1976): 529-533.

Rucker, T.D. Around and beyond UCAS: the road to economic survival for community pharmacy. *Journal of the American Pharmaceutical Association*, NS17 (May 1977): 292-296.

Rucker, T.D. How to survive in a sea of government programs. *American Journal of Pharmacy*, 149 (July-August 1977): 106-112.

Rucker, T.D. Reimbursement policy under drug insurance: administrative expediency or economic validity? *American Journal of Pharmacy*, 150 (July/August 1978): 107-118.

Rucker, T.D., Janis, L. and Bennett, M. Prescriptions ordered by podiatrists for ambulatory patients: an exploratory study. *Drug Intelligence and Clinical Pharmacy*, 12 (December 1978): 720-727.

Rucker, T.D. Third-party drug programs: an overview. *Pharmacy Management*, 151 (January 1979): 26-28.

Rucker, T.D. and Visconti, J.A. *How effective are drug formularies? A descriptive and normative study.* Washington: American Society of Hospital Pharmacists Research and Education Foundation, (1979).

Rucker, T.D. Prescription drug coverage: insurance or prepayment? *Pharmacy Management*, 151 (July/August 1979): 171-173.

Rucker, T.D. and Visconti, J.A. Relative drug safety and efficacy: any help for the practitioner? *American Journal of Hospital Pharmacy*, 36 (August 1979): 1099-1101.

Rucker, T.D. and Grover, R.A. Coverage of OTC preparations under prepayment programs. *Pharmacy Management*, 151 (November/December 1979): 254-257.

Rucker, T.D. Prescription drug benefits under national health insurance–a blue ribbon proposal. *Pharmacy Management*, 152 (January/February 1980): 23-28.

Rucker, T.D. The top-selling drug products: how good are they? *American Journal of Hospital Pharmacy*, 37 (June 1980): 833-837.

Rucker, T.D. and Morse, M.L. The Medicaid drug program in Louisiana: critique of the Hefner-Pracon study. *American Journal of Hospital Pharmacy*, 37 (October 1980): 1350-1353; 38 (March 1981): 304.

Rucker, T.D. Effective formulary development: which direction? *Topics in Hospital Pharmacy Management*, 1 (May 1981): 29-45.

Rucker, T.D., Duche, G., and Clasen, T.E. Clinical pharmacy: a strategy for community practitioners. *Contemporary Pharmacy Practice*, 5 (Winter 1982): 21-26.

Rucker, T.D. Prescription drug insurance: a traditional or trustee role? *Pharmacy International*, 3 (June 1982): 196-198.

Rucker, T.D. Formularies: conceptual and experiential factors related to drug product selection. *Drug Information Journal*, 16 (July; September 1982): 115-121.

Rucker, T.D. Superior hospital formularies: a critical analysis. *Hospital Pharmacy*, 17 (September 1982): 465-524.

Rucker, T.D. Drug utilization review: moving toward an effective safe model. In: *Society and medication: conflicting signals for prescribers and patients*, Morgan, J.P. and Kagan, D.V. (eds.). Lexington, MA: Lexington Books, D.C. Heath and Co., (1983): 25-51.

Rucker, T.D. Selected problems in drug nomenclature. *Journal of Clinical Computing*, 12(1/2) (1983): 31-34.

Rucker, T.D. Putting reimbursement policy back on the track. *Hospital Pharmacy*, 18 (August 1983): 404-405.

Rucker, T.D. Computerization of prescription data with particular reference to drug nomenclature. *Journal of Clinical Computing*, 13(2/3) (1984): 28-34.

Rucker, T.D. Micro/Macro strategies for improving hospital formulary performance. *Clinical Research Practices and Drug Regulatory Affairs*, 2(3) (1984): 295-312.

Rucker, T.D. The role of formularies and their relationship to drug product selection. In: *Generic drug laws: a decade of trial–a prescription for progress*, Goldberg, T., Devito, C.A., and Raskin, I.E. (eds.). National Center for Health Services Research, US Dept. HHS, Washington, (June 1986): 465-485.

Rucker, T.D. Prescribed medications: system control or therapeutic roulette? IFAC Monograph: *Control aspects of biomedical engineering*, Nalecz, Maciej (ed.). Oxford, England: Pergamon Press, (1987); 167-175.

Rucker, T.D. Pursuing rational drug therapy: a macro view à la the USA. *Journal of Social and Administrative Pharmacy*, 5(3) (1988): 76-85.

Schifrin, L.G. Economics and epidemiology of drug use. In: *Clinical Pharmacology*, Melmon, K.L. and Morrelli, H.F. (eds.). New York: Macmillan Pub. Co., (1978): 1084-1109.

Siecker, B.R. Pharmacy economics and principles of uniform cost accounting. *Journal of the American Pharmaceutical Association*, NS15 (December 1975): 678-682.

Siecker, B.R. The uniform cost accounting approach for pharmacy pricing decisions. *Journal of the American Pharmaceutical Association*, NS17 (April 1977): 208-212.

Siecker, B.R. *Uniform cost accounting approach for pharmacy–UCAS.* Washington: American Pharmaceutical Association, (1979).

Silverman, M. and Lee, P.R. *Pills, profits and politics.* Berkeley, CA: University of California Press, (1974).

Silverman, M. and Lydecker, M. Prescription drug pricing by hospital pharmacies. *American Journal of Hospital Pharmacy*, 31 (September 1974): 870.

Silverman, M. *The drugging of the Americas.* Berkeley, CA: University of California Press, (1976).

Silverman, M. The epidemiology of drug promotion. *International Journal of Health Services*, 7(2) (1977): 157.

Silverman, M. and Lydecker, M. *Drug coverage under national health insurance: the policy options.* National Center for Health Services Research, DHEW Pub. No. (HRA) 77-3189, (1977).

Silverman, M. Who needs drug insurance. *Hospital Formulary*, 13 (February 1978): 138.

Silverman, M. and Lydecker, M. (eds.). *Proceedings of the national conference on drug coverage under national health insurance.* National Center for Health Services Research, DHEW Pub. No. (PHS) 78-3208, (1978).

Silverman, M. Pharmacy, society, and upcoming federal legislation. *California Pharmacist*, 27 (October 1979): 38.

Silverman, M. and Lee, P.R. The revolution in drugs. And, Future strategy: prescriptions for action. In: *The Nation's Health*, Lee, P.R., Brown, N. and Red, I. (eds.). San Francisco: Boyd and Fraser, (1981).

Silverman, M. and Lydecker, M. The promotion of prescription drugs and other puzzles. In: *Pharmaceuticals and Health Policy*, Blum, R. and Blum, E. (eds.). New York: Holmes and Meier Publishers, (1981).

Silverman, M., Lee, P.R., and Lydecker, M. *Pills and the public purse.* Berkeley, CA: University of California Press, (1981).

Silverman, M., Lee, P.R. and Lydecker, M. *Prescriptions for death: the drugging of the third world.* Berkeley, CA: University of California Press, (1982).

Silverman, M., Lee, P.R. and Lydecker, M. Drug promotion: the third world revisited. *International Journal of Health Services*, 16(4) (1986): 659.

Smith, M.C. and Wilkinson, W.E. Automation of vendor drug claims. *Journal of the American Pharmaceutical Association*, NS10 (September 1968): 501-505.

Smith, M.C., Mikeal, R.L. and Wilkinson, W.E. Studies in the automation of vendor drug claims. *Journal of the American Pharmaceutical Association*, NS12 (April 1972): 156-165.

Smith, M.C. Pharmacy and national health insurance. In: *Pharmacy in health care and institutional systems*, Lecca, P.J. and Tharp, C.P. (eds.). St. Louis, MO: C.V. Mosby, (1978): 13-46.

Stolley, P.D. and Goddard, J.L. Prescription drug insurance for the elderly under Medicare. *American Journal of Public Health*, 61 (March 1971): 574-581.

Strom, B.L., Stolley, P.D., and Brown, T.C. Drug antisubstitution studies: estimation of possible savings by repeal of antisubstitution laws. *Drugs in Health Care*, 1 (Fall 1974): 99-103.

Wertheimer, A.I. (ed.). *Proceedings of the international conference on drug and pharmaceutical services reimbursement.* National Center for Health Services Research. DHEW Pub. No. (HRA) 77-3186, (1977).

Wolfe, S.M., et al. *Worst pills, best pills.* Washington: Public Citizen Health Research Group, (1988).

REFERENCES

1. Given the provisions of drug coverage under the Medicare Catastrophic Health Insurance Amendments of 1988, it seems impossible that a similar claim could be made for the current legislation.

2. In the early 1970s, Medicare coverage was expanded to include several million disabled persons and their dependents who qualified for monthly benefits under Social Security. This group has an utilization rate for prescribed drugs that exceeds that of aged individuals.

3. A similar recommendation today would assign this duty to HCFA.

4. Office Technology Assessment. *Prescription drugs and elderly Americans: ambulatory use and approaches to coverage for medicare.* Washington: U.S. Congress, (October 1987): 68 pages.

5. Avorn, J. and Soumerai, S.B. Improving drug-therapy decisions through educational outreach: a randomized controlled trial of academically based "detailing." *New England Journal of Medicine*, 308 (June 16, 1983): 1457-1463.

6. Ray, W.A., Schaffner, W., and Federspiel, C.F. Persistence of improvement in antibiotic prescribing in office practice. *Journal of the American Medical Association*, 253 (March 22/29, 1985): 1774-1776.

7. Richards, J.W. third-party prescription programs: cost containment issues and strategies. *American Pharmacy*, NS25 (July 1985): 28-35.

8. Soumerai, S.B., Avorn, J., Ross-Degnan, D., and Gortmayer, S. Payment restrictions for prescription drugs under Medicaid. *New England Journal of Medicine*, 317 (August 17, 1987): 550-556.

9. USP. *Guide to select drugs.* Rockville, MD: United States Pharmacopoeial Convention, (1975).

10. USP. *USP DI–Drug information for the health care professional*, (2 vol.). Rockville, MD: United States Pharmacopoeial Convention, (1988).

11. USP. *USP DI–Advice for the Patient.* Rockville, MD: United States Pharmacopoeial Convention, (1988).

12. AMA Division of Drugs. *AMA drug evaluations*, (5th ed.). Chicago: American Medical Association, (1983).

13. Rucker, T.D. Commentary on: A.M. Lee, Constraining costs on pharmaceutical programs: lessons from abroad. In: *Impact of Public Policy on Drug Innovation and Pricing*, Mitchell, S.A. and Link, E.A. (eds.). Washington: The American University, (1976): 188.

14. Anon. HCFA guide to DESI drugs. *Drug Store News–Inside Pharmacy*, 9 (April 1987): 31-37.

15. Lee, P.R. The task force on prescription drugs. *Drug Information Journal*, 11 (January/March, 1977): 7-10.

16. The TF emphasized that DUR represented a continuing process of claim evaluation and noted how this function differed from the traditional one of claim administration. The concept may be confusing to some because in recent years investigators have employed various handles, such as drug use evaluation and drug usage review, to discuss the basic quality assurance process. The TF, howev-

er, failed to admonish us that the major objective of DUR is to go out of business, i.e., to become so successful in the retrospective mode that review procedures would be incorporated in clinical decision making and patient treatment. Finally, DUR effectiveness may be jeopardized to the extent that inept politicians and zealous administrators depend upon this educational process to offset deficiencies in reimbursement policy.

17. *The Washington Post.* (April 28, 1972).

18. USP. *USP DI–Drug information for the health care professional*, (Vol. II). Rockville, MD: United States Pharmacopoeial Convention, (1988): Appendix III.

19. Health and Policy Committee, American College of Physicians. Improving medical education in therapeutics. *Annals of Internal medicine*, 108 (January 1988): 147.

Chapter 2

Health Policy Initiatives
and the Utility of Economic Research

Robert A. Freeman

INTRODUCTION

In a previous work, I noted that economic analyses of pharmaceuticals (meaning also the areas of health-related quality of life research and outcomes management research) have a number of broad uses in the marketplace (Table 2.1).[1] The driving force behind their application is to respond to a changing, more cost-conscious market by providing persuasive, comparative information to decision makers about the costs and outcomes of therapeutic alternatives. The intended effect is to influence positively the utilization of an individual company's prescription drug product(s). As a consequence of this effect, most pharmaceutical manufacturers currently regard the application of economic research as a competitive marketing strategy, albeit tactical in nature, since it is product-specific in scope and supports the immediate business objectives of the firm. As a preface, I would aver that the use of economic research to influence deliberations on public health policy issues is an untapped resource for most pharmaceutical companies.

Abuses and inconsistencies have occurred in the design, execution, and reporting of specific economic analyses used solely for competitive marketing purposes.[2] Consequently, one might expect that formal guidelines for a standardized methodology (or methodologies), as well as a

The author thanks Pat McKercher and Rachel Tasch for suggestions and comments and Claudia Kovitz for editorial assistance. The comments and opinions expressed herein are not necessarily those of Searle.

Previously published in *Journal of Research in Pharmaceutical Economics*, Vol. 4(4), 1992.

TABLE 2.1. Uses of Economic Analysis

Marketing Services
- Product differentiation
- Price determination
- Product planning

Medical/Regulatory Affairs
- Price/reimbursement negotiations
- Justify existing and new indications

Public Affairs
- Establish the value of therapy
- Influence public health policy

code of ethics for pharmaceutical industry-sponsored research, will be proposed in the near future. Activity is already relatively far along in Ontario, Canada, and Australia.[3,4] However, as long as no explicit regulations exist, compliance with standards and codes of conduct will largely be voluntary, and some degree of inconsistency and abuse is likely to persist.

The lack of regulatory oversight is not suggestive of malfeasance or lack of interest on the regulatory agencies' part; rather, health policy concerning the use of prescription drugs is confined largely to the establishment of criteria and standards for safety and efficacy for approved therapeutic indications, not for the relative cost-effectiveness of products or other economic criteria. Therefore, unless other nations' regulatory systems are modified, as in the cases of the Province of Ontario and Australia, economic data is largely precluded or proscribed from active consideration as a criterion for marketing approval or subsequent listing on a national formulary. Alternatively, in those countries where prescription drug prices are regulated once marketing approval is granted, an increased interest in considering economic analyses in the rate-setting process has begun although regulatory guidelines are not formally in place.

Historically, regulatory agencies have relied on the sponsoring organization or its contractual agents to assume authority and responsibility for the integrity and quality of research performed in this area. It should also be noted that although regulatory agencies do not formally consider economic analyses as part of the marketing approval process for new prescription drugs, the use of economic analysis in product marketing is regulated under the agencies' legislative charters to ensure truth in advertising and other promotional activities.

The purpose of this chapter, however, is not to deal exclusively with the conduct of economic research within the context of product support strategies; rather, the main objective is to discuss the utility of economic research in the context of public health policy as it pertains to the regulation and control of prescription drug products. Regardless, some economic background is of significant import since the domain of health policy per se is both product specific (tactical) and strategic with regard to laws and regulations within and across national borders.

CORPORATE RESPONSE
TO PUBLIC POLICY INITIATIVES

In general, pharmaceutical companies are intimately concerned with developing, evaluating, and implementing strategies to influence public policy formation. Most strategic initiatives are responses to a deteriorating economic or sociopolitical environment and are not particularly aggressive. However, this type of response is not unique to the pharmaceutical industry; it is widespread throughout all sectors of the economy.

The key point to be made is that a company's strategic responses are made at very high levels within an organization, and the locus of the health economics function, whether it be in a medical or marketing division, is not inherently conducive to influencing policy decisions of the firm. In fact, the corporate entity usually responsible for formulating, translating, and disseminating policy statements of the corporation to its various constituencies is the public affairs (or an equivalent title) division, which is often distantly removed from the health economics activity. Moreover, the formulation of a corporate response to public policy initiatives often occurs through a process of consensus building at the industry's trade association level. Again, participation in these industrywide deliberations is typically at the senior levels of corporate management with subsequent elocution by the public affairs group.

ORGANIZATIONAL ISSUES

Those professionals working within the health economics field in the pharmaceutical industry should not take umbrage at this observation and accompanying discussion. Our individual and collective responsibilities have been to support the product-specific needs of our sponsoring division in particular and the company in general, and only recently has the potential value of this type of research as an instrument of policy change become recognized at senior (i.e., corporate or divisional) management levels.

I would also envision that a certain level of resistance to an expanded role would surface among some professionals and managers working within the discipline since much of the body of policy work is intangible and not always directly linked to business or product development objective–the accomplishment of which serves as the basis for remuneration and professional advancement. Moreover, those health economics units located in medical affairs divisions are largely removed from corporate policy making, and involvement in shaping health policy initiatives is not part of their recognized function or mission.

From a personal perspective, I have found it difficult to refocus from product-support activities to broader health policy issues within a finite time period. The proper balance between health policy support and product support is difficult, at best, to manage from the standpoint of allocating professionals' time and a department's financial resources.

There is also a tendency, I believe, within the organization to stereotype the professionals who undertake this type of research. Because of their relatively high theoretical and analytical training and because their function is often closely linked to clinical research and other product support activities, health economists are frequently viewed narrowly as researchers, analysts, or other fact gatherers.

It is often difficult to break away from this initial categorization, but in time, a broader role definition is attainable, especially as the discipline becomes more ingrained in the culture of the organization and more visible at upper management levels. Again, my observations should not be viewed as pejorative; my recommendation, however, is that health economics professionals should look at the ultimate value of the information they produce and its ultimate translation and dissemination, rather than focus exclusively on the successful completion of a series of individual research projects, whether they be product-support studies or health-policy analyses.

Briefly, a number of informal surveys have reported that the primary locus of health economics activity has been in the marketing division, followed closely by the medical affairs division.[1,5,6] My own personal bias favors location at a corporate, rather than divisional, level since such a location affords an opportunity for worldwide access to divisions and affiliates. The downside, of course, is a general lack of vested authority to influence internal divisional or affiliate affairs and, consequently, decision making. The relative advantages and disadvantages of organizational loci are summarized in Table 2.2.

POLICY ISSUES AFFECTING PRESCRIPTION DRUGS

As mentioned earlier, health policy concerning prescription drug products has historically dealt with ensuring safety and efficacy in approved therapeutic indications. Even the European Community's (EC) move toward harmonization of standards for pharmaceutical products is largely concerned with relatively technical issues involving good manufacturing practices, good clinical practices, and the free movement of goods across members' borders. To a great extent, the EC's directives are mainly concerned with policies to promote the free trade of pharmaceutical products as commodity items rather than with standards defining clinical outcomes or patient benefits.[7]

As discussed in a later section, reimbursement and pricing policies are still highly nationalistic throughout most of the industrialized world, although some harmonization of pricing levels in Europe is expected in the intermediate term as decisions concerning prescription drug pricing and reimbursement become more transparent in the EC. As such, the value of economic analyses is largely country specific and, in turn, product specific within the context of a nation's reimbursement and pricing policies. I suspect this will remain the case in the near future, since I have seen no evidence of EC initiatives or directives concerned with economic or quality of life assessment issues. This is not to say, of course, that consortia of academicians and other researchers are not working toward increased standardization. The comments refer to formal actions of the EC only.

TABLE 2.2. Organizational Issues

Location of Function	Advantages	Disadvantages
Marketing	Linkage to product support; visibility	Tactical, not strategic; short-term focus
Medical/ regulatory	Linkage to RCT and dossier preparation	Budgets; priority
Corporate	Access to other divisions; strategic	Lack of authority

A number of companies have begun to realize that in the absence of regulatory standards to evaluate economic analyses, the policy-making process can be influenced formally or informally within certain countries. Most companies recognize the benefit of providing economic information informally in registration and pricing dossiers. The more astute, progressive companies are recognizing the value of influencing the standards and criteria by which regulatory bodies assess economic studies. If successful, one company's strategy can, in effect, become the standard for the industry. In essence, economic research has become a competitive policy strategy in addition to its immediate utility as a tactic to support a particular product's price or reimbursement.

To a certain extent, the pharmaceutical manufacturers, as well as regulators, are on the early stages of the learning curve in understanding the application of economic analysis in pharmaceutical policy. For instance, it is most difficult to know, in the absence of explicit guidelines, where to place economic analyses in a national pricing or reimbursement dossier. In fact, the management of the local corporate affiliate, as well as that of the commission, will not always be able to offer clear guidance, especially when the submission of economic data is occurring for the first time.

For those companies bravely considering submission in a national or a Committee for Proprietary Medicinal Products (CPMP) registration dossier for marketing approval, should the economic information be a part of the clinical file or a part of the administrative section? Moreover, what are the practical implications of submitting this type of information in a CPMP submission? Specifically, can national financial data always be withheld from the overall CPMP review process? Admittedly, these are largely tactical questions (and to an extent already answerable), but they are presented as an epexegesis to the overall issue of standardization of methodologies, interpretations, and reporting.

In summary, even in countries where economic analysis has a more accepted role in technology assessment, guidance from regulatory authorities is not always forthcoming or consistent. For the present, one singular approach does not seem feasible for all countries, even for those countries sharing a common border, language, and culture.

A TOPOLOGY OF ECONOMIC ANALYSES

The terms Anglophone and European have been used by Klein to describe the topology of economic analyses.[8] Under the Anglophone rubric, economic analyses are intended to justify restricting access to individual pharmaceutical products or classes of therapy. This framework is said to be common to the United States, Canada, the United Kingdom, and Australia, where aggressive positive and negative formulary management systems are commonplace. Under the European model, economic analyses are employed to justify inclusion of products and are considered the operant framework in Sweden, the Netherlands, Germany, and Denmark. It is difficult to generalize the applicability to countries in which economic analysis is best described as emerging in acceptance and application (e.g., France, Spain, Italy, and Japan).

As expected, the Anglophone model typically focuses on the payers' perspective, whereas the European model has a broader societal perspective that includes both the payers' and the patients' (society) perspectives. In some countries, health-related quality of life measurement is necessary and sufficient evidence, perhaps more so than economic analysis, to justify approval for new indications and to support price negotiations. While the topology may oversimplify the framework for understanding the intent or objective of economic analyses, it is useful to introduce a number of concerns I have regarding overall policy implications of economic research.

SPECIFIC POLICIES AND CONCERNS ABOUT METHODOLOGIES

As a preface to the discussion on research issues, a fundamental question should be raised: Does research affect policy, or does policy affect research? One school of thought would argue that health services research (of which health economics is a subset) does not directly influence policy since policymakers do not share the empirical basis for rational decision making that researchers value. Rather, they are influenced by intuition, political reality, and a desire to do what is "right." Research findings are considered only post hoc if the findings support the policymakers' set of beliefs and values.

The other side, of course, would argue that if research outcomes are presented in a format that is acceptable and understandable, then policy initiatives can be influenced by health services research. The value of health services research per se is of importance when it focuses attention on the magnitude of a problem of societal concern.

I raise the question not to proffer an answer, but to address the fundamental question of assessing where we are in the state of the art of conducting economic research, translating it into meaningful and relevant information, and effectively disseminating its results. Moreover, a continuous reassessment of the value of economic research must be undertaken to determine its ultimate, realistic value to the firm. As mentioned, the organizational placement of the function and its integration with strategic and operational planning (business and product research and development) are essential in influencing positively the formation of corporate strategy and in determining its incremental value to the firm.

Value as a Criterion for Decision Making

As noted, economic analysis of pharmaceuticals has added the variable of cost-effectiveness into the traditional equation of a product's safety and efficacy. Frankly, I am somewhat ambivalent about the degree to which economic information should be considered in the overall equation. The Anglophone model causes me more concern than the European model in that the former advocates restricting access based on economic criteria while there is lack of consensus on methodological standards.

My concern is not assuaged by the presence of well-conceived a priori assumptions about the base case scenario at the core of economic analyses and its relevant sensitivity analyses. I am also concerned that a consensus on standards will emerge prematurely in reaction to perceptions of widespread methodological abuses and inconsistencies. Instead, I would prefer a gradual evolution of options to guidelines to standards.

The Choice of an Alpha Level

The next point is controversial, especially for clinicians and biometricians. Clearly, there is a preference for use of the randomized clinical trial (RCT) as the proposed gold standard for economic and health-related quality of life assessment. On this point, I certainly concur with advocating the performance of meta-analyses on existing RCTs germane to a comparative therapeutic question. While recognizing the need to remove the costs of protocol-driven procedures from the analysis, one still works with either the evaluable cohort or the intent-to-treat cohort, modifying either or both to approximate actual clinical practice. Indeed, there are even national preferences for the use of one cohort over the other. This situation impedes the development of a coherent standardized approach.

While this strategy is a reasonable and acceptable one for performing economic analyses, I express concern that the alpha level for judging clinical efficacy is not ipso facto an appropriate level for making policy decisions. I am concerned that an alpha level of 0.05 (or more stringent levels) is being assumed to be the appropriate level for what is basically an administrative decision, the appropriate level for which is probably much lower than that for a judgment involving severe consequences for the occurrence of a Type 1 error. I do not know what the appropriate level should be for decisions of this type. Instinctively, I suspect it should be less stringent than the level used to assess safety and efficacy in clinical trials. While sensitivity analyses allow for the relaxation of modeling assumptions for the base case scenario in an economic analysis, perhaps some attention should be given to the placement of a confidence interval around the estimates of economic parameters in the context of guiding administrative policy decisions. Alternatively, one could construct best case and worst case scenarios to present with the base case.

Experimental Designs

Policymakers prefer to have information about the use of prescription drugs for all relevant indications, approved and unapproved. RCTs are frequently designed to measure safety and efficacy for a limited number of indications, notably those that are more prevalent and clinically significant. Some resolution will be necessary to allow carefully designed clinical studies or retrospective analyses as alternatives to the RCT. The main problem with relying on the RCT is, in essence, external validity or generalizability. This is also the case when one considers the wide range of variability from country to country in defining standards of acceptable medical practice and the design of RCTs and clinical studies.

A concluding note to the RCT issue is the subject of the ethics of undertaking clinical research that has the assessment of economic outcomes as the primary objective. Not being an ethicist, I defer commentary to those more qualified to speak on the issue. It does seem likely that there would be ethical issues involved in the performance of research that would focus attention on an outcome such as average length of a hospital stay associated with alternative therapies. Ethics aside, what are the more practical implications of obtaining informed consent in conducting RCTs that focus mainly on economic outcomes? I would think that institutional review boards and protocol review committees would experience dissonance in reviewing protocols of this type in addition to the potential for patients to be reluctant to participate in a trial with explicit economic outcomes as the main study objectives.

Economic and Quality of Life Outcomes

Finally, one remaining major area of concern is the use of the quality-adjusted life year (QALY) as a main outcome of drug therapy. QALYs are a measure of the number of years of life gained as the result of drug therapy adjusted (in effect, discounted) by the health-related quality of life associated with incremental survival. QALYs are, in effect, endpoints associated with therapeutic interventions. The general consensus is that QALYs are better employed in chronic than acute conditions. The overriding reservation expressed in some quarters is the acceptance of the concept by decision makers who are not economists by formal training. The measurement of QALYs is perceived as somewhat arcane, and their utility in policy-making is not abundantly clear.

Ontario, for example, proposes to screen prescription drug products across therapeutic categories for inclusion (exclusion) in the provincial formulary based on the following QALY criteria: [4]

QALY Valuation	*Type of Product*
<20,000$/QALY gained	A
20,000 - 100,000$/QALY gained	B-D
>100,000$/QALY gained	E

From the results of a comparative RCT, a dominant product is placed in Category A; addition to the formulary is virtually assured. Categories B, C, and D offer increasing incremental costs and lessening therapeutic gains in relation to the standard therapy. Category E suggests a comparably less effective product that costs more than standard therapy and would not likely be added to the formulary. While the Ontario draft guidelines offer a degree of flexibility on some research issues, I am not certain that the QALY is very meaningful to clinicians and other decision makers without significant educational efforts; hence, some resistance might be predicted.

QALYs have become a relatively accepted norm in the research community for approximating the utility of drug therapy, especially in countries using the Anglophone model of decision making. They are not without controversy, however, in terms of measurement and theoretical security; i.e., QALYs are not, in effect, utility measures, and there are legitimate differences of opinion on analytic paradigms.

REIMBURSEMENT/PRICING POLICY ISSUES

Perhaps the most immediate policy issue to which health economics is being applied is worldwide pricing. Kolassa has estimated that within ten years the worldwide pricing environment for pharmaceuticals will show: (1) a continual decline of price growth; (2) harmonization of price regulation systems and program evaluation methods; (3) mandatory cost-benefit analyses to gain approval or use; and (4) a need to "sell price" as a positive component of the drug product or to justify the price charged.[9] Further, he summarizes the current systems of pricing policies:

- Policies encouraging generic drug products
- Prices based on cost
- Negotiated prices
- Formularies
- Mandatory rebates, price cuts
- Indexing
- Tendering/bidding
- Cost-benefit analyses
- Reference prices
- Patient cost sharing

In virtually all of Kolassa's examples, the value of economic research in influencing policy is straightforward. They range from documenting the value of therapeutic intervention to applied macro- and microeconomic strategies. Whether the applications are tactical, product-specific activities, or corporate strategies to effect policy formation and change will depend, in part, on the continued maturation of the discipline and the gradual institutionalization within the industry.

Finally, this is not to say that either strategies or tactics based on economic analysis will ensure premium pricing outcomes for pharmaceutical manufacturers. There are and will continue to be instances where the reimbursed price of a particular prescription drug, even a therapeutic breakthrough, will be below its economic value due to overriding economic or political factors.

SUMMARY AND CONCLUSIONS

The ultimate caveat is that economic analysis is only one part of a complex, dynamic decision-making process, and it is our responsibility both to maintain and advance its presence in rational public policy deliberations. I would contend that health economics should be nurtured and repositioned within the pharmaceutical industry. For this to happen, those professionals and managers in the economics function must learn to think and act strategically. While the pressure to remain accountable in supporting prescription drug products will remain, the ultimate value of the economics function within the firm is in the accomplishment of corporate business goals, which include both commercial and policy objectives.

I would suggest that the following steps would enable the health economics function to contribute more effectively to formulating health policy initiatives:

- Create and nurture additional formal alliances with corporate public affairs, strategic planning, business development, and product planning and development;
- Focus creative thinking on translating and disseminating information based on economic research beyond tactical needs, focusing instead on broader policy implications;
- Educate our internal constituencies (marketing, medical, public, and regulatory affairs) on an ongoing basis about public policy issues and their implications for the firm; and
- Incorporate economic planning into the long-range planning process, operational planning (e.g., annual marketing and product development plans), and other developmental planning processes of the firm.

Finally, the worldwide market for pharmaceutical products will become more challenging. Those firms that can respond quickly and decisively to the changing marketplace by influencing or responding actively to major policy issues will compete more effectively than firms that cannot. Again, the health economics function has contributions to make, but the discipline must mature and learn how to contribute incrementally to the success of the firm.

REFERENCES

1. Freeman R.A. Organizational issues in outcomes management research. J Pharmacoepidemiol 1991;2(2):59-67.

2. Hillman A.L., Eisenberg, J.M., Pauly, M.V., Bloom, B.S., Glick, H., Kinosian, B., and Schwartz, J.S. Avoiding bias in the conduct and reporting of cost-effectiveness research sponsored by pharmaceutical companies. N Engl J Med 1991;324:1262-1265.

3. Anon. Guidelines for the pharmaceutical industry on preparation of submissions to the Pharmaceutical Benefits Advisory Committee: including submissions involving economic analyses (draft). Australian Pharmaceutical Benefits Advisory Committee, 1990.

4. Anon. Guidelines for preparation of economic analysis to be included in submission to Drug Programs Branch for listing in the Ontario Drug Benefit For-

mulary/Comparative Drug Index (draft). Ministry of Health, Drug Programs Branch, October 1991.

5. Fifer S.K. Staffing of pharmacoeconomic units in pharmaceutical firms. San Francisco, CA: Technology Assessment Group, Inc., 1991.

6. Zitter M. How manufacturers are organizing for outcomes research: a survey by the Center for Outcomes Evaluation. San Francisco, CA: The Zitter Group, 1991.

7. Taylor D. The evolution of Europe's pharmaceutical market. Scrip 1991; 1591(Feb 15):10.

8. Klein R. Traditions of social insurance. In: Teeling Smith G, ed. Measuring the benefits of medicines: the future agenda. London: Office of Health Economics, 1989.

9. Kolassa M. Pharmaceutical price regulations, potential new regulations and how to survive them. Unpublished.

Chapter 3

The Technology Trust Fund: Paying for Medical Technology

Robert A. Freeman
Rachel F. Tasch

INTRODUCTION

For many private insurance programs, publicly financed sickness funds, and national health care financing systems, the introduction of new medical technologies presents a challenge: while new technologies can offer substantive improvements in patient care and potential efficiencies in medical care delivery, medical technology is frequently at an aggregate cost that places the programs' financial integrity at risk. Further, new medical technologies enter the market at relatively high rates, and coverage decisions are often made under pressure from patients and medical care providers and with incomplete information.

The decision to reimburse providers for using new medical technologies or to permit the acquisition of new technologies is made in an environment clouded by uncertainties associated with the technologies' expected utilization in both approved and unapproved indications, the standards for appropriate use, the extent of eventual diffusion within the medical community, and the actual market price and its impact on health care expenditures. Moreover, while health care providers and administrators are somewhat aware of the impending availability of specific new technologies, the actual date at which market entry occurs and its relationship to the program's operational budget cycle are additional uncertainties.

This work is based on a presentation delivered before the annual meeting of the International Society for Technology Assessment, Helsinki, Finland, July 1991.

Previously published in *Journal of Research in Pharmaceutical Economics*, Vol. 4(2), 1992.

Health care delivery is clearly technology driven, and there are no obvious signs of a reversal or slowing in this trend. Historically, physicians have been rapid adopters of new prescription drugs, devices, and medical/surgical procedures. The acquisition of new equipment by hospitals and other health care organizations to remain at the cutting edge of high-tech medicine is also reflective of the trend favoring rapid technology diffusion and adoption. Decisions to adopt a specific technology are often made in the absence of definitive research outcomes describing relative effectiveness and associated cost implications for both intended and unintended uses. Gastric freezing for treating peptic ulcers and hyperbaric oxygen therapy for cognitive disorders in the elderly are illustrative of therapies once commonplace and now discredited after further evaluation.

Clearly, some technological advances (laparoscopic general surgery and cimetidine, for example) have made it possible to shift the locus of medical care delivery away from the resource-intensive inpatient care setting to less intensive outpatient services or to home settings without reducing the overall quality of care. However, technology in the aggregate is relatively expensive to acquire and maintain, and the pressure to contain costs has an adverse impact on the operational budgets of many clinical service managers. While the overall financial impact of any particular medical technology may be cost savings, our traditional health care accounting systems, which are more or less based on identifying and assigning costs to departments or centers, are impediments to decision making based on the criterion of overall economic impact. This is because fiscal responsibility for any particular component of health service delivery is vested at a departmental level and not at a system level.

The role of consumers in technology adoption and diffusion is less definitive because consumers generally do not have access to adequate information related to the availability and clinical efficacy of specific new technologies. However, the results from consumer survey research suggest that consumers demand access to and availability of the latest technological advances.[1] Evidence also suggests that consumers are willing to pay for unfettered access and availability and are unwilling to accept rationing of or other restrictions on access to technology.[2]

In essence, the administrators of health care financing systems and health care delivery systems are confronted by two technology-driven constituencies: physicians and other providers who demand the best technology available for patient care; and consumers who demand access to the latest medical technologies in general and, on occasion, to specific technologies about which they have obtained information from the lay press, friendship networks, or consumer advocacy groups. Beyond the obvious need to satisfy these constituencies, where appropriate, health services administrators and researchers are faced with an obligation to assess technology and to determine equitable coverage and reimbursement decisions.

This chapter contains a presentation of a conceptual framework for financing the coverage of new medical technologies. While the content is concerned primarily with financial issues, we contend that technology assessment is a sine qua non of rational medical decision making. Formalizing the technology assessment process within an organization is beyond the scope of this discussion, although we would argue that meaningful financial planning cannot occur with out a structured approach to technology assessment by both the public and the private sector.[3] Strict reliance on evidence from randomized clinical trials completed prior to market entry as the sole criterion for coverage decisions is myopic in the long run for reimbursement decisions and for clinical decisions. Accordingly, both medical care providers and administrators of financing schemes in partnership with manufacturers have an ongoing obligation to conduct further technology assessments of the drug, device, equipment, or diagnostic as it is used in actual clinical practice.

Finally, we have chosen to construct our example around new prescription drugs because of the high frequency of drug use, the extensive amount of technology assessment conducted prior to market approval, and the pervasiveness of drugs in both ambulatory and institutional medical practices worldwide. Moreover, the financial and scientific commitment of the pharmaceutical industry in sponsoring ongoing evaluations of its products is unique in medical technology assessment and, consequently, facilitates the orderly dissemination of information into the technology assessment process.

We present our model within the context of the traditional accounting/ financial reporting systems as they presently exist. These rely on identifying and assigning costs and revenues (where appropriate) to departmental accounts of budgets defined by the type and locus of medical care service provided. Recognizing that accounting systems only slowly change, we have chosen to work within that framework to create, in essence, a new line item account to which the costs of technology assessment, acquisition, and maintenance may be initially budgeted and assigned during a current fiscal cycle. We also recognize that financial reporting systems as well as terminology vary on a country basis; therefore, we attempt to maintain internal consistency and parsimony in the use of terminology rather than present varying examples of such usage.[4]

THE CONCEPTUAL MODEL

We propose that a technology trust fund (TTF) be established as a recurring account in the financial statements of health care organizations and financing systems for the purpose of managing the expenditures associated with the acquisition, evaluation, and diffusion of a set of medical technologies during a current fiscal cycle. The TTF would be constructed as a risk-sharing arrangement among medical care providers, manufacturers, consumers, and the health care financing system. In this case, the risk shared by the parties is the financial risk of losses due to overutilization of the technologies, inappropriate utilization of the technologies, and the administrative costs of technology assessment.

The ultimate objective of the TTF is to manage the diffusion of new medical technologies into the health care delivery system and finance the system in an orderly, efficient manner without disrupting the financial operations of key departments within the system (e.g., physician services, pharmacy services, and inpatient services). In practice, the TTF would serve as an escrow account funded by direct contributions from or deferred reimbursements to each of the aforementioned partners. The exact amount of funding, along with its source, would be determined by the expected or actual price of the technology, start-up costs (primarily training costs, installation costs, and costs associated with replacing obsolete technology, where relevant), maintenance costs, and costs associated with current or planned technology assessment projects.

As envisioned, the TTF would contain sufficient financial resources to manage efficiently the technology adoption and diffusion process within the system and to prevent the curtailment of planned expenses in departmental budgets associated with the introduction of new technology. Accordingly, at the completion of the current budget cycle, the fiscal responsibility for managing the new technology would be transferred to the appropriate clinical budget(s). While the TTF is envisioned as a recurring fund account, monies associated with specific medical technologies would be entering and leaving the fund as their incorporation into ongoing clinical operations was achieved.

Due to the disparate nature of new medical technologies and their associated costs, we envision that the TTF would have at least the following accounts: a drug fund, a device fund, a diagnostic fund, a medical/surgical procedure fund, and a major equipment fund (Figure 3.1). Unique line items within each fund account would be used to describe the specific technologies constituting each fund type.

Should the new technology be overutilized or inappropriately utilized, the risk-sharing provisions would penalize financially the source of the

FIGURE 3.1. Drug Component of the TTF

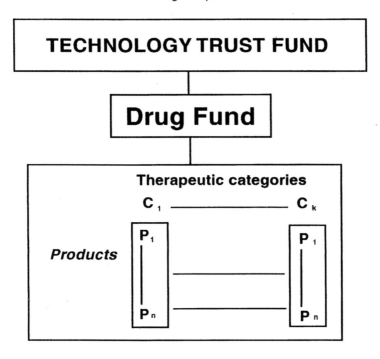

overutilization/inappropriate utilization to the degree it was responsible for the variance. (Note: We use the term variance in the traditional sense, referring to a deviation that is controllable.) For instance, physicians would be at risk financially if the technology were overprescribed or prescribed suboptimally, assuming that standards or guidelines for appropriate use can be promulgated and incorporated into the physicians' practices in a timely manner. The manufacturer of the technology would be at risk of not receiving full reimbursement of its market or negotiated price if the technology were marketed inappropriately or if the technology were found to be ineffective relative to existing technology in a general population. It is recognized that effectiveness and safety in large patient populations may not be known with relative certainty for several years after the product is introduced. Consequently, it may be necessary to conduct an observational clinical study (e.g., postmarketing surveillance study or open-label comparative drug study) or to perform a meta-analysis of existing clinical trials and studies before the product diffuses widely in the market.

The financing system would also be at risk for failing to estimate accurately a technology's expected utilization and associated costs. Failure to apply established actuarial methods for patient populations or subpopulation groups at risk would likely lead to underestimates of a technology's utilization and, consequently, inadequate resources for funding its coverage or acquisition.

In a case where the new technology was found to be cost saving or cost-effective in comparison to existing technology–should this be a relevant criterion–adjustments to future TTF contributions could be made by reducing contributions for the next fiscal cycle, freezing contributions, or granting rebates from the current TTF's surplus. In any event, as there are penalties for overutilization of specific medical technologies, there should also be financial incentives for the adoption and diffusion of technologies found to offer substantive patient care benefits and economic efficiencies.

Finally, we recognize that the costs of technology adoption and diffusion will not likely be mitigated by this or any other conceptual model. We assume that aggregate expenditures for new technology will increase annually, and our emphasis, therefore, is on affecting the rate of increase in expenditures or costs. Our model is based on the management of the marginal costs of technology adoption and diffusion.

AN EXAMPLE

For simplicity, assume T is a new prescription drug in a novel therapeutic category and is expected to enter the market during time t. In this example, we limit the creation of the TTF to one set of technologies only: new prescription drug products with regulatory approval for marketing limited to the treatment of condition X. However, product T is known to have other recognized therapeutic indications (Y, Z) for which regulatory approval will be sought in subsequent years. Additionally, indication W is a disease for which product T can be prescribed, but T is considered to be both inappropriate and unwarranted for treatment of W. Hence, we present a fairly typical example of a new technology approved narrowly but with a known number of unapproved indications and, for this example, one inappropriate indication. Additionally, there are n drug products in therapeutic category G that are indicated for the treatment of conditions X, Y, and Z.

The TTF may be created as follows, using the following assumptions and symbols:

Given that

1. *n* products within category *G* are approved for treating disease condition *X*.

2. Conditions *Y* and *Z* are treated by the *n* drugs in therapeutic category *G*.

3. Drug product *T* will be prescribed for unapproved conditions *Y* and *Z* in addition to condition *X*.

4. Some physicians will prescribe products in *T* for *W*, an inappropriate indication, but not preventable a priori.

5. Prevalence of *Z* > prevalence of *Y* > prevalence of *X*, and prevalence of *X* = prevalence of *W*.

6. The price (P_T) of *T* > the prices of all *n* products in *G* (P_G).

Then,

7. For approved indication *X*, assuming 20% of all *X* will be treated by *T* during *t*,

   expected costs $(C_1) = P_T \times 0.20(X)$, and

8. For unapproved indications *Y* and *Z*, assuming 10% of all *Y* and *Z* will be treated by *T* during *t*,

   expected costs $(C_2) P_T \times 0.10(Y + Z)$, and

9. For inappropriate indication *W*, assuming 5% of all *W* will be treated by *T* during *t*,

   expected cost $(C_3) = P_T \times 0.05 (W)$.

Also,

10. The cost of displacing category *G* by category *T* in treating conditions *X*, *Y*, *Z*, and *W* $(C_4) =$

    $MD\$ \times (0.2X + 0.1(Y + Z) + 0.5W)$

Where,

   MD\$ = cost/physician visit (\$) × number of visits to replace *G* with *T* and,

   (. . .) = expected utilization of *T* in conditions *X*, *Y*, *Z*, and *W*.

Therefore,

11. The expected cost (T_c) of new technology T during time t is given by
$T_c = C_1 + C_2 + C_3 + C_4$.

The amount budgeted to the TTF is the total sum from Equation 11, which is the marginal cost of product T during time t.

At this point, we do not recommend an all-inclusive rule for the identification and assignment of exact amounts into the TTF account by source of funding. The scheme for the TTF's cash flows, however, is presented in Figure 3.2, followed by a plausible scenario.

SCENARIO

Suppose, in this example, that the program views the utilization of product T for an inappropriate indication (W) as an unacceptable risk in terms of patient outcomes and economic consequences. The potential contributors to the occurrence of this risk would be the physicians who prescribe the product for the indication and, perhaps, the manufacturer, whose marketing practices may explicitly or implicitly encourage the use of the product for the unaccepted indication.

FIGURE 3.2. TTF Financial Cycle

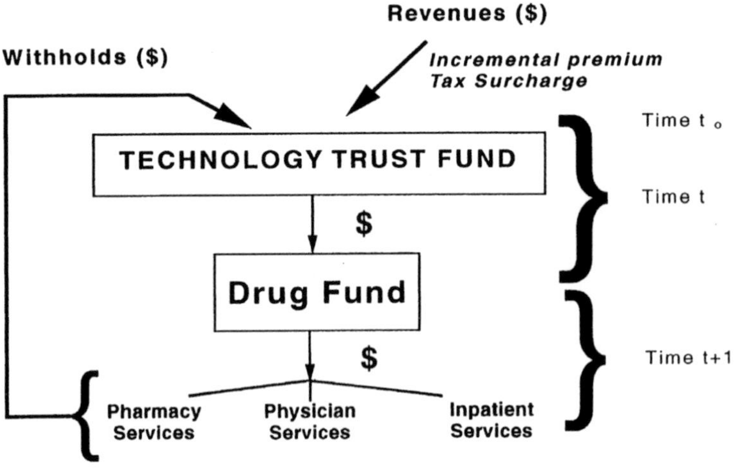

To this point, we have an estimate of the magnitude of the risk, which is from Equation 9 and from the part of Equation 10 that is directly attributable to W. In fact, the magnitude of the risk is approximately 25% of the expected use in the approved indication X. (It is, of course, a smaller magnitude if conditions Y and Z are deemed appropriate for reimbursement, especially since the prevalences of Z and Y are greater than X).

It may be appropriate to withhold, for example, an equivalent percentage of expected reimbursement from the provider community and the manufacturers of the technology as a risk-sharing amount for inappropriate utilization. This withhold is, in effect, a surcharge, a portion (if not all) of which would eventually return to the provider(s) and the manufacturer(s) if the risk did not materialize at the end of time t.

In the case of unapproved uses Y and Z, it is clear that prescribing category T for these indications, while clinically appropriate, could have dire consequences for the financial integrity of the program. As noted, Y and Z exceed X in patient volume, and market penetration of these populations by a more expensive technology than existing category G amplifies the need for careful forecasts of potential utilization in these conditions since the manufacturer cannot promote directly for these uses. Diffusion can and will occur, primarily through dissemination in the medical literature and by professional and collegial networks. Clearly, the program's administrators will have to accept responsibility for underestimating potential utilization in these conditions, as will the medical community.

Therapy G is assumed to be used appropriately in treating conditions X, Y, and Z. Prescribing G for condition W is assumed not to occur; therefore, prescriptions for G are assumed to be appropriate. Also, expenditures for G are allocated to the pharmacy services budget and can be predicted within $\pm 10\%$ of actual utilization during the course of cycle t. As noted, the use of G will decrease as T diffuses in the medical community, thereby creating a temporary budget surplus in pharmacy services since the marginal cost of adding drug T to the program's budget is contained in the TTF. It would be possible, therefore, to withhold a portion of this operational surplus as a contribution to the TTF.

An alternative to the manufacturers' surcharge that was mentioned previously would be to apply a sliding scale of rebates or other volume-based withholds that are engaged only when predetermined thresholds are exceeded in the aggregate or in specific indications. Also, the establishment of a predetermined number of grant awards for technology assessment of the therapy used in treating these conditions would be a viable alternative to withholds, although the logistics of such a mechanism appear problematic administratively and, perhaps, legally.

To this point, we have not discussed the responsibility of the consumer in sharing the financial risks of overutilization or inappropriate utilization. We would encourage, where practicable, that the consumer share some of the financial costs of the risks associated with technology adoption and diffusion. In competitive markets for health insurance, this responsibility could be met by assigning a modest incremental charge for technology assessment in the premium structure, with the resultant revenues transferred to the TTF. While relatively uncommon, the practice does occur in managed health care organizations whose premium structures contain a separate charge for quality assurance.[5]

In markets where the consumer's share of health insurance costs approaches zero, a state-financed TTF, may be worthy of consideration, and for private insurance schemes, a premium surcharge could be considered. Admittedly, with the exception of the Netherlands and the U.S., it is not commonplace for insurers or sick funds to undertake directly sponsored technology assessment research. Regardless, consumer demand does play a role in technology diffusion and should be a part of the equation either through incremental premium surcharges or other appropriate schemes.

As noted in Figure 3.2, there is no explicit relationship between the TTF and clinical services budgets during time t. In other words, the TTF is responsible for managing the costs associated with the new technologies although the service delivery per se occurs at the clinical service level. At the end of time t, however, fiscal responsibility for the new technology would be allocated to the appropriate service department(s), and the functional manager(s) would be held accountable for achieving appropriate cost and service goals and objectives in subsequent periods.

It is acknowledged, however, that a one-year period may be insufficient to manage complex technologies, and exceptions could naturally be made to extend the time frame required for an orderly incorporation of the technology into standard medical practice. In the case of therapeutic breakthroughs, for example, the information base is quite sparse in comparison to what is known about more established therapies. In fact, the cost of acquiring definitive information about breakthroughs can be expected to be quite high, in economic terms, in relation to the cost of obtaining and processing information about new products within therapeutic areas that are well understood. We propose that the marginal cost of information about novel technologies is substantially higher than the marginal cost of information related to new products within a therapeutic category that is relatively mature in terms of the number of products available and their comparative effectiveness.

One ramification of this issue that is worthy of note is the economic cost to the program when the new product is not effective clinically in terms of absolute as well as relative frequencies of therapeutic failure. The magnitude of the cost is, of course, a function of the number of patients for whom a treatment failure occurs and the prevalence of the condition. One could expect the cure rates for antibiotics, especially novel antibiotics, to be quite high in comparison to those of other therapeutic categories, notably those that are primarily palliative therapy in chronic conditions (e.g., nonsteroidal anti-inflammatory drugs). It may be desirable, therefore, to add an amount to the TTF to take into account the probability that treatment failures do occur and that economic costs associated with differential rates of therapeutic failures among products within the same therapeutic class may be significant.

DISCUSSION

On the surface, it would appear that the creation of the TTF is nothing more than an accounting ploy that shifts costs into a new line item rather than a concentrated effort to assist managers in the control of technology-related costs. In reality, the creation of a new account for the assignment of costs associated with technology acquisition can be used to address major technology policy issues actively.

The creation of the TTF presents a structure by which technology planning can be undertaken with increased priority and visibility within and external to the health care delivery and financing system. Under this scheme, clinical services managers, financial analysts, technical personnel, and other decision makers can address the status of therapeutic needs, emerging technology trends, potential impact on patient care, and expected costs and utilization. In addition, a dialogue can be created early in the decision-making process with manufacturers of technology to determine the timing of the product's availability and adequacy of supply, the manufacturer's marketing practices and its provision of value-added services, start-up resource requirements, and other distributional matters. By using the outcomes of these deliberations and negotiations, health services managers can translate these findings to cost projections, cash flow requirements, capital requirements, and other financial parameters, thereby obtaining a preliminary assessment of the economic pact of the new technology on the system and its relative components.

The above discussion should not be interpreted as suggesting that this planning process does not occur in any particular nation's health care institutions and financing agencies; indeed, discussions of this nature are routine. We suggest, however, that the discussions are highly compartmentalized in their conduct and, therefore, isolated from considerations of the perspective of the entire system, as reflected by the hierarchical management structure of most complex health care organizations and financing agencies. (We note that capital expenditure projects would be an obvious exception to this general observation.) Simply, we offer this mechanism as a method of facilitating financial and tactical planning.

Finally, the TTF will require both strategic and tactical management. While the structure and constitution of the fund's oversight function will be dependent on the corporate and/or national cultures of a particular insurer, sick fund, etc., it would seem obvious that a matrix organization comprised of clinicians, health services administrators and researchers, and consumers would be required to ensure that appropriate medical technology is available and accessible to patients and clinicians at an affordable price.

SUMMARY AND CONCLUSION

We have been deliberately ambiguous as to specific recommendations for managing the logistics of the TTF. A discussion of specifics would be premature at this time. The key issue, in our opinion, is that the problem of financing new medical technologies is at the breaking point, and other alternatives for its management should be brought to the debate.

The proliferation of new technologies, along with their costs, has been a major contributor to health care inflation. In some instances, operational budgets of health care plans, both public and private, have been disrupted, and painful decisions have had to be made between acquiring new technologies or maintaining basic health care services. By creating a TTF, we have focused the consumers' attention (as well as that of the body politic) on the budgeting of technology expenses, and we incur an additional risk to medical care decision making by raising the public's consciousness of the amount we spend for technology and the choices we make.

We recognize that a TTF will not likely result in a decrease in expenditures for medical technology. Our model is an attempt to manage efficiently the marginal cost of technology diffusion during the time when little is known about the technology's effectiveness in actual medical practice. In effect, we have proposed a cost minimization strategy to which more formal quantitative models can be applied.

REFERENCES

1. Jennett B. Assessment of clinical technologies. Int J Technol Assess Health Care 1988;4:438.

2. Ginzberg E. High tech medicine and rising health care costs. JAMA 1990; 263:1820.

3. Perry S, Pillar B. A national policy for health care technology assessment. Med Car Rev 1990;47:408.

4. Glasser WA. Paying the hospital: the organizational dynamics and effects of differing financial arrangements. San Francisco, CA: Jossey-Bass, 1987.

5. Zapka JG, Rapoport J, Shamos E. Technology decisions in health maintenance organizations. GHAA J 1987;(Sum):79-91.

Chapter 4

Medicaid Drug Cost Containment: An Economic Perspective

John A. McMillan
Charlotte A. Jankel

INTRODUCTION

The joint state and federal Medicaid program was enacted in 1967 under Title XIX of the 1965 amendments to the Social Security Act. By providing first-dollar coverage of health care costs, the mission of Medicaid was to eliminate financial barriers to mainstream medical care for the indigent and medically needy. In the years since the program's inception, expansion in eligibility and scope of coverage and advances in medical technology have dramatically increased the costs of accomplishing this mission, and most states are now wrestling with these rising costs.

Currently, all states provide some form of Medicaid drug coverage, budgets for which range from $4.2 million (Alaska) to $458 million (California).[1] Mechanisms to prevent excessive or unnecessary use and thus contain rising drug costs were an inevitable response to the increasing budgetary pressures facing Medicaid. However, minimizing the cost of excess demand while not impeding the provision of needed care has not been an easy balance to achieve: "The Medicaid dilemma lies in the incongruence of controls and the overarching legislative goal of Medicaid. It is difficult to ensure access to care while creating mechanisms to regulate its use."[2]

There is a lack of consensus on the "ideal" constraint, and Medicaid drug program managers, attempting to control burgeoning budgets, have employed a multitude of interventions that have targeted both supply and demand aspects of drug use.

Previously published in *Journal of Research in Pharmaceutical Economics*, Vol. 5(2), 1993.

The purpose of this chapter is to evaluate, from the perspectives of efficiency and equity, the suitability of various methods of controlling drug program costs within the Medicaid population. It will be argued that although traditional cost-containment measures are effective, they will continue to have varying degrees of success in accomplishing Medicaid's mission and that nonmarket approaches may provide the most equitable answer to the cost-containment dilemma.

A normative discussion of Medicaid drug cost containment must first address the basic question of whether drug coverage should be provided at all. The most effective and predictable means of controlling drug cost is to exclude drug coverage; however, without drug coverage, the indigent Medicaid population would face a financial barrier to needed therapy. Empirical evidence supports this contention. A study of indigent patients terminated from Medi-Cal suggested that inability to pay for medications resulted in patients stretching medication supplies by lengthening dosing intervals and discontinuing relatively inexpensive medications, a possible cause of associated adverse health consequences.[3,4] Similarly, 35% of medically stable patients terminated from a Veteran's Association Medical Center outpatient setting as a result of budget cuts either reduced or stopped prescribed medications due to financial pressures.[5] Exclusion of drugs, the most widely used therapeutic approach, is incompatible with the equity-based mainstream care concept of Medicaid's mission. Equity aside, drugs are a relatively small component of the overall Medicaid budget (7.9% of 1991 Medicaid expenditures), yet as a class of medical care, drugs often provide more cost-effective treatment than institutional alternatives.[6,7,8] Since it may be wiser to pay for some degree of drug treatment than for preventable hospitalization, exclusion of drug coverage is not likely to be a cost-effective option from the perspective of the Medicaid system. Equitable methods to contain Medicaid drug costs, therefore, become desirable management tools.

SUPPLY-SIDE EFFORTS

The opportunity to constrain drug costs via supply-side intervention rests with the simple economic endeavor of limiting the amount (price) Medicaid will pay for goods and services purchased on behalf of the beneficiary. Since they do not directly affect the patient, supply-side efforts equitably restrict the cost of all drug use if judiciously designed and implemented so as not to inhibit access through provider alienation.

Supply-side constraints have been incorporated into Medicaid drug programs from the outset, restricting the prices of goods and services at the provider level by limiting reimbursement for both product (e.g., maximum allowable cost) and service (e.g., dispensing and physician fees). Through these constraints, Medicaid simply purchases needed health care for its beneficiaries at a lower cost. Additionally, as the level of constrained reimbursement approaches the economic cost of product/service provision, provider incentive to promote use and to gain excess profits in an imperfectly competitive market is reduced.

Provider-targeted supply-side constraints of various forms remain in effect in most Medicaid programs. The degree to which constraints targeting providers can be effective is limited by providers' economic costs, reimbursement below which would result in reduced access through loss of participation, a result contrary to Medicaid's goal.

Recent supply-side efforts, such as the rebate mechanisms mandated by the Ominbus Budget Reconciliation Act of 1990 (OBRA90), have shifted toward the drug manufacturer, the final supply-side avenue for savings.[9] Given the current level of provider reimbursement and the fact that drug prices are currently under attack at the industry level, the attainable benefits of supply-side constraint have probably been realized. Beyond these efforts, additional supply-side intervention, short of direct government provision of the drug needs of the poor, is not likely to significantly affect Medicaid drug budgets.

DEMAND-SIDE EFFORTS

Demand-side constraints have a long history in both public and private-sector health care plans and remain a primary focus of Medicaid's drug cost-containment efforts. Although demand-side constraints vary in operational complexity and degree of predictability of savings achieved, they fall into two general categories:

1. *Economic- or market-based constraints* **indirectly** exert cost-containment pressure through the price-quantity relationship at the recipient level.
2. *Non-market-based constraints* rely upon **direct** intervention at the aggregate and/or recipient level in the decision to provide coverage for a given drug or condition.

To identify which and to what degree specific demand-side mechanisms can provide equitable cost containment under the mission of Medicaid, it is necessary to discuss the theoretical basis upon which these mechanisms depend.

Critics of full insurance coverage generally express concern over its inefficiency as represented by a predicted increase in utilization over that observed under self-insured conditions, a prediction supported by empirical evidence (e.g., the investigations conducted by the Rand Corporation).[10] This phenomenon, termed *moral hazard,* results from an effective marginal unit price reduction to the patient. As a simple example (moral hazard is a well-developed concept in the economic literature), Figure 4.1 depicts an individual's demand curve (*D*) to be other than perfectly inelastic (downward sloping, a necessary assumption) and, for simplicity, a linear function of price.

The individual's demand curve depicted in Figure 4.1 shows that Q_1 units of health care would be purchased at price P_1 (at total cost $P_1 * Q_1$) and Q_5 units at zero price. Assuming diminishing marginal utility of drug use, the specific prescription drugs that the patient would be willing to purchase at a higher price should represent those that offer the most personal utility, i.e., those perceived as most necessary to restore or maintain good health from the patient's perspective. The area under the demand curve therefore represents the maximum expenditure the patient would be willing to bear if each specific unit was incrementally purchased at the maximum price he would be willing to pay for that specific unit.

FIGURE 4.1. Insurance and Drug Demand

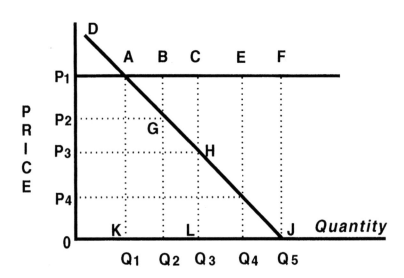

Under total insurance (market price P_1 to the insuring body, but zero price to the consumer), an individual's demand results in expenditure area *AJF*: *more* than he or she would ever be willing to pay for this same care. Full coverage in the face of homogenous market price P_1 therefore allows the consumer to purchase his or her desired zero price quantity (Q_5), thereby gaining a *consumer surplus* of patient-specific value (area *AJK*). But since the price ($P_1 * Q_5$) must be paid by the insuring body for the quantity demanded, area *AJF* represents the expenditure in excess of value received, the value of other goods and services whose purchase must be foregone to pay for the increased use–a *welfare cost* to society.

As the proportion of insurance coverage increases, the welfare cost resulting from moral hazard increases at an increasing rate.[11] The incremental utility of marginal purchase decreases, thus the marginal cost of increased use is being transferred from other uses to buy units that are of less and less value to the consumer.

Economic (Indirect) Mechanisms

Economic- or market-based demand-side cost-containment efforts seek to manipulate the patient's effective point-of-service price to reduce excessive use, a potential component of the moral hazard associated with insurance.

As just discussed, the welfare cost of moral hazard is generally held to represent economic inefficiency. However, in the provision of insured care to the Medicaid population, not all of the welfare cost (in the classical sense) resulting from insuring patients is bad. In fact, bearing some degree of the potential welfare cost is expected, even desirable, if Medicaid is to succeed in enhancing health care access, thereby increasing the population's consumption of care to the level of need.

Need has been defined as "a normative professional medical judgment concerning the quantity of medical services that [a population's] members ought to consume over some specified period of time."[12] In Figure 4.2, a vertical indicator depicts the needed quantity of drug treatment (Q_n) to be greater than Q_1, the suboptimal level of care that the indigent would consume without drug coverage, but less than Q_{max}, the amount of care the patient would demand if provided drugs free of charge.

If the patient's drug use was equitably subsidized for his particular demand such that his portion of drug cost was P_n (which could be "0" if Q_n coincided with Q_{max}) of full cost P_1, the patient would be induced to purchase the needed quantity of care Q_n. This results in an estimated welfare cost symbolized in magnitude by area *ABC,* the minimum cost that must be transferred from other societal uses to promote consumption of needed care for the individual. Area *CFGH* plus the resulting consumer

FIGURE 4.2. Welfare Cost and Medical Need

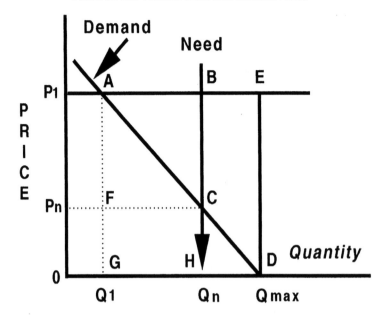

surplus (*ACF*) represents the maximum value that the recipient places on the additional ($Q_n - Q_1$) units of care. However, given a legislative commitment to provide the needed level of care, the value to society of the additional ($Q_n - Q_1$) units is implicitly greater (by area *ABC*). Therefore, the welfare cost necessary to promote consumption of needed care (represented in Figure 4.2 by area *ABC*), a measure of inefficiency in an economic sense, has been implicitly deemed a socially equitable price of meeting the mission of Medicaid. The cost of legislating medical equity may necessarily reflect economic inefficiency in the traditional sense.

But should drug coverage be provided without constraint? Figure 4.2 also shows that if drug coverage was unconstrained, the patient would consume ($Q_{max} - Q_n$) more units of care than is needed, resulting in a true inefficiency cost represented as *BCDE,* the undesirable welfare cost of utilization in excess of need. The attempt to promote Medicaid drug utilization commensurate with need must incorporate constraints to partition only the welfare cost of excessive use. To be compatible with Medicaid's mission, demand-side interventions must limit unnecessary or excessive drug use without reducing consumption of needed therapy simply for budgetary reasons. As discussed below, it is questionable whether economic-based mechanisms provide the most equitable approach to accomplishing this mission.

1. *Deductibles.* Health insurers frequently constrain use by imposing a deductible mechanism upon the insured. As a simple illustration, Figure 4.1 shows a demand function for a patient who would consume Q_1 units of care under self-pay conditions and Q_5 units of care under full coverage. However, if a deductible of magnitude ($Q_3 * P_1$) was imposed, the patient would have to pay his resulting welfare cost component (area ACH, more than he would ever be willing to pay out-of-pocket for the first Q_3 units of care) to receive Q_5 units under subsequent full insurance coverage. In theory, the patient would choose to pay the deductible only as long as the consumer surplus (HJL) gained from additional consumption under full coverage of incremental use exceeds the welfare cost component (ACH) of the deductible that he or she would have to pay.

A deductible is not a desirable mechanism for containing Medicaid drug costs for three reasons. As a financial barrier to care, the deductible is not compatible with Medicaid's mission. Many of the poor could not pay the deductible; thus, mainstream and needed care might not be obtained. Second, the deductible promotes an all-or-none consumption pattern.[13] A deductible may result either in consumption of the same amount of care as in the case of no insurance (Q_1) or in consumption of the same amount of care as in the situation of full coverage (Q_5). The patient either chooses not to satisfy the deductible and purchases as if uninsured or chooses to satisfy the deductible and purchases as if under full coverage. The deductible, therefore, either inhibits purchase of drugs offering high patient utility (those for which the patient would pay a price close to the market price) or insures therapies of less utility (those lower on the demand curve and thus not highly valued), an undesirable result. Finally, a deductible requires the Medicaid recipient to weigh the utility loss of the moral hazard implicit in the deductible against the consumer's surplus to be gained under insurance once the deductible is covered. The recipient's ability to make such a decision would likely be limited given his or her level of drug knowledge.

2. *Other Types of Coinsurance.* Another means of reducing use might be to require patients to pay a fixed percentage of drug cost (percentage coinsurance) or a fixed fee per prescription (copayment) as an alternative to full coverage. The effect of either method on purchasing behavior can be considered in terms of the proportion of market price that the patient is ultimately required to pay. As indicated in Figure 4.1, if full coverage was replaced with either a copayment or percentage coinsurance mechanism such that the patient's share of the cost was P_2 of full price P_1 per unit of care, use would fall to Q_2, and welfare cost would shrink to AGB from AJF.

By imposing a per-unit cost across all purchases, these types of coinsurance constrain in an incremental manner, imposing less patient cost than deductibles on high utility first-purchase prescriptions, but becoming a greater deterrent as consumption expands to products of lower marginal utility. This is more desirable from the standpoint of providing the Medicaid patient access to therapy because there is less tendency to force consumption to either extreme.

As with the deductible, however, other forms of coinsurance may conflict with the mission of Medicaid because they impose a reduced–but nonetheless positive–financial cost on all units of drug use within the indigent population. The cumulative financial requirement of coinsurance schemes may force individuals in high use categories to forego needed treatment.

The cost-sharing variants briefly discussed above offer potential for cost savings in Medicaid drug programs by limiting the manner and degree to which drug coverage controls the point-of-purchase price to the enrolled population, a point supported by empirical evidence in poor populations.[14] As previously stated, to be consistent with the mission of Medicaid, constraints should avoid imposing monetary costs on needed drugs and should be structured such that high utility first-unit purchase is not affected. To varying degrees, however, these mechanisms are incompatible with this mission due to the imposition of positive monetary cost on first-unit use. Lacking the ability to discriminate between appropriate and inappropriate use at the point of purchase, these cost-sharing mechanisms can potentially result in the foregoing of needed care.

By imposing costs on the enrollee, deductibles and other coinsurance measures rely on the patient's demand function to reduce consumption under price pressure. Such mechanisms exert pressure at the point of purchase, thus affecting compliance without discriminating essential from excessive use.[15,16] Individual drug demand does not address drug therapies as a homogeneous set of products. Under price pressure, it is likely that the patient will not reduce consumption of all drugs equally, but will choose specific products to forego. As reported in the Rand Health Insurance Experiment, prescription drug expenditures declined as a function of cost sharing. However, the decline was predominantly due to reduction of the number of prescriptions purchased as opposed to actions to reduce the average prescription price, e.g., purchasing fewer dosage units than prescribed, but both decisions differ from the treatment prescribed by the physician.[17]

Theory and empirical findings indicate that the demand curve for any patient cannot be relied upon to identify health needs accurately or to perform utility comparisons of drugs. A study of drug utilization response to the institution of a copayment for South Carolina Medicaid enrollees demonstrated a differential reduction in drug use across therapeutic categories. Of concern was the observation that an immediate and significant reduction in the level of expenditures occurred for all drug categories except analgesics and sedatives/hypnotics. Additionally, a reduction in cardiovascular drug use was observed over the long term.[18] These findings indicate that patients facing price pressure through coinsurance mechanisms may forego treatment of life-threatening conditions such as hypertension.

Legislation requires physician agency on behalf of the patient to prevent adverse health consequences resulting from informational asymmetry. Because patient-targeted price constraints circumvent physician agency, the resulting decisions made by patients may ultimately not be in their own best interests or that of Medicaid. The cost of adverse health consequences resulting from the foregoing of needed therapy is an undesirable possibility.

The economics of demand-side cost-containment measures are therefore complicated by several often overlooked factors. First, individual drug demand represents demand for a diverse set of products, each with a satiation point (generally assumed away in classical economic analyses). Second, economics assumes that price is indicative of utility, i.e., that drug prices reflect their ability to produce or maintain good health. However, as evidenced by the large drug price differentials between some life-sustaining drugs (e.g., digoxin, which is relatively inexpensive) and many costly agents of a palliative nature, individual drug prices are likely to be poor comparative indicators of health "value." Furthermore, deductibles, co-payments, and percentage coinsurance schemes rely upon the patient's own perception of health care (drug) value to reduce purchases. Cost-containment measures that manipulate the point-of-sale price may force the patient to rebundle his or her purchasing in response to price. One can only hope that in the rebundling the patient will make the correct choices. But the patient should not be the rationing mechanism for the Medicaid program. Possessing imperfect information, the enrollee may choose to forego valuable drug treatment for insidious health problems such as hypertension to purchase drugs of potentially less therapeutic benefit, incorrectly alter therapeutic regimens by reducing dosage to their satiation level, or substitute other, more costly services. The long-term cost to the system resulting from these actions could be great.

Nonmarket (Direct) Mechanisms

Although it is an unpopular subject in the medical literature and it is a label that is not usually attached to a cost-containment mechanism, rationing–in its most general sense–lies at the heart of any cost-containment effort. Whenever the cost of unconstrained consumption exceeds allocated funding and efforts to restrict consumption to funding boundaries are employed, the result is a rationing, or forced sharing, of the health resources that can be purchased. As previously discussed, economic- or market-based constraints defer the rationing decision to the consuming individual through his or her demand curve. This may be equitable from the perspective of the patient's perception of utility, yet possibly inequitable from the perspective of sound medical judgment. Often, it is incompatible with the mission of the program. Rationing is most often perceived in the strict nonmarket sense of directed allocation of health resources to specific individuals based on prioritized medical need. The Oregon experiment notwithstanding, such a strict operational version has yet to become generalized to a population such as Medicaid due to the incompatibility of this mechanism with the common view of health care as a basic right. However, all nonmarket mechanisms currently in use employ this approach to some degree.

Nonmarket mechanisms directly affect drug use by limiting therapeutic choices either to those perceived to provide the greatest utility per unit cost or to specific drug entities that are appropriate in kind and quantity for the intended use. Nonmarket mechanisms, therefore, offer the advantage of directly targeting the possibly imperfect agency of the gatekeeping health professionals, the basis for excessive or inappropriate drug therapy in many cases.

In contrast to economic-based constraints that rely upon an uninformed patient decision to forego, alter, or not seek prescribed therapies, the designs of nonmarket steering or limiting mechanisms rely upon expert medical assessment of the comparative utility of treatment options. Compared with purely economic constraints, reliance upon informed medical opinion in the decision-making (rationing) process gives nonmarket approaches a greater potential for providing equitable cost containment commensurate with medical need. However, efficiency and equity concerns apply to nonmarket constraints as well.

Nonmarket efforts seek to optimize the amount or value of care provided within the budget limitations of the program. Although optimality implies a singular solution, nonmarket constraints fall into two extreme categories: those seeking optimal allocation (rationing) in a societal sense (efficiency) and those seeking optimality at the individual level (equity). Since economic efficiency may be gained largely at the expense of individual equity, no single nonmarket mechanism can simultaneously satisfy the mission of the Medicaid program and the cost-containment needs of its administrators. As a result, nonmarket compromise mechanisms have evolved.

1. *Formularies.* Restricted formularies seek to shift demand to what are generally perceived by medical authority to be more efficient drug choices.

Individual drugs or entire classes of drugs may be excluded from formulary coverage if expert medical opinion determines the cost of such drugs to exceed the aggregate benefits. This is an attempt to achieve efficiency, i.e., optimal allocation (rationing), from the societal perspective.

In a review of the literature on Medicaid formularies, Jang concluded that formulary restriction generally resulted in shifts to alternative drugs and/or other, more expensive services, thus generating illusionary savings when the effects of the formulary were viewed only from the use results of the specific drug.[19] This is not unexpected given the often desired goal of restricting use to less costly agents. Although formulary restriction may not be the complete answer to cost containment, it may be useful for targeting specific drugs and/or drug classes for which less expensive (and potentially equally effective) alternative drugs exist. For such circumstances, formulary exclusion may be economically efficient. However, efficiency must be balanced with equity. In most cases, imposition of societal formularies will be inequitable for some individuals. For example, if formulary exclusions leave the physician nothing with which to treat a condition unresponsive to preferred therapies, the affected enrollee is then prohibited from receiving mainstream care. It therefore seems possible and desirable to strike an efficiency-equity balance in formulary management by incorporating mechanisms to limit rather than to exclude some drugs that may be needed by, and singularly effective for, statistically outlying patient groups. In either case, administrators must be careful that the administrative costs of formulary management do not overwhelm the savings.

2. *Utilization Review/Prior Approval.* Aggregate or macrolevel drug utilization review (DUR) is still in its infancy as a cost-containment mechanism and is currently functioning more as an expenditure-tracking mechanism than as a measure to control costs. DUR is, nonetheless, a valuable tool with which to identify drug use patterns indicative of inappropriate or excessive use. However, the art of medicine relegates assessment of therapeutic appropriateness to the individual or microlevel, more appropriately designated drug regimen review (DRR). DRR is an attempt to attain individual optimality (equity). The resource-intensive nature of individual regimen review within large patient populations such as Medicaid may be equitable, but it is likely to be highly inefficient as a cost-containment mechanism. However, individualized review in a limited sense provides a valuable mechanism for managing restricted-use drugs within a flexible Medicaid formulary as previously suggested. Prior-approval restrictions currently in place within many states require individualized medical justification for use of specific drugs, an operational example of an efficiency-

equity compromise blending macrolevel formulary constraint and individualized flexibility.

Economic/Nonmarket Composite Mechanisms

Although inequitable for many individuals and generally incompatible with the mission of the program, economic constraints are efficient in the sense that once they are imposed, no administrative carrying costs are required of the Medicaid program. In contrast, many nonmarket constraints favor equity at the expense of efficiency. Therefore, cost-containment strategies have been developed to capture what are perceived to be the efficiency attributes of both economic and nonmarket approaches and the equitable aspects of the latter. The most visible of these is a composite effort: the prescription (episode) limit or cap.

The episode limit, or cap, places a specific numeric limit on the number of cost-free or subsidized prescriptions allowed the Medicaid eligible within a specified period, usually one month. Caps represent a composite of economic and nonmarket constraint that appears consistent with Medicaid's mission and circumvents the weaknesses of generalized cost-sharing methods.

In general, caps provide for restricted reimbursement and thus limit use only with respect to prescription numbers above a specified limit. The patient may restrict his or her use to the limit (a nonmarket effect), but marginal use above the numeric limit results in out-of-pocket cost to the patient. This is cost-sharing in the sense that total cost is shared by the patient only if consumption exceeds the limit. Because high-utility, first-purchase use is unconstrained, patients are not likely to forego their most needed therapies. Caps are therefore equitable for those individuals whose needs fall at or below the limit. Second, the welfare cost of insured use due to upward use "creeping" in the region below the limit is less per incremental unit of consumption than in the upper use region; welfare cost increases at an increasing rate as use expands along the demand curve.[11] Constraining items of lower utility (i.e., those further out along the demand curve) is more efficient, provided the drug's location on the demand curve correctly reflects its relative utility in maintaining or restoring health.

Due to varying drug needs across the subgroups comprising the Medicaid population, however, strict adherence to a specific prescription limit would prevent those (particularly the aged and medically needy) whose conditions require prescriptions in excess of the limit but who cannot afford the cost from obtaining needed therapy, potentially resulting in adverse health consequences. A possible illustration of this potential is provided by Soumerai and colleagues. In their study, the regimens of multiple drug users—predominantly female, elderly, or disabled–were affected most when a monthly limit of three paid prescriptions was imposed in New Hampshire.[20] In a follow-up study, Soumerai and colleagues found an approximately twofold increase in the rate of nursing home admissions among the chronically ill elderly when a monthly limit of three paid prescriptions was imposed in New Hampshire, an effect that disappeared when the limit was removed 11 months later.[21] Because nursing home patients were exempt from the cap, however, the authors could not determine the extent to which the increased rate of nursing home admissions was related to adverse health consequences or to enrollee efforts to obtain alternative care in unconstrained settings, both possible causative factors.

These results should not serve as a general indictment of caps, but as an indication that design of a constraint framework must consider the degree of restriction and the resulting patient response. Was a limit of three prescriptions so severe as to result in adverse health consequences, or was the constraint so narrow in scope that the unconstrained nursing home setting was perceived to be the utility-maximizing alternative?

How might a limit process be altered to accommodate variations in need? Given the informational disparity and utility variation in marginal prescription use across various disease groups, a variable limit structure addressing the differing levels of need across disease states seems a more equitable solution. But the categorical "sets" of disease states with the statistical distribution in number of drugs appropriate to each have yet to be identified. In addition, a variable limit mechanism poses significant concerns from the standpoint of efficiency. Due to changing health status, an individual may fall into multiple limit levels within a single constraint cycle, but it is doubtful that such changes in limit status could be disseminated to providers in a timely manner.

One possible solution is a simple prescription limit coupled with exemption mechanisms. This, in effect, creates a variable limit by determining exceptions to the limit in an individualized manner based on need. This combination also removes the cost-sharing component of the limit mechanism with respect to needed drugs. In the study by Soumerai and colleagues, the availability of an exemption mechanism was not addressed. Equitable service provision can be approached through exemption processes that provide for emergency exemption for the high-volume user who faces unanticipated acute drug need and through long-term exemption for individuals who legitimately demonstrate chronic need in excess of limit. In contrast to deductibles, copayments, and percentage coinsurance, numeric episode limits–coupled with appropriate exemption mechanisms–provide the advantages of:

- Unconstrained high-utility first-unit use with selective restriction of lower utility drugs.
- Imposition of nonmonetary "process" costs of time and search effort on the enrollee and his agent.
- Short-term (emergency therapy) and long-term (chronic need) exemption based on the informed decision of the patient's agent rather than the patient's potentially irrational demand function.

From the perspective of the individual enrollee, a prescription limit coupled with exemption pathways for emergency and chronic use appears to be an equitable demand-side mechanism with which to control Medicaid drug program costs.

This approach is not without criticism or room for further improvement. The nonmonetary cost of the exemption process may constrain patients who perceive the value of a prescribed drug to be lower than the nonmonetary costs imposed but for whom high-volume drug consumption may be necessary. The exemption process may also place such a burden on physicians as to force imperfect agency through inconvenience. In addition, an exemption process selectively affects the medically needy who must go through the process for each drug above the limit. This process is dependent upon a patient's ability to act in his or her own best interests and pursue exemption. The search process may be particularly difficult for many individuals, such as the elderly, who may not be physically able or sufficiently informed to pursue exemption. As a result, patients requiring many drugs may forego needed therapy.

CONCLUSION

Due to the rising cost of health care and the limitations on funding, cost containment is likely to be an issue of permanent concern for public health insurance programs such as Medicaid. Supply-side intervention in the form of limitations (through market leverage) on reimbursement of product cost and service fees to providers and manufacturers is an important and probably permanent component of the aggregate cost-containment effort. However, supply-side effectiveness is limited by provider/manufacturer costs, necessitating employment of demand-side approaches to the problem.

Although empirical evidence may demonstrate a given economic constraint to be superior in reducing expenditures within the framework of its application, no single demand-side economic constraint process is inherently more effective than another in reducing drug use. Economic constraints such as co-payments or percentage coinsurance schemes can be designed to be of such minimal magnitude as to offer little or no containment pressure or to be so costly to the patient as to promote use approaching that under self-pay conditions–the very conditions such programs have been developed to combat. Although demand-side economic mechanisms such as co-payments can be effective in controlling costs, their use should be minimized in indigent-targeted programs due to the inability to ensure medically justifiable, need-based care for these populations.[22] While they demonstrate a wide range of efficiency-equity balance among themselves, nonmarket demand-side approaches, as a class, offer a need-based cost-containment approach that is more equitable for Medicaid drug recipients than economic-based methods. The nonmarket constraint options do not sufficiently overlap to preclude coexistent use; thus, it is likely that most nonmarket options can be employed simultaneously.

The episode limit or cap, coupled with proper exemption mechanisms (an economic/nonmarket composite approach), appears to be the best single efficiency-equity compromise if demand-based approaches are necessary. However, greater efficiency and equity can be obtained by combining the limit mechanism with a formulary variant such as a prior-approval mechanism that offers individual assessment of need. In this manner, some degree of unjustified therapy associated with sublimit consumers could be contained, thereby reducing the welfare cost that would otherwise go unchecked within the unconstrained window of the limit mechanism.

REFERENCES

1. National Pharmaceutical Council. Pharmaceutical benefits under state medical assistance programs. Reston, VA: National Pharmaceutical Council, 1990.

2. Barrilleaux CJ, Miller ME. Decisions without consequences: cost control and access in state Medicaid programs. J Health Polit Policy Law 1992; 17:97-118.

3. Lurie N, Ward NB, Shapiro MF, Gallego C, Vaghaiwalla R, Brook RH. Termination of Medi-Cal benefits: a follow-up study one year later. N Engl J Med 1986;314:1266-8.

4. Lurie N, Ward NB, Shapiro MF, Brook RH. Termination from Medi-Cal–does it affect health? N Engl J Med 1984;311:480-4.

5. Wicher JB, Fihn SD. Withdrawing routine medical outpatient services: effects on access and health. Clin Res 1985;33:269A.

6. U.S. Department of Health and Human Services. Health Care Financing Administration. 1992 HCFA statistics. HCFA Pub. No. 03333. 1992.

7. Geweke JF, Weisbrod BA. Some economic consequences of technological advance in medical care: the case of the new drug. In: Helms, RB, eds. Drugs and health. Washington, DC: American Enterprise Institute, 1981.

8. Feldstein PJ. Health care economics. 3rd ed. New York: John Wiley and Sons, Inc., 1988.

9. Omnibus Budget Reconciliation Act of 1990 (OBRA90). (PL 101-508, 5 Nov. 1990).

10. Newhouse JP, Manning WG, Morris CN, Orr LL, Duan N, Keeler EB, Leibowitz A, Marquis MS, Phelphs CE, Brook RH. Some interim results from a controlled trial of cost sharing in health insurance. N Engl J Med 1981;305:1501-7.

11. Pauly MV. A measure of the welfare cost of health insurance. Health Serv Res 1969;281-92.

12. Jeffers JR, Bognanno MF, Bartlett JC. On the demand versus need for medical services and the concept of "shortage." Am J Public Health 1971;61:46-63.

13. Pauly MV. The economics of moral hazard: comment. Am Econ Rev 1968;58:531-7.

14. Beck RG. The effects of co-payment on the poor. J Hum Resources 1974;9:129-42.

15. Muller C. Drug benefits in health insurance. Int J Health Ser 1974;4:157-70.

16. Siu AL, Sonnenberg FA, Manning WG, Goldberg GA, Bloomfield ES, Newhouse JP, Brook RH. Inappropriate use of hospitals in a randomized trial of health insurance plans. N Engl J Med 1986;315:1259-66.

17. Leibowitz A, Manning WG, Newhouse JP. The demand for prescription drugs as a function of cost sharing. Soc Sci Med 1985;21:1063-9.

18. Reeder CE, Nelson AA. The differential impact of copayment on drug use in a Medicaid population. Inquiry 1985;22:396-403.

19. Jang R. Medicaid formularies: a critical review of the literature. J Pharm Market Manage 1988;2(3):39-61.

20. Soumerai SB, Avorn J, Ross-Degnan D, Gortmayer S. Payment restrictions for prescription drugs under Medicaid: effects on therapy, cost, and equity. N Engl J Med 1987;317:550-6.

21. Soumerai SB, Ross-Degnan D, Avorn J, McLaughlin T, Choodnovskiy I. Effects of Medicaid drug-payment limits on admission to hospitals and nursing homes. N Engl J Med 1991;325:1072-7.

22. Nelson AA, Reeder CE, Dickson WM. The effect of a Medicaid co-payment program on the utilization and cost of prescription services. Med Care 1984;22:724-36.

Chapter 5

Public Policy and Drug Costs: Legitimate and Bastard Options

T. Donald Rucker

INTRODUCTION

All societies must eventually confront the issues of limited resources and opportunity costs when purchasing prescribed medications. The matter of public policy and legitimate forms of cost containment within this area is so complex that several weeks could be spent just defining the problem and proposing various control options. To meet time and space limitations, it is necessary to invoke two major shortcuts. First, the question of compensation for retail pharmacy and drug wholesalers will be excluded. (If you wish to consider my views about reimbursement for these providers, a list of more than ten publications can be supplied.) Second, the focus for this discussion–analysis of alternative reimbursement policies for drug product cost–will be simplified. If a viable pharmaceutical manufacturing industry in the free world represents an important goal, however, Canadians and Americans must do a better job of differentiating between socially justifiable and haphazard methods of paying for pharmaceutical preparations.

This chapter has been developed around a single underlying theme: current policy often imposes economic constraints on drug use that are more appropriately pursued elsewhere. To illustrate this impact, we turn to the expenditure equation provided in Figure 5.1. This formula reminds us

This paper was presented at the Symposium on Bioequivalence and Interchangeability of Pharmaceutical Products held at the University of Montreal, Canada, on April 23, 1991.

Previously printed in *Journal of Research in Pharmaceutical Economics*, Vol. 4(1), 1992.

that total program outlay is determined by average prescription charge multiplied by the average number of prescriptions used plus an administrative cost.

Many health insurance schemes impose various controls on utilization while giving superficial attention to the expense of program administration and the true economic cost of provider contributions. Because of pressures to keep taxes and/or insurance premiums under control, suboptimal results are likely to occur. This finesse model has a great deal of political appeal.

If one elects to move toward an optimizing solution, revision in program design is needed that will focus on each component: minimize administrative cost, permit scientific/clinical factors to guide drug use, and limit reimbursement of all providers to methods that reflect justifiable economic criteria. This new approach, however, requires that taxes and/or insurance premiums fluctuate to accommodate the optimizing features associated with the three components in the expenditure equation.

The remainder of this discussion will be limited to three important issues:

1. What are the economic/administrative principles that portend optimizing results in shaping reimbursement policy?
2. What are the payment formulas for drug products where welfare losses seem to outweigh social benefits?
3. What are the reimbursement choices that promise results superior to those listed as nonoptions?

While optimization is an elusive goal in an imperfect world, it may be useful to recall that problems created by man are also subject to resolution via diligent attention from this same source.

BASIC PRINCIPLES

Payment methods for pharmaceutical products are derived from the underlying philosophy and objectives of public policy; therefore, it seems essential to pause and make explicit those administrative and economic factors that should govern the more technical specifications subsequently manifest in particular payment formulas. Public debate and legislative action seem to focus more on the latter than the former. In any case, my purpose here is to suggest a foundation that will assist in classifying payment schemes as either viable or nonviable social options. If consensus

FIGURE 5.1. The Expenditure Equation

$$\text{Total Program Cost} = \bar{x}\,R_x\,\$ \times \bar{x}\,\#\,R_x + \text{Administrative Cost}$$

	Taxes/Premiums	Mean Cost of Prescriptions ($)	Mean Number of Prescriptions	Administrative Cost
Current policy	Keep stable	Flexibility or ad hoc controls	Numerous controls on utilization	Ignore
Revised policy	Adjust periodically	Minimize TEC	Scientific/clinical factors first	Minimize

can be achieved regarding those principles that society ranks highest, the task of formula development will be facilitated.

Table 5.1 enumerates those objectives that seem likely to lead to an optimal reimbursement policy. This brief survey begins with attributes whose genesis lies primarily in the administrative model. The term equity implies that the payment of all vendors–manufacturers, drug wholesalers, and retail pharmacies–be derived from the same conceptual foundation. Thus, if neutrality is obtained, one type of provider would not be subject to the discipline of marketplace pricing or government fiat while another had its remuneration frozen for months or years by third-party programs.

The term simplicity connotes that both the method of provider payment and insurance coverage, if any, should be sufficiently simple so that vendors can understand the basis for compensation and their obligations to patients and insurance programs. The principle of indirect control admonishes us that the regulatory model traditionally leads to complex and static guidelines as well as the risk of the agency being co-opted by the very industry it purports to supervise. All other things being equal, therefore, indirect means seem preferable whenever similar outcomes can be achieved.

Program/policy integrity under a capitalistic system depends on the voluntary cooperation of a large number of suppliers in the private sector. Practices that tend to erode voluntary cooperation, such as inadequate compensation or delayed payment, should be avoided. The next characteristic–supporting rational drug therapy–represents an essential objective if drug therapy is to maximize its contribution to patient health status. Unfortunately, many drug insurance programs adopt across-the-board controls on utilization where cost-containment stipulations do more to distort than support therapeutic considerations.

The final criterion on the left side of the ledge–the monitoring function–reminds us that an effective and efficient evaluation component should accompany any efforts to change reimbursement policy and continu-

TABLE 5.1. Basic Principles to Guide Reimbursement Policy for Pharmaceutical Products and Prescribed Medications Classified by Two Constructs

Administrative Emphasis	Economic Emphasis
Equity	Adequacy
Simplicity	Conservation
Indirect controls	Incentive structure
Program integrity	Flexibility
Rational drug therapy	Precision
Monitor outcomes	Validity

ally assess the economic health of pharmaceutical providers as new methods are adopted. However, as long as return on invested capital holds at the average or above the average level of all manufacturing, there is no a priori reason for fearing the flow of capital to nondrug sectors or negative results associated with changes in pharmaceutical research and development.

The first criterion for satisfying economic objectives is that reimbursement must be adequate. This means that payment levels must be consistently sufficient to cover the true economic cost, which includes a reasonable profit, of an efficient producer who supplies goods/services that are essential for maximizing patient health status. While this standard raises a host of operational issues concerning efficiency and therapeutic contribution, it also proclaims that third-party insurance programs–public or private–must forsake attempting to solve their fiscal problems by shifting them to providers of drug products or even to patients.

The second principle, conservation, reminds us that neither insurance program funds nor patient income should be employed to procure drug products and related services that do not yield user benefits that are at least equal to the cost of those products and services. Moreover, methods generated internally by pharmaceutical firms that lead to contrived demand distort the basic principle that prescribing should be a function of illness, on the one hand, and clinical decision making carried out in an environment of enlightened neutrality, on the other.

The next criterion reminds us that a prudent reimbursement policy requires a comprehensive set of incentives that simultaneously reward producers who supply useful therapeutic entities in an efficient manner while discouraging the use of resources that violate the principles of conservation.

The fourth element in our economic model, flexibility, acknowledges that payment formulas must be responsive to competitive and inflationary pressures, shifts in demand due to changing patterns of illness, and the availability of new products with superior therapeutic credentials. Flexibility also implies that buyers may wish to shift resources from the treatment model to the preventive model (or nonhealth sectors) when more positive cost-effectiveness and cost-benefit ratios seem apparent.

The term precision implies that cost and benefit judgments pertaining to adequacy, conservation, incentives, and flexibility be made with confidence. Thus, a uniform cost accounting system developed for manufacturers, drug wholesalers, and community pharmacies, respectively, seems essential for collecting appropriate cost data for parties on both sides of the economic equation.

The last element on our economic agenda pertains to validity. Reimbursement within a provider category should not yield uneven results because of a producing unit's size, geographic location, political connections, or ability to beat the system. If program integrity is an important goal on the administrative side, validity represents its counterpart when economic factors are introduced.

NONOPTIONS

While the principles outlined above for moving toward an optimal reimbursement policy require further study, it is time to consider payment methods that fail to satisfy one or more of these standards. Table 5.2 provides a list of strategies that seem to qualify as nonoptions.

The first method, relying on market pricing, does satisfy the criterion of adequacy, but it fails to meet most of the remaining requirements. Drug product prices, like airline fares and hospital charges, are best described as chaotic. Drug product prices, even in the multiple-source sector, seldom closely approximate the true economic cost of production. Rather, they serve as vehicles for promotion, deals, and obfuscation. Moreover, they fuel profit patterns that exceed those levels that they would be expected to obtain under more competitive conditions. The model reimbursement program proposed below, however, would place no limits on profitability because the opportunity to make a financial killing by bringing new, breakthrough products to the marketplace constitutes an important component of a positive incentive system.

Government ownership of pharmaceutical manufacturers has been listed as a nonoption for two cogent reasons. First, alternative intervention

TABLE 5.2. Nonoptions in Constructing Reimbursement Policy for Pharmaceutical Products

Market pricing

Government ownership

Political/consumer jawboning

Utilization controls

Mandated rebates

Price/profit controls

Patent modification

Negotiation with government agency
based on cost-plus

strategies are likely to be more effective and efficient. Second, nationalization of business enterprises throughout most of the world has usually been an economic disaster. This measure represents an option of last resort.

Political jawboning occurs when a government official or agency admonishes the provider to lower prices. Consumer chastisement occurs when an activist group uses the media for a similar purpose. While both procedures periodically exhibit some success, results tend to be ephemeral because they seldom affect underlying imperfections in organizational behavior and resource allocation that lie at the heart of the problem. Moreover, inordinate amounts of media resources seem to be wasted in pursuing such nonsolutions.

Utilization controls are illustrated by across-the-board limits applied by insurance programs to restrict the maximum number of prescriptions a patient may receive per month and/or the number of days' supply allowed on a given prescription. Restrictions of this type can most often be traced to underbudgeting and/or a fluid reimbursement policy. Consequently, the administrator pursues controls within his or her jurisdiction to demonstrate his or her contribution in bringing the program back into fiscal alignment. Since utilization limits of this type fail to affect the basic economic problem and seldom qualify on therapeutic grounds, they have been classified as a nonoption. If questions concerning appropriate utilization of prescribed medications arise, they should be addressed within a therapeutically oriented drug utilization review program where cost-containment problems can be explored once prescribing has been achieved within the drugs of choice model.

Mandated rebate provisions have been enacted by the U.S. Congress for Medicaid drug programs in an attempt to capture the more favorable prices often available to hospitals and other volume purchasers in the private sector. Further, pricing formulas have been specified for multiple-source products and to estimate the actual transaction cost at which community pharmacies procure pharmaceutical items. Because pharmaceutical firms with market power can circumvent rebate programs, engage in external and internal cost shifting, and control firm revenue by bringing new products to market at prices closer to extortion than cost recovery, most rebate provisions and formulas to limit procurement expenses provide, at best, a superficial means for dealing with a complex problem. If profit controls are advocated as an alternative solution, many pharmaceutical companies have enough subsidiaries and accountants to render such efforts largely ineffective. Profit restrictions also conflict with at least two of the desired objectives supporting an optimizing system: a positive incentive structure and the validity of compensation among providers.

The next nonoption, patent modification, has attracted considerable attention from economists who seek an impersonal means of inducing more price competition among suppliers in the marketplace. A common proposal requires that the innovator firm, after seven to nine years of patent protection, be forced to cross-license the product (for a royalty) to other companies. As more suppliers enter the market, a downward pressure on price can be expected. However, mandatory cross-licensure is likely to be accompanied by one or more of the following consequences:

1. Total receipts of the innovative firm may not fall significantly since royalty income will tend to offset decreased sales revenue.
2. If receipts do fall, the incentive structure advocated above will be impaired.
3. Although reduced patent life will militate toward more effective price competition, many firms can be expected to increase promotional outlays to gain market share.

Thus, the basic problem of misallocation of resources seems more likely to be shifted than minimized by cross-licensure.

Our final strategy is one based on negotiation, where a government agency certifies the actual cost of pharmaceutical production and determines an allowable rate of return on invested capital. Since an unbiased assessment of such methods is not currently available, price/profit negotiation has been placed on the "avoid" side of our ledger for several reasons. First, indirect methods should be proven ineffective before more direct forms of intervention are attempted. Second, over the long run, no government agency seems likely to match the sophisticated economic/accounting talent that can be deployed by most large pharmaceutical firms. Third, implementation of the negotiation model per se does not necessarily vitiate a firm's control over its demand curve and the corresponding misallocation of resources associated with these activities.

In summary, the ultimate goal of reimbursement policy should not be to restrict prices or profits, but to ensure that pharmaceutical firms use resources efficiently in their quest to bring even more therapeutically valuable products to market. Policy alternatives classified as nonoptions offer a superficial means for pursuing this objective.

REIMBURSEMENT REFORM

Perhaps you have already read more about pharmaceutical economics and public policy than seems relevant to the issues of bioequivalence and product interchangeability. However, the vacuum created above must be filled. We now turn to our final task of outlining strategies to reshape reimbursement policy for pharmaceutical products. These proposals are presented in Table 5.3.

Adoption of a uniform cost accounting system would ensure that economic issues are discussed on a level playing field. Since many firms in the pharmaceutical industry obtain revenue from over-the-counter preparations, veterinary products, and nonpharmaceutical operations, as well as overseas subsidiaries (and vice versa), a common system for recording joint costs and allocating overhead seems essential if several of the recommendations in Table 5.3 are to be implemented successfully. The uniform costing system is also required to help evaluate the economic merit of any new options that may appear on the legislative table from time to time.

The second component in construction of a national reimbursement policy is that legislation be enacted to make bundling and all other forms of price obfuscation illegal. Further, discriminatory pricing would be prohibited unless price reductions are proportional to the decreased cost associated directly with increased volume. In short, all buyers would be confronted with an explicit, one-price policy from each firm.

The third component on our reimbursement agenda calls for a special tax of 90% to be levied on reinvested earnings generated by all firms that qualify as pharmaceutical manufacturers. If drug companies cannot finance desired research and development projects out of the reduced levels of cash flow, they will be forced periodically to raise capital from equity or debt markets. This form of impersonal adjudication seems preferable to the self-perpetuating biases of the current system, where a major by-product is often excess capacity and product duplication sans significant thera-

TABLE 5.3. Selected Strategies for Developing National Reimbursement Policy for Pharmaceutical Products

- Mandate adoption of a uniform cost accounting system

- Outlaw bundling and prohibit discriminatory pricing unless reductions are proportional to decreased cost associated with increased volume

- Levy tax of 90% on reinvested earnings for all firms that qualify as pharmaceutical manufacturers

- Make illegal all forms of persuasion/education conducted directly or indirectly by pharmaceutical firms

- Develop comprehensive scientific programs to supply information about pharmaceutical products to health professionals and patients

peutic contribution. It also seems better than enduring the bureaucratic impediments often manifest when a government agency attempts to regulate the R&D function.

The next strategy calls for a mechanism to eliminate all forms of industry-sponsored persuasion/education. These efforts to enhance producer sovereignty artificially inflate drug product costs by an average of 25%. As a result, such outlays appropriate around $7 billion a year from American patients that could be reallocated for the purchase of other goods and services with far more favorable cost-benefit ratios. More important, promotional efforts represent one of the three major contributors to that pandemic disease, irrational drug therapy, a welfare loss that easily costs society an additional $10 billion per year.

No single firm, however, should be expected to commit economic suicide by unilaterally terminating promotional/educational activities. Curtailment could be accomplished by disallowing such expenses as a cost of doing business in calculating the corporation net income tax or by convening a government-industry conference to specify certain expenditures that subsequently would become illegal.

The final item on our reimbursement agenda has nothing to do with reimbursement. However, the previous step eliminated the major source of drug information furnished to health professionals: inputs provided by industry sponsorship. It is necessary to reconstitute this function, albeit on a much reduced level, by organizing a professional/scientific body to supply comparative information on the therapeutic and economic properties of pharmaceutical preparations. This national drug education foundation would hire some 2,500 drug information specialists to provide objective data to health practitioners, develop a therapeutic formulary for voluntary application, and provide a variety of additional educational services that seem cost-effective in pursuing the overall goal of rational drug therapy. Since the foundation could probably operate on $325 million a year, net savings attributable to the purchase of pharmaceutical products should exceed $6.5 billion. (Indirect savings associated with better prescribing, dispensing, and consumption practices could be much larger.) Continuous financing for this drug information body could be assured simply by levying a 1% excise tax on product sales, a reduction of 95% in the implicit tax currently imposed by pharmaceutical suppliers.

DISCUSSION

This bolus approach to revamping reimbursement policies governing pharmaceutical products can, of course, be expected to precipitate disquietude among industry executives as they become prisoners of marketplace economics, as well as consternation among legislators whose cooperation will be required to enact a statutory framework to achieve this end. The net result of these proposals is intended to allow drug product prices and profits to vary, subject only to the one-price policy advocated above and the competitive pressures generated by firms in the industry. Moreover, on the supply side, product pricing will be influenced heavily by manufacturing efficiencies and the nature of monopoly power associated with patent protection. Suppliers who bring marginal pharmaceuticals to the market will receive marginal returns because promotional techniques will not be available to override prescribing decisions that focus on the drugs of choice. However, firms whose R&D operations yield breakthrough products can rely on patent protection coupled with formulary listing to generate premiums beyond the level of anticipated economic profits. "Excessive returns" of this type should be recognized as proof that capitalism is working. Further, they are a small price to pay under any insurance scheme, since increased revenues here are associated closely with benefits received by patients.

A major advantage of this proposal is that while market price of pharmaceutical products will structure purchase decisions, this process should not be subject to additional cost-containment efforts by third-party programs. Further savings cannot be realized by tampering with reimbursement formulas without eroding the productive contributions of the industry. It is assumed that questions pertaining to bioequivalency and therapeutic interchange can be resolved on their scientific/clinical merits because reimbursement policy is now carrying the ball on the economic front. When a suboptimal reimbursement policy governs, however, experience confirms the likelihood that insurers will focus on utilization controls as the primary vehicle for cost containment.

While the net economic gains associated with these proposals seem positive, an administrative/political hurdle remains. Public health insurance programs operate within the confines of a fiscal straitjacket called a budget. This instrument is characterized by rigidity, compromise, and a strong propensity for cost shifting. These features, however, conflict sharply with the pricing flexibility prescribed for our revisionist reimbursement policy.

If progress is to be recorded, it seems essential that government-sponsored health insurance programs forsake preoccupation with inflation and budget limits by pursuing techniques that lead to maximum efficiency in production and distribution of pharmaceutical products. This is the true economic issue in any reimbursement policy. However, political leaders have perfected numerous methods to avoid confronting the fundamental issues of our society. Unfortunately, no drugs are undergoing clinical trials to treat this ubiquitous malady.

Time will permit only one concluding observation on this complex proposal. The economic features put forward here discriminate against pharmaceutical manufacturers as a sector of the economy. Why shouldn't drug products be priced and marketed with the same freedom afforded goods and services generally? The answer to this question seems obvious. Useful pharmaceutical preparations play a key role in improving the health status of citizens throughout the nation. In short, they have a much higher personal and social utility than most consumer goods, especially expensive perfumes, luxury automobiles, and even beer. If perchance they do not, then a symposium on bioequivalence and interchangeability of pharmaceutical products, marketing certification by the Food and Drug Directorate, and health insurance coverage all represent a dissipation of resources where patients and taxpayers sustain an unneeded burden.

SELECTED BIBLIOGRAPHY

Davis K, et al. Health care cost containment. Baltimore, MD: Johns Hopkins University Press, 1990.

Eastman HC. The report of the Commission of Inquiry on the Pharmaceutical Industry. Ottawa, Canada: Supply and Services Canada, 1985.

Lexchin J. The real pushers. Vancouver, Canada: New Star Books, 1984.

Medawar C. The wrong kind of medicine. London, England: Consumers Association.

Mitchell SA, Link EA, eds. Impact of public policy on drug innovation and pricing. Washington, DC: American University, 1976.

Pollard MR. Managed care and a changing pharmaceutical industry. Health Aff 1990;9(3):55-65.

Rucker TD. Drug information for prescribers and dispensers: toward a model system. Med Care 1976;14:156-65.

Rucker TD. Economic problems in drug distribution. Inquiry 1972;9(9):43-50.

Rucker TD. Public policy considerations in the pricing of prescription drugs. Int J Health Serv 1974;4(1):171-9.

Rucker TD. Role of the pharmaceutical industry in a dynamic health care system. Drugs Health Care 1975;2(2):86-95.

Rucker TD. Reimbursement policy under drug insurance. In: Silverman M, Lydecker M, eds. Proceedings of national conference on drug coverage under NHI. Washington, DC: National Center for Health Services Research, 1978:121-8 (PHS 78-3208).

Schifrin LG. Economics and epidemiology of drug use. In: Melmon KL, Morrelli HF, eds. Clinical pharmacology: basic principles of therapeutics. New York: Macmillan Publishing Co., Inc., 1978:1084-109.

Schwartzman D. Innovation in the pharmaceutical industry. Baltimore, MD: Johns Hopkins University Press, 1976.

Silverman M, Lee PR, Lydecker M. Pills and the public purse. Berkeley, CA: University of California Press, 1981.

PART II:
INTERVENTIONS AND CONTROLS

Certainly, the burgeoning interest in pharmaceutical economics results in large part from efforts to control the costs of pharmaceuticals and efforts by the marketers of these products to resist that pressure.

This section begins with a chapter by Stuart and Yesalis. Although it reviews the results of an experiment now 15 years old, readers will be aware that there is a rebirth of interest in capitation and the Iowa project remains to date the only one of its kind.

Baum et al., describe a technique for incorporting severity of illness measures in analysis of the cost-effectiveness of treatment. This chapter is followed by reports of two types of interventions aimed at reducing Medicaid expenditures for medications–prior authorization for NSAID prescriptions and utilization review of diabetes medication.

This section concludes with a study showing that formulary restrictions, while reducing prescription charges in a Medicaid program, probably resulted in increases in expenditures for other medical services.

Chapter 6

The Iowa Pharmacy Capitation Experiment: Economic Incentives and Provider Performance

Bruce Stuart
Charles Yesalis

INTRODUCTION

The empirical literature on the effects of capitation payment on provider behavior consists primarily of case analyses of the experience of individual health maintenance organizations (HMOs). While a sufficient number of such studies have been conducted to establish some general patterns of provider response to capitation incentives, the case study approach is inherently limited when it comes to identifying causal relationships. The most celebrated example of this concerns hospital utilization. There is nearly universal consensus among health services researchers that hospitalization rates are lower in HMOs than in traditional fee-for-service plans, but there is little agreement on the relative importance of such factors as enrollee selection bias, hospital bed constraints, and the style of medicine practiced within HMOs.[1-3] Isolation of the individual contribution of each factor requires either highly controlled experimental conditions or multivariate analysis of the experience of many plans operating according to similar capitation rules. These requirements are difficult to meet in practice.

The pharmacy capitation experiment operated by the State of Iowa in 1981 provides a unique opportunity to assess the economic performance of a relatively large sample (n = 347) of independent health care providers practicing under a single plan with common administrative procedures for client enrollment and provider payment. During the experiment, over one-third of Iowa's pharmacies were prepaid using fixed monthly capitation rates for drug products prescribed to Medicaid outpatients. This chapter

Previously published in *Journal of Research in Pharmaceutical Economics*, Vol. 2(2), 1990.

reports the findings of a multivariate statistical analysis of pharmacy costs and profitability under that experiment. Our research has both a broad objective and a narrow objective. The immediate aim of this paper is to identify those characteristics of pharmacies and their Medicaid clientele that are most strongly predictive of favorable economic performance under the capitation plan. The second and broader purpose is to raise theoretical questions about how health care providers behave under risk contracts involving small enrollment panels. We hope these questions will encourage new lines of research in this growing area of policy concern.

The following section of the chapter contains a brief description of the Iowa program, its history, and its capitation rating methodology. The theoretical basis for our research and study hypotheses are presented next. Particular attention is given to the hypothesized effects of enrollment volume, case mix, length of contract, and ownership characteristics on pharmacy performance under the plan. Because the State of Iowa required that participating pharmacies submit pseudo claims for all services rendered to capitated Medicaid enrollees during the experiment, there is an excellent data base available for cost analysis. Following a description of that data base are sections devoted to statistical estimation issues and empirical findings. The chapter concludes with an examination of the study's implications for other capitation plans that place small, independent health care providers at risk.

BACKGROUND

In 1977, the State of Iowa established a two-year pilot program in two rural counties (n = 12 pharmacies) to test the feasibility of using capitation as a method of paying pharmacists under the state's Medicaid plan. The pilot program was designed to address persistent problems of cost escalation and payment delays with the fee-for-service (FFS) system. Under the FFS system, pharmacists were paid an amount sufficient to cover the average acquisition costs of drugs dispensed plus a fixed professional fee. In the pilot program, the capitation rate was a preset monthly amount per Medicaid enrollee that varied according to the aid category of the patient. The rates were established by extrapolating past drug use and cost trends in the two counties to the coming year. The pharmacist was prepaid 90% of the monthly projected per capita cost. The remaining 10% was held by the state in an escrow account to be shared by the state and the participating pharmacies according to a prearranged formula based on pharmacy savings over the estimated FFS cost of treating the capitated enrollees.

Medicaid patients living in the two pilot counties were given the opportunity to choose a pharmacy from which they would receive all outpatient pharmaceutical services during the upcoming month. At the beginning of each month, the 12 participating pharmacies received checks based on the number and category of Medicaid patients who had selected them. If a pharmacy could provide covered services at a cost less than the total capitation allotment, it earned a profit over and above what it would have received under the FFS system.

To assure participation, the pharmacists were guaranteed that they would fare as well, economically, under capitation as they would have under the FFS arrangement in effect for the remainder of the state. For those pharmacies whose costs exceeded their capitation amounts, supplemental payments were made from the escrow account to cover the difference.

The state was encouraged by the results of the pilot project and extended the experiment to an additional 30 counties, representing roughly one-third of the state.[4-8] The expanded capitation program commenced on 1 April 1981 and was scheduled to last one year. The basic characteristics of the expanded program were the same as in the pilot counties, but with a more sophisticated capitation rating methodology. Instead of being prepaid 90% of the estimated FFS costs each month, the pharmacists received 80% up front, with the remainder going in an escrow account to be used for supplemental, emergency,* and bonus payments.** The capitation rates were derived from regression coefficients in a multivariate analysis of prior year Medicaid drug utilization and expenditures with recipients' age, sex, and nursing home residence status used as explanatory variables. These base rates were further adjusted to allow for inflation, seasonal variation in use of services, and the presence of a copayment feature instituted by the state.[9]

As in the pilot project, pharmacists who participated were guaranteed that their Medicaid revenue would remain at least equal to what they would have been paid under the FFS system for the drugs actually dispensed to members of their enrollment panels. Additional features of the expanded study included a modification of the claims filing procedure, an improved communications system for transmitting patient eligibility sta-

---

*These are fee-for-service payments made to another pharmacy for emergency drug services provided to a capitation pharmacy's patient.

**These were payments made to pharmacies that experienced costs below their capitation amounts in a particular quarter. The amount paid equaled one-half of the balance in the pharmacy's escrow account after emergency and supplemental payments had been made.

tus, a special provision for excluding high utilizers from the capitation program, and the preparation and distribution of educational materials to pharmacists.

The expanded capitation program operated for just nine months. It was canceled on December 31, 1981 amid controversy regarding the question of whether capitation was saving the state any money.[10,11] Stuart and Yesalis subsequently determined that a flaw in the rating methodology produced windfall gains for pharmacies with the smallest panel sizes, and that this, together with higher than expected administrative costs, had produced a budget overrun under the experiment.[12] The apparent end of the story came with the publication of research findings by Yesalis et al. that revealed little change in drug use levels or pharmacist dispensing behavior in the capitated counties compared to the remainder of the state.[13,14]

ANALYTICAL APPROACH
AND STUDY HYPOTHESES

We have reanalyzed the Iowa capitation data. The studies by Yesalis et al. used a methodology employing randomly selected experimental and control groups in which the county was the unit of analysis (capitation counties were matched with other Iowa counties that remained on the FFS system).[13,14] Although sound in principle, this approach suffers from the practical disadvantage that it cannot identify the factors that trigger change in pharmacy behavior. Assume, for instance, that the response to capitation varies by type of pharmacy (perhaps large retail pharmacies are more attuned to the economic potential that capitation offers). Because each county contains both small stores and large stores, the aggregate differential in economic performance between capitated and noncapitated counties will understate the true impact of the payment system, if not miss it altogether. Our approach differs in two respects. Instead of treating the county as the unit of analysis, we analyze performance at the level of the pharmacy itself. Instead of asking whether the presence of capitation motivates pharmacies to change their behavior, we focus on differences in the intensity of the motivation for change faced by pharmacies operating in the capitated counties.

Much has been written about the structure of financial incentives under capitation payment schemes.[1-3,15] It is generally assumed–although the proposition has never been formally tested–that providers react to the economic uncertainty inherent in all capitation contracts in a consistent fashion whether the contract subjects them to down-side risk (the probability of loss), up-side risk (the probability that potential earnings will not materialize), or some combination of the two.* The risk structure of the typical IPA or network HMO capitation contract is symmetrical in that providers face both up-side and down-side risks.[16] In up-side-only risk contracts, such as that employed by the State of Iowa, the distribution of possible financial outcomes is truncated at the participating provider's break-even point. Nonetheless, the basic economic incentive to develop cost-efficient patient management practices is present under both types of contracts, as are the incentives to practice preferred risk selection and perhaps to reduce the quality of care.

By incentive, we simply mean the presence of some inducement to action. The term implies nothing about the strength of the inducement nor the conditions under which providers will be moved to act in the hypothesized direction. Thus, to argue that the capitation form of payment creates incentives for economy (and some untoward behaviors as well) is actually saying very little.

Our working assumption is that providers respond to the economic incentives associated with capitation in proportion to the magnitude of their potential returns under the contract. If the net return is perceived to be low, we hypothesize that little effort will be made to achieve it. If it is high, providers will adopt behaviors that increase their chances of seeing the gain (or reduction in losses) materialize. A corollary to this hypothesis is that provider performance should be a function of the determinants of the potential net return. These determinants include the scope of services covered by the capitation contract, the size of the enrollment panel, the provider's capacity to control utilization and service costs, and the duration of the contract. The link between each of these factors and provider performance is explored briefly in the following paragraphs, first from a general theoretical perspective and then from the standpoint of those capitated pharmacists in Iowa.

---

*There is, of course, a very large literature devoted to the general theory of choice under uncertainty. To date there have been no attempts to apply that theory to the decisions of health care providers contemplating capitation contracts. It is of some interest to note that betting experiments conducted by psychologists and economists have consistently shown that individual risk preferences are neither linear nor transitive.[17] Contrary to conventional wisdom, the evidence appears to suggest that people are motivated more by up-side than by down-side risk. If the utility functions of capitated providers mirror these preferences, then carrots rather than sticks may produce greater cost savings.

Contract Coverage

For any voluntary capitation arrangement to succeed, providers must be convinced that the capitation rate is sufficiently high to cover their expected unit costs, i.e., the anticipated expense of providing each enrollee with the services called for in the contract. The relationship between the capitation rate and the scope of coverage is important in two respects. It seems clear that higher capitation rates (relative to expected costs) will encourage greater participation both in terms of the number of providers willing to sign initial agreements and in terms of their subsequent willingness to accept new enrollees. It is less obvious how the scope of coverage/ capitation rate relationship will influence the behavior of providers after they sign up.

The standard economic model of profit maximization predicts that capitated providers will minimize unit costs of production no matter what the coverage is. The theory that providers are motivated by target income expectations suggests that economizing behavior may wane as the margin between costs and revenues grows.[18] Many capitation arrangements now use class rating (the Medicare AAPCC formula is one example). The presence of multiple rate classes further complicates predictions of provider behavior because profit margins will typically differ from class to class.*

Regardless of the behavioral theory one subscribes to, there is another dimension to the coverage/capitation rate relationship that must be considered. Every legitimate capitation system assigns higher rates to more comprehensive service packages, and every class rating system assigns higher rates to the more expensive classes. Rates follow expected cost. In an arithmetical sense, the potential for cost savings also follows expected cost. What makes this important behaviorally is that the financial incentive to seek cost savings is thus a positive function of the capitation rate. We do not mean to suggest by this that providers foreswear their professional ethics for economic gain when they sign capitation contracts. We simply mean that they are likely to work harder to achieve savings when there is a significant gain to be had or a significant loss to be avoided.

---

*Class rating schemes typically price each ratable risk at a constant percentage or multiple of the average per capita historical cost within a given market area (the county in the case of the AAPCC). It would be highly unusual for any provider to have costs that matched the average in every rate class. This means that rate class margins for the typical provider will vary by class of enrollee, with high margins in some and perhaps unit losses in others. Aside from selective enrollment practices, most providers would likely find it difficult to develop class-specific cost control strategies.

The notion that cost savings may follow the capitation rate is a notable consideration in class rating plans where the average payment rate received by capitated providers is highly sensitive to the composition of the enrollment panel. Class rates may reliably reflect current differences in the fee-for-service cost of treating members of each rate class, but the payoff for economizing behavior falls disproportionately on those providers with the most expensive case mix. With 20 rate classes and substantial diversity in panel composition among participating pharmacists, the Iowa experience presents an excellent opportunity to examine this "size-of-the-carrot" hypothesis.

Enrollment Volume

Among providers contemplating capitation contracts, the anticipated size of the enrollment panel, like the level of the capitation fee, is a key factor in the participation decision. Once the contracts are signed, panel size becomes important for other reasons. The degree of credibility that capitated providers can assign to their enrollee's utilization and cost experience under risk contracts is directly related to panel size. Enrollment volume determines whether revenues will be sufficient to cover the fixed costs that providers incur when negotiating capitation contracts and implementing administrative changes necessitated by the payment arrangement. Volume also affects the profit that providers can expect to receive from practice management decisions that reduce the variable cost of patient care.

According to the law of large numbers, capitated providers with small enrollment panels are subject to greater random fluctuation in enrollee costs over time than providers with large capitation panels. Our analysis of the Iowa data, for example, found that pharmacies with fewer than 30 panel members faced a monthly per enrollee cost variance twice that of pharmacies with more than 250 members. The random "noise" associated with month-to-month cost variation can make it difficult for providers to track the returns from their cost-containment efforts. Consequently, practices with small panels may be less willing to undertake such activities.

A first principle of finance is that investment decisions should be evaluated on the basis of total profits and not just on the rate of return. A project may generate a high profit rate but only insubstantial earnings. This same logic can be applied to capitation contracts. The difference between the capitation rate and the provider's potential average unit cost may be high, but with few enrollees these measures will not be worth undertaking. The number of enrollees necessary to induce changes in practice patterns will vary from provider to provider. In order to tell whether volume matters, it is necessary to have a sample of capitated providers that reflects substantial variation in panel sizes. The Iowa capitation experiment meets this criterion. Among the nearly 350 pharmacies that participated, quarterly enrollment ranged from one to over 1,500.

The Potential for Cost Reduction

There is an immense literature dealing with the ways that health care providers contain costs under risk contracts. It will suffice here to note that the case study approach used in most empirical analyses of provider performance under risk contracts is unsuited to assessing the importance of such organization-level traits as firm size and ownership. The Iowa experience presents an opportunity to examine one organizational characteristic of growing importance in health care markets—namely, the chain operation.

In Iowa, as elsewhere, the market for retail prescription drugs is dominated by competition between independent pharmacies and large chains of wholly-owned or franchised outlets. The chains have a significant economic advantage in drug acquisition cost and can generally sell products cheaper; the independents tout professional services and personal pharmacist-patient relationships. Two features of chain operations lead us to hypothesize that they should outperform independents under an identically structured risk contract. The first reason is enrollment volume. Aggregate enrollments among the outlets of any given chain exceeded that in all but the largest independent pharmacy. If volume matters, as we argue above, then it should matter more to chain pharmacies. The second reason is the centralized administrative support that chains can offer their local managers in terms of help in coping with the business and professional practice challenges associated with risk contracts.

Time and Experience

Capitation can be an important stimulus to economic performance, but it takes time and experience to develop successful strategies for cost management. The framers of the Iowa capitation experiment anticipated that pharmacists would respond to the plan's economic incentives by questioning physician prescribing patterns and, where appropriate, substituting less expensive prescription drugs or even over-the-counter products. But old habits are not easily broken. The transition from thinking in fee-for-service to capitation terms entails a learning curve of unknown shape. We do not know whether to expect an abrupt or a gradual response; we just expect that treatment costs should decline (relative to fee-for-service levels) as capitated providers learn the ropes.*

DATA

The data for this study consist of a three-period panel of observations of individual pharmacy experience over the nine months of the Iowa capitation experiment. The 347 pharmacies that participated yielded a total of 895 quarters of usable information. Because some pharmacies joined late and others dropped out, we chose the pharmacy quarter as the unit of analysis.**

The data originated in the Medicaid Management Information System (MMIS), the Medicaid eligibility files, the Master Drug Pricing File, and the quarterly supplemental payment and escrow account reports, all of which were supplied by the Iowa Medicaid program or the fiscal intermediary, System Development Corporation, to the research team of Yesalis et al. at the University of Iowa.[13,14] The specific data file used in the current study was produced by the University of Iowa researchers, but not analyzed by them. It contains pharmacy-level information by quarter on capitation revenue, enrollment volume and enrollee mix, and utilization and drug cost data from the pseudo claims.

Our analysis is based on parameters either selected directly or developed from this file. These are described in Table 6.1. The dependent variables comprise two measures of utilization cost savings under the capitation plan (COSTSAVE and SAVERATE) and two measures of capitation-related profits (PROFIT and PROFRATE).***

The measure of utilization cost savings generated by each pharmacy was calculated by subtracting the fee-for-service equivalent cost of drugs

---

*Our ability to test time-dependent response is limited in that the experiment lasted only nine months. However, there is reason to assume that the participating pharmacists believed the capitation payment system would be continued if it proved successful.[10] Thus, the measured response should be a reasonable indicator of behavioral changes associated with a more permanent capitation system.

**See the section on estimation issues for a discussion of the statistical implications of this decision.

***The utilization cost savings and profit measures are expressed in both dollar and percentage terms. On the whole, the percentage measures are superior indicators of performance in that they standardize for differences in case mix among pharmacies (i.e., a 10% saving per enrollee, per quarter requires more dollar savings for a pharmacy with an expensive case mix than for one with a less expensive mix). However, small dollar variations among pharmacies sometimes translated into huge percentage differences, creating an outlier problem in the regression analysis.

actually dispensed by that pharmacy to capitated enrollees during a particular quarter (ACTCOST) from the pharmacy's expected costs projected on the assumption that it was still being paid on a fee-for-service basis (EXPCOST). By the terms of the capitation agreement, EXPCOST is equal to the *average* capitation rate faced by each pharmacy, which varies according to the characteristics of its enrollee panel.* While these expected costs are not based on the experience of a control group of noncapitated pharmacies as in the earlier evaluations of the Iowa experiment, they represent a sound baseline for measuring differences in economic performance among the capitated pharmacies themselves.**[13,14]

The two measures of capitation-related pharmacy profits employed in

---

*The average capitation rate is the product of two factors: the class rates and the proportion of panel members in each rate class. As noted previously, the Iowa rate book contained 20 classes based on gender, institutional status (in a nursing home or not), and five age groups. Each class was assigned a relative expense weight using a standard linear regression procedure with monthly drug costs per Medicaid eligible as the dependent variable. The parameter coefficients of the rating factors (the explanatory variables in the equation) indicate the dependent effect of each factor on monthly drug expenses, holding all other factors constant. These weights were added to the constant term in the equation to derive base-level expected costs per enrollee, per month, within each of the 20 rate classes. The base level costs were then projected forward to reflect market level increases in drug acquisition costs. What makes the Iowa capitation rating experience exceptional is the relatively high degree of total variance in individual drug expenses explained by the rating factors ($R^2 = .26$). In other class-rated capitation plans, the explained variance is typically in the 2% to 5% range.

**Yesalis et al. reported an average savings of 3% in drug ingredient costs per enrollee, per quarter, in the experimental (as compared to the control) counties.[13] This is approximately half the estimated cost savings of $1.65 per enrollee, per quarter, calculated using the method described here (Table 6.1). The difference can be explained in part by the fact that our method included savings attributable to reductions in dispensing fees as well as drug ingredient costs. Part of the difference may also be due to an artifact in the selection of control counties for the experiment. These counties had higher than average Medicaid drug expenses prior to the experiment. The disparity is not material in either event. Our interest lies in explaining how panel composition and pharmacy characteristics influence economic performance among capitated pharmacies. For this purpose, it is more important that the capitation rating methodology accurately discriminate cost differences due to individual characteristics (see previous note) than that it predict the rate at which costs change over time. Even if COSTSAVE and SAVERATE overestimate the true level of savings, on average, the error will show up in the intercept or constant terms in our regression equations but will not bias the parameter coefficients of the individual explanatory variables.

TABLE 6.1. Model Variables, Definitions, and Mean Values

Variable	Definition	Mean Value
EXPCOST	Projected fee-for-service cost (including dispensing fee) per enrollee, per quarter, weighted to reflect each pharmacy's average quarterly capitation rate)	$23.84
ATCOST	Fee-for-service equivalent cost of drugs dispensed per enrollee, per quarter (including dispensing fee)	$22.19
ENROLL	Number of enrollees per pharmacy per quarter	144
COSTSAVE	Difference between actual and expected cost per enrollee: EXPCOST – ACTCOST	$1.65
SAVERATE	COSTSAVE expressed as a percentage of the expected cost, EXPCOST	6.9%
PROFIT	Quarterly pharmacy receipts in excess of fee-for-service reimbursement amounts	$3.49
PROFRATE	PROFIT expressed as a percentage of EXPCOST	17.4%
CHAIN	Dummy variable = 1 if second pharmacy is part of a chain; 0 otherwise	.2483
QTR2	Time dummy = 1 if second quarter observation; 0 otherwise	.3333
QTR3	Time dummy = 1 if third quarter observation; 0 otherwise	.3333

this study (PROFIT and PROFRATE) are based on the difference between capitation revenue and what the pharmacy would have been paid for the prescription medicines it actually dispensed to Medicaid enrollees under the FFS system. A pharmacy's capitation profits incorporate both the returns from cost-effective case management as reflected in COSTSAVE and any bonus payments received in accordance with the profit-sharing arrangement developed for the experiment.

Our choice of explanatory variables includes measures of enrollment panel size (ENROLL), case mix complexity as reflected by average expected cost per panel member (EXPCOST), two dummy variables indicating length of experience under the plan (QTR2 and QTR3), and a dummy variable indicating whether the pharmacy is independently owned or part of a chain operation (CHAIN). A survey administered by the University of Iowa collected additional information on participating pharmacies, including annual prescription sales volume, number of pharmacists, and whether the store is owner-managed. Unfortunately, fewer than one-fourth of the pharmacies contacted responded to the survey, and the data could not be used directly in this analysis.*

ESTIMATION PROCEDURES

The cost and profit models were estimated with ordinary least squares multiple regression equations of the form:

$$Y_i = \beta X_1 + u_1$$

where Y_1 represents the dependent variables and X_1 is the vector of explanatory variables described above. The appropriateness of the ordinary least squares (OLS) estimator may be questioned on grounds that the error terms u_1 for each pharmacy are likely to be correlated across the three calendar quarters. Correlation among the disturbances will produce downwardly biased standard errors, thereby increasing the chance of Type I error. Tests for the presence of autocorrelation produced negative results, most likely because pharmacy performance, at least on a quarter-to-quarter basis, contained a very strong random element (this can be seen in the low R^2s shown in Tables 6.2 and 6.3). As a further test for autocorrelation, we used a maximum likelihood estimator developed by Fuller and Battese to estimate a set of time-series, cross-section (TSCS) regressions for a subsample of pharmacies that participated throughout the three quarters of the experiment.[19] The findings for the two estimation techniques were virtually identical. The standard errors in the TSCS regressions were somewhat higher, but this could be due to the small sample size.

In classical regression, the independent variables are assumed to explain changes in the dependent variable, not vice versa. If there is reason to believe that the dependent variable also influences one or more explanatory variables, then the OLS estimator will produce biased results. This is an important methodological concern in evaluating provider performance in capitation plans where providers exercise control over the size and composition of their

---

*A set of preliminary regression equations was estimated for the 80 pharmacies for which a complete set of survey data was available. None of the three additional variables just described was statistically significant in explaining variance in pharmacy profits or cost savings under capitation. While it would have been valuable to have additional pharmacy characteristics as explanatory variables, the loss does not appear to be serious.

TABLE 6.2. Regression Results for Cost Savings Equations

Independent Variable	COSTSAVE (t-statistic)	SAVERATE (t-statistic)
Intercept	−1.43* (−1.62)	−7.21 (−1.18)
EXPCOST	.11¥ (4.81)	.52¥ (3.21)
ENROLL	.003 (1.46)	.02 (1.51)
CHAIN	3.00¥ (3.75)	13.41† (2.41)
QTR2	−.73 (−.91)	−10.44* (−1.86)
QTR3	−1.42* (−1.76)	−13.02† (−2.32)
R^2	.04	.02
F/DOF	7/888	4/888

* Significant at $p < .10$
† Significant at $p < .05$
¥ Significant at $p < .01$

enrollment panels.* In the Iowa case, Medicaid recipients (or the state itself) made the pharmacy selection. Although there were probably instances of informal pharmacy recruitment, the structure of the experiment effectively eliminated selection bias in program enrollment. The fact that the ENROLL and EXPCOST variables are exogenous means that there is little chance of simultaneous equation bias in the OLS parameter estimates.

STUDY FINDINGS

The results of the four regressions are summarized in Tables 6.2 and 6.3. On the whole, the predictive power of the models was rather low. The coefficients of determination for the four regressions range from .02 to .13.

---

*If a provider selects only enrollees believed to represent a low risk of needing service, then the cost and profit outcomes for that provider will not represent a true measure of response to capitation incentives.

TABLE 6.3. Regression Results for Profit Level Equations

Independent Variable	PROFIT (t-statistic)	PROFRATE (t-statistic)
Intercept	−1.5¥ (3.96)	22.51¥ (12.73)
EXPCOST	.08¥ (7.46)	−.20¥ (−4.22)
ENROLL	−.004¥ (−4.90)	−.02¥ (−6.01)
CHAIN	2.20¥ (6.08)	11.66¥ (7.23)
QTR2	.25 (.67)	.43 (.27)
QTR3	−.06 (−.16)	−.68† (−.42)
R^2	.10	.13
F/DOF	19/888	26/888

* Significant at p < .10
† Significant at p < .05
¥ Significant at p < .01

This is not surprising given the high degree of variability in prescription drug utilization patterns among individuals and the small enrollment panels for many pharmacies involved in the experiment. The fact that the dependent variables COSTSAVE and SAVERATE are specified as differences rather than as absolute values undoubtedly contributed to the low R^2s in these two equations.[20]

As can be seen in Table 6.2, the utilization cost savings equations produced consistent results whether the impact variable was defined in dollar (COSTSAVE) or percentage (SAVERATE) terms. The hypothesis that pharmacies with more expensive case mixes (and hence higher average capitation rates) work harder to achieve resource savings appears to be supported by these results. For the average pharmacy, a $1.00 increase in the projected cost per enrollee per quarter (EXPCOST) was associated with an 11¢, greater cost saving (COSTSAVE) and a 52% higher rate of savings (SAVERATE). The coefficients are highly significant in each case.

The estimates provide limited support for the notion that panel size drives cost savings behavior. The coefficients for ENROLL are positive, as hypothesized, in both the COSTSAVE and SAVERATE equations, but they fail to achieve conventional levels of statistical significance. The relationship is actually stronger than these findings indicate. Because chain pharmacies had more enrollees, on average, than independent pharmacies, the explanatory power of ENROLL is diluted by the inclusion of the dummy variable CHAIN in the estimating equations.

The ability of chain pharmacies to adapt to the economic incentives presented by capitation appears to be confirmed by these results. We find that the average chain outlet was able to service its Medicaid enrollees for $3.00 less per quarter (a 13.41% greater cost savings) than its independent counterparts, while holding case mix and enrollment volume constant. It is important to emphasize that these cost differences capture only savings attributable to case management (i.e., changes in prescription volume and product mix). They do not reflect any economies associated with differences in drug acquisition cost or pharmacy overhead. Given that chains are known to have a cost advantage in these areas, our estimates probably understate the true cost differences between the two types of retail pharmacy operation.

The COSTSAVE and SAVERATE regressions offer no evidence of a learning curve as pharmacies adjust to capitation. Indeed, the parameter coefficients of the two time dummies QTR2 and QTR3 suggest that pharmacy performance levels declined as time passed. Some, but by no means all, of the negative time effects may be due to rising drug ingredient costs over the course of the capitation experiment. A more likely explanation is that druggists became confused by the payment mechanics associated with supplemental and bonus payments and simply lost interest in the plan when it became clear that the experiment would not be continued.[10]

The profitability results shown in Table 6.3 tell an interesting story. As expected, the chain outlets generated higher profits from capitation than independent pharmacies ($2.20 more per enrollee per quarter, or nearly 12% higher profit rates). Otherwise, the PROFIT and PROFRATE findings appear to bear little relation to the cost savings results. The most fascinating anomaly is the sign reversal on the enrollment variable (ENROLL). If pharmacies with large enrollment panels produce greater utilization savings, how is it that profits per enrollee decline with panel size? The answer lies in the bonus payments that Iowa paid to pharmacies with favorable cost experience. On a per-enrollee basis, the largest payments went to pharmacies with the fewest enrollees–not because these pharmacies were more efficient, but simply because they were prone to greater random variation in utilization patterns. The unintended consequence of this flaw in the bonus payment system was that such pharmacies were rewarded when, by chance alone, their enrollees filled few or no prescriptions during a particular quarter.[12] Another consequence of the flawed bonus payment system can be seen in the EXPCOST coefficients in Table 6.3. There is a strong positive relationship between the average level of capitation rates (as reflected in EXPCOST) and the dollar profits (PROFIT) earned by the capitated pharmacies. This is consistent with the findings in the COSTSAVE and SAVERATE equations. However, when profits are measured on a rate-of-return basis (PROFRATE), the relationship is again reversed. This sign change occurs because the largest bonus payments in percentage terms went to pharmacies with small panels of enrollees concentrated in the highest capitation rate classes.

Once these structural payment anomalies are explained, the behavior of capitated pharmacists become clearer. The combined regression results describe a pattern of economic performance consistent with three of the four study hypotheses. Those pharmacies with larger panel sizes and higher average capitation rates reflecting more complex case mixes do appear to work harder to achieve the potential economic rewards associated with capitation.* The organizational benefits of chain operations are also apparent. Only the learning curve hypothesis is unsupported by these results, and that may well be due to the shortness of the experiment.

The fact that the average pharmacy in the experimental counties achieved prescription cost savings estimated to be about $1.65 per enrollee, per quarter (see Table 6.1), suggests that capitation had the intended effect of promoting economizing behavior. However, it is important to emphasize who achieved these savings. Given the parameter coefficients in the regression equations, we can attribute the entire savings (and then some) to the responses of pharmacies with larger panel sizes, more complex case mixes, and affiliation with a chain. The rest—fully a third of the pharmacies in the capitated counties—posted no gains whatsoever. This is consistent with a principal theme of our research: it is the intensity of the motivation, rather than the presence of capitation itself, that leads providers to change their practice patterns.

---

*Because the data file analyzed in this chapter does not contain individual prescription level data, we are unable to determine how the capitated pharmacies achieved their savings. Yesalis et al. detected no statistically significant changes in the quality of pharmacy prescribing patterns associated with the expanded capitation experiment, where quality was measured by the type and quantity of drugs prescribed as well as by the presence of drug combinations known to produce adverse interactions.[13] This would suggest that the observed savings were due to efficiency improvements.

CONCLUDING COMMENTS

The special features of the Iowa pharmacy capitation experiment make it difficult to extrapolate these findings to other settings. However, the questions raised by this research have broad applicability. As payers in both the private and public sectors expand capitation contracts beyond the traditional venue of health maintenance organizations, the issue of what drives providers to economize takes on added importance. Basing future capitation schemes on accepted dogma has its risks.

For instance, conventional wisdom holds that capitated providers must be placed at risk of financial loss in order to generate incentives for economizing behavior. We were able to show that under one set of circumstances carrots had the same effect as sticks. Or, take the question of panel size. It has long been recognized that enrollment volume is a critical actuarial factor in the design of capitation contracts. Our work suggests that it may be an important motivational factor as well. One final example should make the point clear. Increasingly, capitation contracts are being written that cover specific, limited types of services (primary physician care is one example; the Iowa capitation program is another). It is tempting to think of single-service risk contract plans as scaled-down HMOs. But if the motivation for cost efficiency is linked to the level of the capitation rate, then such contracts are unlikely to produce commensurate resource savings.

REFERENCES

1. Luft H. Health maintenance organizations and the rationing of medical care. Milbank Mem Fund Q 1982;60(2):268-306.

2. Welch W, Frank R, Diehr P. Health care costs in health maintenance organizations: correcting for self selection. In: Scheffler R, ed. Advances in health economics and health services research. vol. 5. New York: JAI Press, 1984.

3. Luft H. How do health maintenance organizations achieve their savings? New Engl J Med 1978;298:1336-43.

4. Yesalis C, Norwood G, Lipson D et al. Use and costs under the Iowa Capitation Drug Program. Health Care Finan Rev 1981;3:127.

5. Yesalis C, Norwood G, Lipson D et al. Capitation payment for pharmacy services: impact on generic substitution. Med Care 1980;18:816.

6. Helling D, Yesalis C, Norwood G et al. Effects of capitation payment for pharmacy services on pharmacist dispensing and physician prescribing behavior: I. prescription quantity and dose analysis. Drug Intell Clin Pharm 1981;15:581.

7. Norwood G, Helling D, Burmeister L et al. Effects of capitation payment for pharmacy services on pharmacist dispensing and physician prescribing behavior: II. therapeutic category analysis; OTC drug usage and drug interactions. Drug Intell Clin Pharm 1981;5:656.

8. Lipson D, Yesalis C, Kohout F et al. Capitation payment for Medicaid pharmacy services: impact on non-Medicaid prescriptions. Med Care 1981;19:342.

9. Joseph H, Burmeister L, Lipson D et al. Pharmacy costs: capitation versus fee-for-service. Q J Business Econ 1983;22(4):41-51.

10. Yesalis C, Levitz G. The life and death of a field experiment: a case study of health care research in a hostile environment. J Health Polit Policy Law 1985;9: 611-28.

11. McCormack J, Stuart B. Report to the Iowa Drug Capitation Review Committee. State of Iowa, Department of Social Services, 1982.

12. Stuart B, Yesalis C. On taking chances with the law of large numbers. Health Ser Manage Res 1988;1(Nov):3.

13. Yesalis C, Lipson D, Norwood G, Burmeister LF, Jones ME. Capitation payment for pharmacy services: I. impact on drug use and pharmacist dispensing behavior. Med Care 1984;22:737-45.

14. Yesalis C, Norwood G, Helling D, Lipson DP, Mahrenholz RJ, Burmeister LF. Capitation payment for pharmacy services: II. impact on costs. Med Care 1984;22:746-54.

15. Luft H. Health maintenance organizations: dimensions of performance. New York: John Wiley & Sons, 1981.

16. Welch W. The new structure of independent practice associations. J Health Polit Policy Law 1987;12:723-39.

17. Machina M. Choice under uncertainty: problems solved and unsolved. Econ Perspectives 1987;1(1):121-54.

18. DHEW. The target income hypothesis and related issues in health manpower policy. Washington: U.S. Department of Health, Education, and Welfare, 1980. HRA 80-127.

19. Fuller W, Battese G. Estimation of linear models with crossed-error structure. J Econometrics 1974;2:67-78.

20. Cohen J, Cohen P. Applied multiple regression/correlation analysis for the behavioral sciences. Hillsdale, NJ: Lawrence Erlbaum Associates, 1975.

Chapter 7

Incorporating Severity-of-Illness Measures into Retrospective Claims-Based Cost-Effectiveness Analyses

Kristina Baum
Lisa Muggeo
Carol Brignoli Gable
Rhonda B. Friedman
Susan Sedory Holzer

INTRODUCTION

In the last two decades, health care providers have been subjected to intense scrutiny as federal and private payers have emphasized cost containment. The pressure to reduce costs while maintaining quality of care has led researchers to examine the cost-effectiveness of a variety of medical therapies. One approach to cost-effectiveness analysis has been the examination of associated outcomes and costs of competing therapies within the confines of a prospective, randomized, controlled trial. Unfortunately, prospective data collection is costly and time consuming, taking years to accomplish. In addition, clinical trials do not fully represent the true diversity of patient conditions and therapeutic regimens.

As an alternative to controlled trials, some researchers have used retrospective claims databases. Retrospective cost-effectiveness analyses provide information on large numbers of diverse patients at a relatively low cost. However, a major drawback associated with claims data is that comorbidities

Previously published in *Journal of Research in Pharmaceutical Economics*, Vol. 5(1), 1993.

and severity of illness may differ between groups of patients. These confounding factors must be controlled to obtain meaningful research results. Researchers have developed a number of severity measurement systems to address patient differences in severity within diagnosis-related groups (DRGs), and these systems have also been used to correlate severity of illness with costs or medical outcomes.[1-13] One of these systems, Disease Staging, has been widely used to measure severity of illness and its impact on hospital costs.[11-13] Disease Staging is well suited for cost-effectiveness research because, as a discharge-based system, it does not require medical chart review or clinical judgment as part of the rating methodology; thus, it can be applied easily to automated medical claims data.

In this paper, we describe the use of Coded Disease Staging and Q-Scale™, a software program marketed by SysteMetrics/McGraw-Hill, to control for patient severity of illness in cost-benefit analyses using retrospective claims data during an acute inpatient hospital stay. We also describe a modification of the method that allows severity of illness to be determined over an extended patient therapy period using both inpatient and outpatient claims data.

METHODS

Coded Disease Staging and Q-Scale

In brief, Disease Staging is a clinical staging methodology covering approximately 400 disease categories that reflect virtually all U.S. hospital discharges. Each disease category is divided into four generic levels of severity, as shown in Table 7.1. Within each stage, substages further refine the level of severity. Related complications of a disease are defined as stages or substages within that disease category, whereas unrelated comorbidities are defined as independent disease categories. Using Coded Disease Staging on a patient with multiple diagnoses will result in these being reduced to the smallest number of independent disease categories, each of which will be assigned a stage, based on severity.

Because disease stages are expressed as ordinal levels that cannot be averaged to describe a patient's overall severity of illness, in 1986 SysteMetrics developed Q-Scale, an empirical software system that projects relative resource use (an indicator of severity of illness) as a function of all of a patient's disease stages. DRG-Scale represents the patient's overall severity relative to the national average within that DRG; TOT-Scale expresses the patient's overall severity relative to the national population of hospital dis-

TABLE 7.1

Stages of Disease

Stage 1:   Conditions with no complications
             or problems of minimal severity

Stage 2:   Problems limited to an organ or organ
             system; significantly increased risk of
             complications

Stage 3:   Multiple site involvement; generalized
             systemic involvement; poor prognosis

Stage 4:   Death

charges across all DRGs. These indexes were developed using empirical analysis of almost ten million hospital discharges throughout the United States and validated on two million randomly selected hospital discharges throughout the U.S. Because these scales are linear, values can be meaningfully averaged across patients, physicians, or providers.

The Coded Disease Staging software and its inclusion of a resource-based severity measure, Q-Scale, are more completely described in the literature.[11-13] For this study, we used the personal computer version of Coded Disease Staging and Q-Scale–EQCEL™ Version 1.5. The software requires input of age, gender, discharge status, and ICD-9-CM diagnosis and procedure codes, all of which are available from automated claims data files. The EQCEL software calculates each patient's disease stage(s) on an ordinal scale of one to four as well as the two Q-Scale severity-of-illness indexes: DRG-Scale and TOT-Scale.

Missing Data

EQCEL software requires input of valid three-, four-, and five-digit ICD-9-CM codes, although many payers do not require this level of ICD-9-CM code specificity from providers. To use the more general codes found in some retrospective claims databases, we needed to increase the code specificity of incomplete three- and four-digit codes in the retrospective data by adding the missing fourth and/or fifth digit(s). To minimize distortion of the data that this manipulation could cause, we constructed an impact algorithm. Given an invalid three- or four-digit code *ABC/ABC.D,* the impact algorithm evaluated all possible combinations of missing digits *D/DE* for overall severity (TOT-Scale) when testing the adjusted code as if it were a principal diagnosis. The algorithm then substituted the missing digits that correlated with the lowest overall severity score. In this way, we consistently minimized the impact of the algorithm on the overall severity measure for each patient. Similarly, when given an invalid five-digit code *ABC.DE* where the *E* digit was unallowable within ICD-9-CM, either the *E* digit was substituted or the code was truncated at digit *D,* whichever yielded the lowest overall severity when testing the adjusted code as if it were a principal diagnosis. We chose this conservative approach of understating stage of disease and overall severity to be consistent with the original development of Disease Staging. When creating the coded staging criteria, Gonnella and colleagues treated lack of specificity in the ICD coding systems and unavailability of certain data items on a typical discharge abstract by conservatively assigning only the stage of disease that could be positively specified from the coding system.[10]

APPLICATIONS: TWO EXAMPLES

Antibiotic Treatment of Acute Inpatient Pneumonia

We recently conducted two cost-effectiveness analyses using severity of illness as a predictive variable. The first application involved an assessment of total hospital charges, length of stay, and length of therapy associated with various antibiotics used to treat pneumonia during an acute hospital stay. We used retrospective hospital discharge claims data from Hospital Data Services, Inc. (HDS) that provided patient-level records of demographic data, pharmacy utilization, length of stay, total charges, and up to ten ICD-9-CM diagnosis and procedure codes for each hospital stay.

Because the data were limited to clearly defined and discrete hospital stays, we found it relatively straightforward to apply Disease Staging in this study. The inability to segregate pneumonia-related charges from comorbidity-related charges mandated that an overall severity-of-illness measure be incorporated into the analysis. We found that the overall severity measure, TOT-Scale, was a significant predictor of total hospital charges, length of stay, and length of therapy in a full factorial analysis of variance (ANOVA) model. There was significant interaction between overall severity and antibiotic for total charges and length of stay in adult patients and three-way interaction among overall severity, antibiotic, and hospital teaching status for length of therapy. In addition, the analysis supports the work of other researchers in that the significantly higher charges and length of stay found in teaching–as opposed to nonteaching–hospitals in this study were not associated with a concomitant higher overall severity of illness in the patients treated in teaching hospitals.[14,15]

Long-Term Nitrate Therapy for Chronic Angina

The second application involved assessing angina health care utilization and total cardiovascular-related charges over the course of one year of therapy comparing nitrate patch therapy to oral therapy. We used retrospective claims data from Physicians Health Plan of Minnesota (PHP) that provided patient-level records of demographic data, pharmacy claims, inpatient hospital claims, and outpatient visit claims. Integrating Disease Staging into this study presented three challenges: identifying principal diagnoses, limiting the number of diagnosis codes, and integrating the outpatient diagnoses into Disease Staging.

Identifying the Principal Diagnosis. Coded Disease Staging requires that a principal diagnosis be specified; however, the PHP database does not designate principal diagnosis. Rather, an inpatient stay is comprised of numerous individual claims for inpatient services, with each inpatient claim having an associated ICD-9-CM code. We therefore had to assign a principal diagnosis for each hospital stay. We chose the most frequently appearing ICD-9-CM diagnosis code within each hospital stay as the principal diagnosis, assuming that the majority of services received by the patient during the hospitalization would be related to the principal diagnosis.

Limiting the Diagnosis Codes. Unlike the HDS database, PHP claims are coded with only a single diagnosis or procedure code; however, each service provided during an inpatient stay has a separate claim. Therefore, after we defined the hospital stay, some patients had extensive lists of diagnosis and procedure codes. Eliminating duplicate codes usually resulted in a diagnosis code set within the Coded Disease Staging limits of 14 secondary diagnosis codes and 15 procedure codes. If the unique code set exceeded these limits, the codes were run through the previously described impact algorithm. Codes were eliminated from the set in order of least impact first until the set was within limits.

Integrating Outpatient Diagnoses. If we had restricted our analyses to inpatient diagnoses only, we could have missed significant comorbidities treated on an outpatient basis. However, Coded Disease Staging has no provision for analyzing outpatient data. We integrated outpatient diagnosis codes by adding them to the inpatient stay before staging. Thus, for patients who had inpatient stays, we reduced the outpatient claims to a unique set that was then added to the inpatient stay code set. If necessary, we ran the consolidated set of inpatient and outpatient codes through the impact algorithm and eliminated codes in order of least impact first. However, recognizing that inpatient diagnoses reflect a higher level of treatment than outpatient diagnoses, a hierarchical order was superimposed on this process so that outpatient codes were eliminated first; thus, the highest impact outpatient code was eliminated before the lowest impact inpatient code.

For patients who had outpatient claims but no inpatient claims, we treated the set of outpatient claims as if they represented an inpatient stay, aggregating the ICD-9-CM codes and assigning the most frequent code as the principal diagnosis. We then created a unique set by eliminating duplicate codes and, if necessary, running the codes through the impact algorithm, as described above.

Patients who had multiple inpatient stays were analyzed using their highest disease stage. We also used the sum of their TOT-Scales because we considered frequent hospitalizations consistent with more severe and/or less well-controlled angina. Interestingly, almost 39% of the patients had no coronary artery related inpatient or outpatient diagnoses during the year, despite having continuous prescriptions for nitrate therapy. Although nitrates can be used on a short-term basis for other conditions, long-term use indicates coronary artery disease. We assumed that claims for coronary-related procedures during the year, as well as continuous nitrate use, indicated an angina diagnosis. However, because many patients had no specific coronary artery related diagnoses, they did not stage into the appropriate Disease Staging disease category. For the purpose of analysis, we created a "Stage 0" for these patients because we believed that their lack of specific coronary artery related diagnosis was consistent with the lowest severity angina.

In this study, both disease stage and overall severity were significant independent variables in a linear regression model ($p = .0001$). Because disease stage confounded coronary artery related costs, it was important to control for disease stage in the analysis. Unlike the study of antibiotic use in pneumonia, however, we did not find interactions between type of treatment and severity of illness as measured by disease stage or overall severity.

DISCUSSION

In a recent editorial in *Medical Care,* Lurie posed a number of questions about the usefulness of using administrative data to assess health outcomes, including whether the accuracy of diagnoses in claims data is sufficient for analysis and identification of comorbidities.[16] These concerns are valid and appropriate. For example, Coffey and Goldfarb have shown that in a comparison of computer staging and hand staging of the same set of complete medical records, up to 22% of the stagings may not match due to coding errors and lack of specificity in the ICD-9-CM system.[17] Problems associated with the specificity of the ICD-9-CM classification system have been well documented.[18-20]

Our extensive experience, combined with that of other researchers using state, federal, and private claims databases to assess outcomes and costs of a variety of therapies, however, leaves us convinced that, despite the limitations inherent in retrospective claims-based research, well-designed studies can provide useful and reliable information.[21-26] Our goal in applying Coded Disease Staging and Q-Scale to retrospective claims data was to achieve an incremental improvement in the control of severity-of-illness confounding in these studies. Whereas in this chapter we describe use of two resource-based measures of severity, a more recent version of EQCEL (2.0) also provides separate indexes for length of stay and mortality risk. We are currently studying the feasibility of incorporating these two additional indexes into cost-effectiveness analyses.

We performed several manipulations to adapt Coded Disease Staging and Q-Scale to retrospective claims data: assignment of principal diagnoses, correction of unacceptable ICD-9-CM codes, integration of inpatient and outpatient claims, and summation of TOT-Scales for patients with multiple hospitalizations. While we believe that our approaches were reasonable and logically justifiable, we have no measure of the extent of error that these manipulations introduced.

In conclusion, we have developed a methodology to apply Coded Disease Staging and Q-Scale in retrospective claims data research to control for patient severity of illness and have applied it to two retrospective studies. In both of these studies, patient severity of illness measures were significant independent variables in the models predicting outcomes and, in one study, there was significant interaction between patient severity and therapy type that would have biased study results if left uncontrolled. The ability to control for patient severity of illness in retrospective claims data addresses one of the major concerns about the use of administrative data for outcomes research.

REFERENCES

1. Horn SD, Sharkey PD, Chambers AF, Horn RA. Severity of illness within DRGs: impact on prospective payment. Am J Public Health 1985;75:1195-9.

2. Hornbrook MC. Techniques for assessing hospital case mix. Ann Rev Public Health 1985;6:295-324.

3. Jencks SF, Dobson A. Refining case-mix adjustment: the research evidence. N Engl J Med 1987;317:679-86.

4. Knaus WA, Zimmerman JE, Wagner DP, Draper EA, Lawrence DE. APACHE–acute physiology and chronic health evaluation: a physiologically based classification system. Crit Care Med 1981;9:591-7.

5. Iezzoni LI. Severity of illness measures: comments and caveats. Med Care 1990;28:757-61.

6. Iezzoni LI, Shwartz M, Moskowitz MA, Ash AS, Sawitz E, Burnside S. Illness severity and costs of admission at teaching and nonteaching hospitals. JAMA 1990;264:1426-31.

7. Thomas JW, Ashcraft MLF. Measuring severity of illness: six severity systems and their ability to explain cost variations. Inquiry 1991;28:39-55.

8. Horn SD, Sharkey PD, Buckle JM, Backofen JE, Averill RF, Horn RA. The relationship between severity of illness and hospital length of stay and mortality. Med Care 1991;29:305-17.

9. Hopkins L. Cost analysis with institutional data. J Pharm Market Manage 1987;2(2):33-47.

10. Alemi FA, Rice J, Hankins R. Predicting in-hospital survival of myocardial infarction: a comparative study of various severity measures. Med Care 1990;28: 762-75.

11. Gonnella JS, Hornbrook MC, Louis DZ. Staging of disease: a case-mix measurement. JAMA 1984;251:637-46.

12. Christoffersson JG, Conklin JE, Gonnella J. The impact of severity of illness on hospital costs. DRG Monitor 1988;6(1):1-8.

13. Epstein AM, Stern RS, Weissman JS. Do the poor cost more? A multihospital study of patients' socioeconomic status and use of hospital resources. N Engl J Med 1990;322:1122-8.

14. Rich EC, Gifford F, Luxenberg M, Dowd B. The relationship of house staff experience to the cost and quality of inpatient care. JAMA 1990;263:953-7.

15. Richards T, Lurie N, Rogers WH, Brook RH. Measuring differences between teaching and nonteaching hospitals. Med Care 1988;26(5 Suppl):S1-S141.

16. Lurie N. Administrative data and outcomes research. Med Care 1990;28:867-9.

17. Coffey RM, Goldfarb MG. DRGs and disease staging for reimbursing Medicare patients. Med Care 1986;24:814-29.

18. Mullin RL. Diagnosis-related groups and severity: ICD-9-CM, the real problem. JAMA 1985;254:1208-10.

19. McMahon LF, Smits HL. Can Medicare prospective payment survive the ICD-9-CM disease classification system? Ann Intern Med 1986;104:562-6.

20. Gertman PM, Lowenstein S. A research paradigm for severity of illness: issues for the diagnosis-related group system. Health Care Finan Rev 1984;(Ann Suppl):79-90.

21. Gable CB, Holzer SS, Engelhart L, Friedman RB, Smeltz F, Schroeder D, Baum K. Pneumococcal vaccine: efficacy and associated cost savings. JAMA 1990;264:2910-5.

22. Holzer SS, Gable CB, Friedman RB. Cost effectiveness of pneumococcal vaccine: implications for managed care. In: The contemporary HMO: managing care in the modern market. Proceedings of the 1991 Group Health Institute. Washington, DC: Group Health Association of America, Inc., 1991. Reprinted in J Res Pharm Econ 1993; 5(1):79-95.

23. Gable CB, Engelhart L, Sarma S, Holzer SS, Smeltz F, Schroeder DA, Friedman RB. Mixed vaginal infections–candidiasis and venereal disease–in Medicaid women. J Res Pharm Econ; 1993;5(1): 69-78. Published as "Rate of venereal disease coinfections in women with vaginal candidiasis: Michigan Medicaid" in Pharmacoepidemiol Drug Safety 1992; 1(3): 125-32.

24. Oster G, Huse DM, Adams SF, Imbimbo J, Russell MW. Benzodiazepine tranquilizers and the risk of accidental injury. Am J Public Health 1990;80: 1467-70.

25. Bloom BS, Fox NA, Jacobs J. Patterns of care and expenditures by California Medicaid for peptic ulcer and other acid-related diseases. J Clin Gastroenterol 1989; 11:615-20.

26. Jick H. Use of automated databases to study drug effects after marketing. Pharmacotherapy 1985;5:278-9.

Chapter 8

Initial Impact of a Medicaid Prior Authorization Program for NSAID Prescriptions

Jeffrey A. Kotzan
John A. McMillan
Charlotte A. Jankel
Anita L. Foster

INTRODUCTION

The Medicaid drug program presented a special problem for the State of Georgia. The program ranked ninth in total expenditures for Medicaid drugs among all states. Total drug costs were $127.5 million in 1989 for 445,000 recipients. The program allocated 10.4% of the total Medicaid budget for drugs, thus ranking third in percentage allocation for drugs behind Mississippi and Tennessee.[1]

Concern over drug program costs is not unique to Georgia. Along with mandates for procurement of pharmaceuticals and drug use review programs, legislation sponsored by Senator Pryor (Arkansas) and included in the Omnibus Budget Reconciliation Act of 1990 (OBRA90) contained provisions for limiting coverage of drugs and for other cost-saving tactics.[2] Among these provisions, prior authorization programs were explicitly addressed. Prior authorization is a process that requires a prescriber to obtain permission to use a drug for the Medicaid patient before it is reimbursed. The legislation listed certain restrictions for prior authorization programs:

1. The state may not subject any new biological or drug to prior authorization for a period of six months after its approval by the Food and Drug Administration.

Previously published in *Journal of Research in Pharmaceutical Economics*, Vol. 5(1), 1993.

2. Prior authorization programs must have a system in place to provide a response for a requested drug within 24 hours.
3. Emergency provision of a 72-hour supply of drugs must be allowed.

Further, the legislation required the Secretary of the Department of Health and Human Services to:

1. Study the impact of prior authorization programs on beneficiary and provider access to prescription drugs.
2. Determine the impact of prior authorization programs on program costs.
3. Make recommendations for reforms of prior authorization programs if needed.

Because prior authorization implies the existence of a restrictive formulary, it is important that a formulary be rational and carefully conceived. Some evidence exists to suggest that formularies may not, in themselves, be an effective means of cost containment. Kozma reported that removal of a restricted formulary for Medicaid prescriptions in a single state was associated with decreased use of other medical services. However, those products included in the restricted formulary were not necessarily selected on the basis of cost and efficacy.[3] In another Medicaid study, Soumerai et al. reported that a formulary that removed coverage for Drug Efficacy Study Implementation (DESI) drugs increased the utilization and cost of other, more expensive drug products.[4] Kreling, Knocke, and Hammel studied the removal of propoxyphene napsylate from a state Medicaid formulary and concluded that lost market shares were directly shifted to other analgesic products without a reduction in overall expenditures.[5] Finally, in a review of the formulary literature through 1987, Jang noted that formulary restrictions for Medicaid drug programs may not lower overall costs. Any savings in a drug program may increase the need for other medical services.[6] Also, some Medicaid recipients may choose to discontinue drug therapy or to pay for the restricted drug.[7] Thus, a carefully planned drug formulary is a requirement for a cost-effective prior authorization program.

A review of the data compiled in 1990 by the National Pharmaceutical Council indicated that 18 states had restricted drug formularies with prior authorization programs in place.[1] The 18 programs were managed with different approaches. Some required an authorization when a pharmaceutical product exceeded a predetermined price or quantity limit. Other programs required authorization when patients exceeded a monthly prescription limit or requested a prescription for a nonformulary drug product.

Before 1990, Georgia required prior authorization for Medicaid recipients who exceeded a six-prescription-per-month limit. Customarily, the pharmacist initiated the process upon dispensing the prescription by completing a form that included a prior authorization number. The forms were forwarded to the physician who completed a short description of the diagnosis, signed the form, and mailed it to the Department of Medical Assistance. The approved forms were mailed back to the physician and pharmacist within a week or so. Since almost all requests for prior authorizations were approved, the dispensing pharmacist assumed little risk in dispensing the prescription before receipt of final approval.

Pharmaceutical manufacturers are generally opposed to prior authorization programs for drugs.[8] Nevertheless, state Medicaid administrators may view them as an effective means of controlling drug utilization and costs. Few current, documented studies are available to assess the financial and health-related effects of prior authorization programs. However, Mississippi and California are notable for their extended experience with prior authorization drug programs.[9] Further study may or may not conclude that prior authorization programs offer an acceptable means of cost containment as new and more expensive drugs are introduced.

On January 1, 1990, the Georgia Department of Medical Assistance implemented a policy that restricted Medicaid recipients to multisource nonsteroidal anti-inflammatory drugs (NSAIDs). Anaprox® was the exception to the multisource limitation. Following a one-prescription-per-year limit, single-source products remained available to recipients through a prior authorization process. Since no other policy changes had been imposed on the NSAIDs for the previous years, the situation presented a natural opportunity to study the economic and medical impact of a prior authorization program for a single therapeutic category.

The overall objective of the research was to determine the utilization of and total costs for NSAID prescriptions before and after implementation of the prior authorization program. The secondary objective was to determine changes in the use of medical services other than prescription drugs. An additional study objective was to determine shifts in prescription utilization among different categories of drug products following implementation of the prior authorization policy.

METHODS

All data analyses were calculated on a mainframe system in a TSO environment using the Statistical Analysis System.[10] Three data sets were provided by Electronic Data Systems Corporation, the claims processor for the State of Georgia. The first file described recipient eligibility and demographics. The second contained prescription records for all drugs dispensed from January 1989 through November 1990 and provided a thorough description of each prescription, including trade name, therapeutic class, and the amount paid.* The third data set, the medical history file, provided a comprehensive description of all other service claims processed during the study. For example, the records contained fields identifying the type of provider and the place where the service was provided.

The recipient file was abstracted to create a data set containing all of the continuously eligible Medicaid recipients over the entire study period. Next, the prescription files were abstracted to isolate the antiarthritic drugs (including NSAIDs), analgesics, and narcotics. This file was merged with the continuously eligible recipient file for all subsequent drug analyses.

The demographics of the continuously eligible NSAID recipients were tabulated, and month-by-month NSAID prescription totals were calculated and compared to the analgesic, narcotic, and non-NSAID antiarthritic products. The last stage of the research included calculation of the month-by-month totals for nondrug services for the continuously eligible recipients. Using the autoregression procedure of the Statistical Analysis System, the monthly totals were then analyzed by time series methods. The autocorrelation models were developed in accordance with those described by Ostrom.[11] These were constructed to determine the elasticity of demand between single- and multiple-source NSAIDs and other services.

RESULTS

Of the 609,924 individuals who received Medicaid benefits during the study period, 237,529 were continuously eligible, and of these, 80,064 received one or more NSAID prescriptions between January 1989 and July 1990. The average age for the continuously eligible NSAID patients was 58.22 years, with a standard deviation of 22.45 years. The majority were black (62.7%), and 80.4% of the total recipients were female.

A total of 10,669,451 prescriptions were dispensed to Georgia Medicaid recipients during the study period. Of that total, 679,761 were NSAID

---

*Data were collected through November 1990 but limited to July 1990 due to the lag between provision of services and submission of claims. Our analyses of other months indicate that greater than 98.5% of all prescription claims were represented for the July 1990 data by including all claims processed through November.

prescriptions. The continuously eligible received the large majority of the NSAID prescriptions—466,465 in total. The 1989 pattern of NSAID prescription use appears in Figure 8.1. Of the continuously eligible patients, 39% received a single prescription in 1989, accounting for 12% of the total prescriptions. However, 3% of these patients received 11 prescriptions during the year, accounting for 11% of the total NSAID prescriptions.

The impact of the prior authorization program is portrayed in Figure 8.2. During 1989, the total monthly volume of single-source NSAID prescriptions remained stable at about 11,000 prescriptions per month. Following implementation of the policy on January 1, 1990, the monthly prescription volume dropped immediately and continued to decline to approximately 1,000 in July 1990. The trend in the monthly prescription volume for the multiple-source NSAID products was almost a mirror image of that seen for the single-source prescriptions. However, it appears that the decrease in single-source products did not correspond to the increase observed for the multiple-source products on a one-to-one basis. The combined monthly prescription volume of single- and multiple-source prescriptions decreased from approximately 23,500 to 18,500 in 1990 (Figure 8.3).

The combined effects of the apparent substitution of multiple-source products for single-source products and the reduction in the total number of NSAID prescriptions led to a gross savings of slightly more than $3 million for the first seven months of the prior authorization program (Figure 8.4). During 1989, the monthly NSAID expenditures for the 80,064 recipients amounted to greater than $700,000. Following policy implementation, that total decreased to about $325,000.

There were additional costs for nonnarcotic analgesics that were associated with the NSAID prior authorization program. During 1989, analgesic prescription costs increased from $123,605 to $140,000 per month and escalated to more than $180,000 during May and June of 1990. The additional costs for the seven months amounted to $193,540 (Figure 8.5). However, not all analgesic products appeared to share equally in the additional prescription volume. The monthly prescription volume for Dolobid® exceeded 200% growth above the prepolicy level, compared to less than 30% growth for propoxyphene hydrochloride and napsylate (Figure 8.6). A similar analysis of the narcotic analgesics identified a modest increase in costs during 1990 amounting to $13,096 for the seven months. However, an analysis of other antiarthritic agents, such as phenylbutazone and allopurinol, uncovered no increase in prescriptions and their associated costs for 1990.

An analysis of nondrug services for the continuously eligible NSAID patients did not reveal significant changes in utilization. The monthly volume of physician claims and their associated costs were remarkably

FIGURE 8.1. 1989 Percentage Prescriptions and Recipient Consumption for All NSAIDs

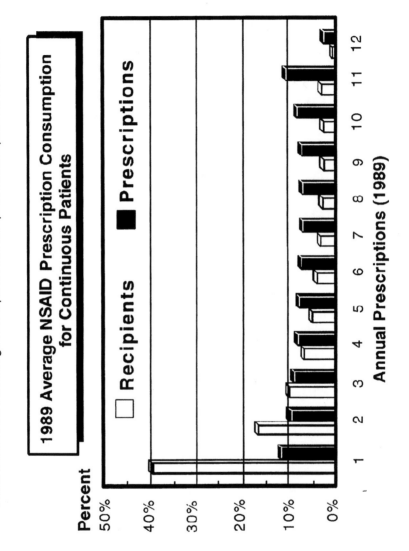

FIGURE 8.2. Single- and Multiple-Source NSAIDs Between January 1, 1989 and July 31, 1990

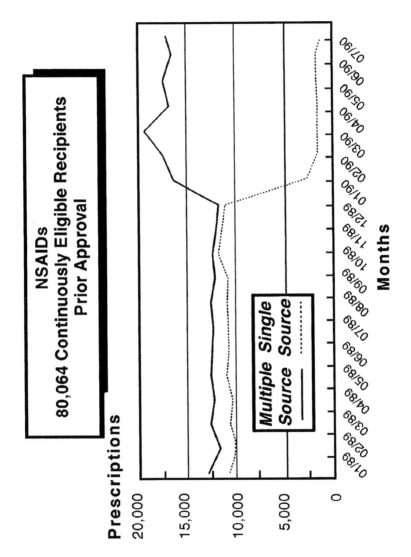

FIGURE 8.3. Total Monthly Prescriptions for Single- and Multiple-Source NSAIDs Between January 1, 1989 and July 31, 1990

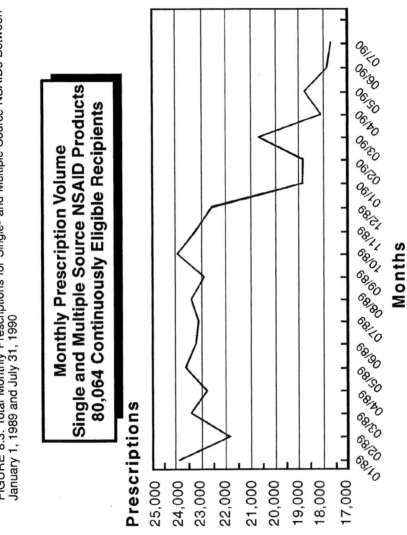

Monthly Prescription Volume
Single and Multiple Source NSAID Products
80,064 Continuously Eligible Recipients

FIGURE 8.4. Total Monthly Prescription Dollars for Nonnarcotic Analgesics Between January 1, 1989 and August 31, 1990 with Ordinary Least Squares Fit of 1989 Totals

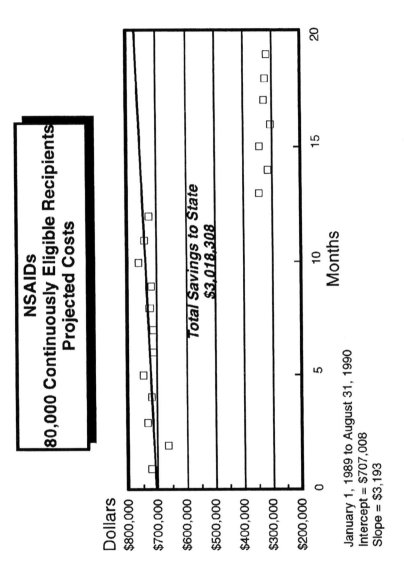

NSAIDs
80,000 Continuously Eligible Recipients
Projected Costs

Total Savings to State
$3,018,308

Dollars

Months

January 1, 1989 to August 31, 1990
Intercept = $707,008
Slope = $3,193

FIGURE 8.5. Total Monthly Prescription Dollars for Nonnarcotic Analgesics Between January 1, 1989 and July 31, 1990 with Ordinary Least Squares Fit of 1989 Totals

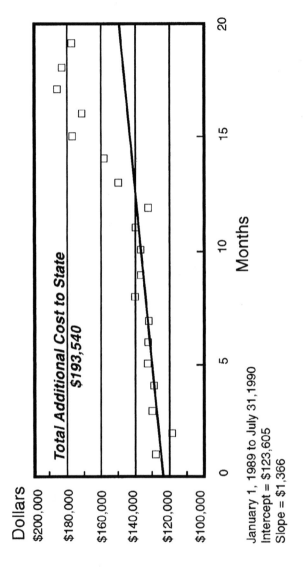

Analgesic Prescription Costs for 80,064 Continuously Eligible NSAID Patients

Total Additional Cost to State $193,540

Dollars

January 1, 1989 to July 31, 1990
Intercept = $123,605
Slope = $1,366

122

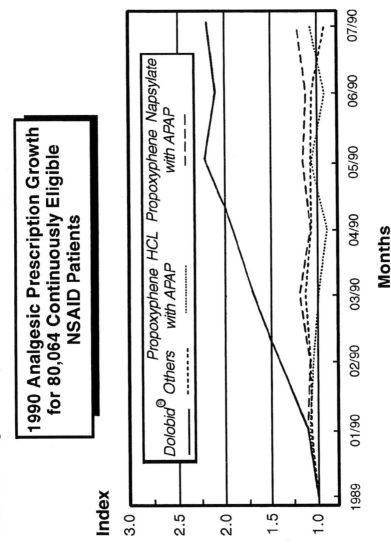

1990 Analgesic Prescription Growth for 80,064 Continuously Eligible NSAID Patients

Base 1989 = 1.0

consistent for the study period. Approximately 25,000 physician claims were submitted each month at a cost of about $2 million. Furthermore, no additional costs were observed in 1990 for inpatient, outpatient, or other categories of medical services for these patients.

The results from the autoregression procedures are provided in Table 8.1. The coefficients of regression (beta values) may be interpreted as elasticities between the matched variables. The -0.541 reported for the first row indicates that for every decrease of 100 single-source NSAID products, an increase of 54 multiple-source NSAID prescriptions was calculated. Similarly, for every decrease in 100 total NSAID prescriptions, an increase of six (-0.059) Dolobid® prescriptions and 14 (-0.138) total analgesic prescriptions was observed. Nonsignificant relationships were reported for the other antiarthritic products. Also, no relationship between the nondrug categories of service and the decrease in total NSAID prescriptions was observed.

The determined statistical relationships appeared to confirm those results previously reported. For example, the change in prescription volume between the single-source and multiple-source products reported in Figure 8.2 resulted in the significant negative coefficient reported between the single- and multiple-source products in Table 8.1. Likewise, the additional utilization and costs of the analgesic prescriptions reported in Figure 8.5 resulted in the significant relationships for analgesic prescriptions reported in Table 8.1.

CONCLUSION AND DISCUSSION

The impact of a drug policy may be measured in both economic and human terms. Does the policy save money and are the recipients injured? Clearly the NSAID policy analyzed here appeared appropriate in terms of economic issues. The $3 million savings for seven months for the continuously eligible recipients, less the increased costs for analgesic and narcotic prescriptions, can be extrapolated to the entire year for all recipients. If the NSAID use in discontinuous recipients is similar to that described in this study, then the projected savings to the program amounted to $7,024,009 for 1990.

The increased costs associated with the administration of the program were not documented as part of this study. The additional prior authorizations associated with the NSAID program added to the existing six-prescription-per-month prior authorization system without adding personnel. Other costs associated with the administration of the Medicaid drug program did not increase in 1990. In fact, the expenditures for the program management division responsible for administering the drug program decreased from $3.8 million in 1989 to $2.8 million in 1990.[12,13]

TABLE 8.1 Autoregression for Montly Total Claims of Selected Drug Categories and Medical Services

Dependent Variable	Regressor Variable	Total R Square	Beta Value	T-Ratio Beta	Probability Beta
No Approval*	Approval Required	0.938	-0.541	-19.800	0.0001
Dolobid©*	Total NSAIDs	0.729	-0.059	-4.736	0.0002
Total Medical Claims	Total NSAIDs	0.177	-0.205	-1.370	0.1893
Other Antiarthritics	Total NSAIDs	0.317	-0.013	-1.749	0.0994
Narcotics*	Total NSAIDs	0.191	-0.042	-2.196	0.0432
Analgesics*	Total NSAIDs	0.479	-0.138	-4.478	0.0004
MD Claims	Total NSAIDs	0.052	0.028	0.233	0.8189

SAS ETS Series, Lag=1, Method=Yule Walker
*significant at 0.05

The second factor used to assess the effects of a policy change relates to possible harm to recipients. An increase in nondrug services used by the continuously eligible NSAID users was not apparent during 1990. It was demonstrated that multiple-source NSAID prescriptions and analgesic prescriptions increased as the single-source NSAIDs decreased; however, no additional physician or institutional costs were observed in the study. Apparently, patients did not seek additional medical attention when confronted with a prior approval requirement for single-source NSAID use. Since about 1,000 single-source NSAID prescriptions were dispensed per month with prior approval, it appears that patients who responded best to these products continued with their therapy. In conclusion, no adverse effects were observed at the aggregate level of analysis.

The study was not without limitations. The project examined a large group of continuously eligible recipients for a 19-month period. The mean age for this group was 58 years at the onset of the study period. The aging factor is confounded by the effects of the policy implementation and the added effect of the aging process. It is reasonable to conclude that the health status of the study population declined as the subjects approached 65 years of age. Another factor that was not included in the study was the number of recipients who may have opted to pay for the prescriptions rather than accept a multiple-source (generic) substitute. However, given the price differential of the single- and multiple-source products and the relative ease of obtaining prior approval, this practice should not be widespread.

It is tempting to interpret the observed inverse relationships as replacement of one product/service for another. However, the autoregression model represented a market level rather than a recipient-by-recipient analysis. Therefore, these results represent relationships among changes in market shares for specific drugs and medical services.

It appears that the policy for the single-source NSAID prescriptions was more successful than those of similar formulary policies previously reported in the literature. Several notable differences between this policy and other recent findings may account for the divergent results. First, the policy targeted very expensive products for which there was no more expensive alternative drug therapy. It is also unlikely that an antiarthritic patient would seek emergency or institutional care as a substitute for single-source NSAID therapy. Further, the therapeutic advantage of the single-source products over the multiple-source products may not be sufficient to provoke the recipient to insist upon the more expensive single-source product. Finally, the formulary restrictions were not an absolute. The prescriber was offered the option of prior authorization. Thus, the program may meet with less professional resistance because the policy allows the prescriber a means of addressing special patient needs.

The long-term impact of prior authorization programs has not been documented. If the drug programs are devised solely on the basis of economic consideration without regard for medical consequences, then it is likely that more expensive services will replace those expensive drugs removed from the formulary. Furthermore, not all categories of drugs appear appropriate for prior authorization programs. Categories without multiple-source substitutes or with major therapeutic differences among products appear unlikely candidates for prior authorization programs. One final note: drug therapy is a cost-effective modality of medical treatment. Therefore, a formulary revision with or without an accompanying prior authorization should be undertaken with extreme caution and after consideration of all possible outcomes.

REFERENCES

1. National Pharmaceutical Council. Pharmaceutical benefits under state medical assistance programs. Reston, VA: National Pharmaceutical Council, 1990.

2. Fed Regist H12467 (26 October 1990).

3. Kozma CM, Reeder CE, Lingle EW. Expanding Medicaid formulary coverage: effects on utilization and related services. Med Care 1990;28:973-6.

4. Soumerai SB, Ross-Gegnan D, Gortmaker S, Avorn J. Withdrawing payment for nonscientific drug therapy. JAMA 1990;263:831-9.

5. Kreling DH, Knocke DJ, Hammel RW. Changes in market shares for internal analgesic products after a Medicaid formulary restriction. J Pharm Market Manage 1988;3(2):65-76.

6. Jang R. Medicaid formularies: a critical review of the literature. J Pharm Market Manage 1988;2(3):39-61.

7. Smith DM, McKercher PL. The elimination of selected drug products from the Michigan Medicaid formulary: a case study. Hosp Formul 1984;19:366-72.

8. Pharmaceutical Manufacturers Association. 1991 annual report. Washington, DC: Pharmaceutical Manufacturers Association.

9. Lederle Laboratories. Medicaid Pharm Bull 1990;4(3).

10. SAS Institute, Inc. SAS/ETS user's guide: statistics. Version 5 edition. Cary, NC: SAS Institute, Inc., 1984.

11. Ostrom CW. Time series analysis: regression techniques. 2nd ed. Newberry Park, CA: Sage Publications, 1990.

12. Johnson A J. Georgia Department of Medical Assistance annual report. Atlanta, GA: Georgia Department of Medical Assistance, 1989.

13. Johnson A J. Georgia Department of Medical Assistance annual report. Atlanta, GA: Georgia Department of Medical Assistance, 1990.

Chapter 9

Effect of Medication Utilization Review on Medicaid Health Care Expenditures: A Case Study of Patients with Noninsulin-Dependent Diabetes Mellitus

David Alexander Sclar
Tracy L. Skaer

INTRODUCTION

An estimated 20 million Americans suffer from diabetes, a chronic, systemic disorder resulting from a variable interaction between hereditary and environmental factors and characterized by abnormal insulin secretion or action.[1] Patients with noninsulin-dependent diabetes mellitus (NIDDM) comprise approximately 90% of the diabetic population.[2,3] In contrast to patients with insulin-dependent diabetes mellitus (IDDM), these patients retain some pancreatic function and can, in the majority of instances, be treated with diet, exercise, and/or oral sulfonylureas.[4,5] The prevalence of NIDDM is highest among African Americans, Hispanics, Native Americans, and women.[6] Diabetes represents a significant risk factor for the development of atherosclerotic coronary artery disease and is a principal cause of peripheral vascular

The authors wish to acknowledge the time and assistance of Jerry F. Wells, RPh, Florida Department of Health and Rehabilitative Services, and James B. Powers, RPh, Executive Director of the Florida Pharmacy Association.

This research was supported by a grant from the Diabetes Research and Education Foundation.

Previously published in *Journal of Research in Pharmaceutical Economics*, Vol. 3(1), 1991.

129

disease (PVD), neuropathy, and retinopathy.[7,8] The expressed goal of sulfonylurea therapy for NIDDM is the achievement and long-term maintenance of a fasting plasma glucose concentration of 115 mg/dL or, at a minimum, of less than 140 mg/dL.[9] Recent pharmacotherapeutic advances in the treatment of NIDDM have included the development of the second generation oral sulfonylureas. These compounds, first introduced in the United States in 1984, are approximately 100 times more potent on a mg per mg basis than the first generation agents.[10-12]

This research sought to investigate the financial utility of a monthly medication utilization review (MUR) program for ambulatory noninsulin-dependent diabetic Medicaid recipients who were prescribed the second generation compound glyburide as the tradename products Diabeta® or Micronase®. The analysis addressed three specific issues. First, to what extent are noninsulin-dependent diabetic Medicaid recipients interested in receiving and disposed toward attending a monthly review of their medication regimen? Second, to what extent does regimen complexity mediate the desire for consultation? Finally, what is the relative influence of MUR participation on an individual's health care expenditure profile?

DATA AND METHODS

Medicaid (Title XIX of the Social Security Act) is a program of medical assistance funded by both the federal government and the states.[13] Florida's Medicaid program served approximately 470,000 recipients in 1987, with $116,229,852 in prescription expenditures.[13] Medicaid recipients age 65 and older are eligible for coverage under both Medicaid and Medicare (Title XX of the Social Security Act). Efforts to merge Medicaid and Medicare paid claims data for cost-effectiveness analyses have been unsatisfactory at best; therefore, to discern actual rather than estimated program expenditures, this research was limited to an investigation of ambulatory noninsulin-dependent diabetic patients for whom Florida's Medicaid program provided complete coverage for health care services.

Data for this analysis were derived from Florida's Medicaid computer records. Patient-level paid claims data for the period from October 1, 1986 through December 31, 1988 were abstracted for patients under 65 years of age who were prescribed glyburide as the tradename products Diabeta or Micronase. Each patient-level file consisted of extensive information on the health services received, including type of service, date of service, amount billed, amount paid, and units (e.g., days) of service. Prescription claims data included information identifying the manufacturer, medication strength, and date a given prescription was filled.

The study population consisted of 3,147 patients identified as filling a prescription for glyburide. Selection criteria for inclusion in the study were:

1. Patients were under age 65.
2. Patients were prescribed and remained on 10 mg of glyburide per day.
3. Patients had no prior experience with oral sulfonylureas.
4. Patients had not utilized insulin in the time frame prior to or post receipt of the initial glyburide prescription.
5. Patient-level data files contained at least three months of data prior to the date the first prescription for glyburide was filled.
6. Patient-level data files contained at least 12 months of data post receipt of the initial glyburide prescription.
7. Patients had not utilized intermediate care (ICF) or skilled nursing facilities (SNF) in the time frame prior to or post receipt of the initial glyburide prescription.

A total of 1,049 recipients satisfied the selection criteria.

The date of service for the first glyburide prescription was used to partition the data into pre and post time periods. The time periods for analysis were specified as prior (the period 0-3 months prior to receipt of the initial glyburide prescription) and post (the period 0-12 months post receipt of the initial glyburide prescription).

Ambulatory Medicaid recipients exercising their initial prescription for 10 mg of glyburide per day were selected for enrollment in an experimental group. These patients were informed of and recruited into a free monthly MUR program. Patients were mailed a computer-generated appointment reminder each month, approximately ten days prior to the completion of each 30-day cycle after receipt of their initial glyburide prescription in the pharmacy. In addition to the selection criteria stated above, MUR enrollees had not transferred their glyburide prescription during the one-year experimental period.

MUR appointments were structured to facilitate a uniform assessment of each patient's experience with his or her respective prescription and nonprescription medication. Pharmacists were provided MUR program questionnaires for use with computerized prescription profiles to review sequentially a patient's regimen and to record inquiries about prescription medication and/or health status. Where the use of nonprescription medication would have resulted in an undesirable physiological effect or a known interaction with current prescription therapy, alternative over-the-counter (OTC) products were to be recommended. Moreover, when deemed appropriate and in keeping with professional practice standards, the pharmacist was to contact the patient's physician(s) to discuss the need for modification within the therapeutic regimen and/or a physician office visit prior to dispensing authorized prescription refills.

The names of recipients enrolled in the experimental group were submitted to the Florida Department of Health and Rehabilitative Services for incorporation into the abstracted analytical data file. Variable coding as to receipt of the MUR intervention was matched with each recipient's patient-level expenditure profile. In this manner, confidentiality was maintained as to the specific level of Medicaid resources expended.

HYPOTHESES

This research investigated the influence of a monthly MUR program on Medicaid health care expenditures for ambulatory patients with NIDDM. A computer-generated MUR appointment reminder mailed to the recipient's residence was viewed as a viable method to promote MUR attendance. Medicaid recipients were hypothesized as being interested in receiving and disposed toward attending a monthly review of their respective prescription and nonprescription medication. It was theorized that as regimen complexity (the number of prescribed maintenance medications) increased, the desire to participate in the MUR program would increase. The first two hypotheses follow directly:

- H_1: Medicaid beneficiaries will attend monthly MUR appointments.
- H_2: MUR attendance is directly related to regimen complexity.

The medication possession ratio (MPR) for glyburide, defined here as the n umber of days' supply of medication obtained per year (365 days), was hypothesized as being higher for MUR enrollees than for controls. A higher MPR was theorized as being correlated with increased prescription expenditures and decreased financial commitments for physician, laboratory, and hospital services. The final two hypotheses were:

- H_3: MUR enrollees will exhibit a higher MPR for glyburide than controls.
- H_4: Medicaid recipients enrolled in the MUR program will exhibit an increase in prescription expenditures and a decrease in physician, laboratory, hospital, and total health care expenditures relative to controls.

STATISTICAL APPROACH

Table 9.1 summarizes the variables collected for analysis. Prior period data regarding the use and cost of Medicaid health care services provided an indirect estimate of the underlying health status of study recipients. The multiple regression model given below was used to discern the incremental influence of demographic characteristics, prior period use and cost of services, MUR participation, and regimen complexity on post period Medicaid health care expenditures (PPE). Results are expressed in 1989 constant dollars.

PPE = $\alpha + \beta_1(AGE) + \beta_2(GENDER) + \beta_3(P\text{-}MD) + \beta_4(P\text{-}RX)$
$+ \beta_5(P\text{-}LAB) + \beta_6(P\text{-}HOSPITAL) + \beta_7(MUR) + \beta_8(COMPLEXITY) + \varepsilon$

Where:

PPE = $ {(POST-PERIOD MD) + (POST-PERIOD RX)
+ (POST-PERIOD LAB) + (POST-PERIOD HOSPITAL)}

RESULTS AND DISCUSSION

Table 9.2 summarizes the demographic, clinical, and financial characteristics of the 1,049 noninsulin-dependent diabetic Medicaid recipients meeting the study selection criteria. Of the 1,049 recipients, 103 were enrolled in the experimental MUR program, while 946 functioned as controls. Women comprised the majority of both the control and MUR categories. The average recipient's age was in the latter forties. Data reveal that recipients enrolled in the MUR program have significantly ($p < 0.05$) higher mean total prior period expenditures and significantly (p M 0.04) lower mean total post period expenditures than controls. Specifically, MUR recipients have significantly ($p < 0.05$) higher mean post period prescription expenditures and significantly ($p < 0.05$) lower mean post period expenditures for physician, laboratory, and hospital services (Figure 9.1).

Table 9.3 details the number of concomitant maintenance medications prescribed for each MUR enrollee and control during the one-year experimental period. A chi-square analysis for homogeneity revealed no significant difference (chi-square = 5.72, df = 3) between groups in the distribution of concomitant maintenance medications.

Hypothesis Testing

The first hypothesis suggested that Medicaid recipients would be interested in receiving and disposed toward attending a monthly review of their respective prescription and nonprescription medication, and, moreover, that

TABLE 9.1. Variables for Analysis

Variable	Definition
Dependent Variable	
PPE	Post period expenditures
Explanatory Variables	
AGE	Patient's age in years
GENDER	1 if female
	0 if male
P-MD	Prior period physician expenditures
P-RX	Prior period prescription expenditures
P-LAB	Prior period laboratory expenditures
P-HOSPITAL	Prior period hospital expenditures
MUR	1 if experimental
	0 if control
COMPLEXITY	Number of concomitant maintenance medications

a computer-generated MUR appointment reminder mailed to a recipient's residence would be a viable method to promote MUR attendance. Data in Table 9.4 document the number of MUR appointments attended per enrollee during the one-year post period. The majority of MUR enrollees (62%) attended between ten and 12 scheduled MUR appointments throughout the post period.

Three suggested modifications in prescription therapy were initiated during MUR appointments by community pharmacists with prescribing physicians. These efforts resulted in one alteration to an existing regimen and two scheduled office visits. In addition, pharmacists, on a regular basis, recommended alternative OTC products to those which recipients were currently employing or intended to obtain.

The second hypothesis held that MUR attendance was directly related to regimen complexity. Kendall's tau-b was used to evaluate the direction and magnitude of the proposed association. Results (tau-b 0.597) indicate that the number of MUR appointments attended per enrollee increased with the number of concomitant maintenance medications prescribed.

The third hypothesis suggested that MUR enrollment would result in a higher glyburide MPR than that achieved by the control group. Results revealed a significant ($p < 0.02$) increase in MUR enrollees' MPR (0.82 ± 0.08) relative to that of controls (0/58 ± 0.07).

TABLE 9.2. Demographic, Clinical, and Financial Characteristics: Mean Comparisons

Characteristics	Control	MUR
	Demographics	
N	946	103
Mean age	48.6	46.4
Gender		
Female	492 (52%)	59 (57%)
Male	454 (48%)	44 (43%)
Mean Prior Period Per Capita Expenditures (3 months)		
Physician	$33.72	$40.43*
Prescription	59.76	83.17*
Laboratory	12.39	2.16*
Hospital	22.45	8.40*
Total	$128.32	$134.16*
Mean Post Period Per Capita Expenditures (12 months)		
Physician	$204.65	$78.73*
Prescription	363.55	482.42*
Laboratory	23.53	9.02*
Hospital	51.73	0.00*
Total	$642.46	$570.17*

*p < 0.05

Multivariate Statistical Results

Table 9.5 presents multiple regression results for PPE in 1989 constant dollars. The final hypothesis suggested that there would be a reduction in PPE for patients enrolled in the MUR program. Results indicate that for MUR enrollees there existed a significant ($p < 0.001$) reduction in PPE of $41.86 over the one-year experimental period. An examination of Tables 9.6 and 9.7 reveals that MUR enrollment is associated with a significant increase in prescription expenditures ($27.69, p M 0.001) and significant reductions in physician ($18.42, $p < 0.001$), laboratory ($1.19, $p < 0.05$), and hospital ($49.94, $p < 0.001$) services after adjustments for age, gender, prior period expenditures, and regimen complexity (Figure 9.2).

FIGURE 9.1. Mean Per Capita Expenditures for Health Services

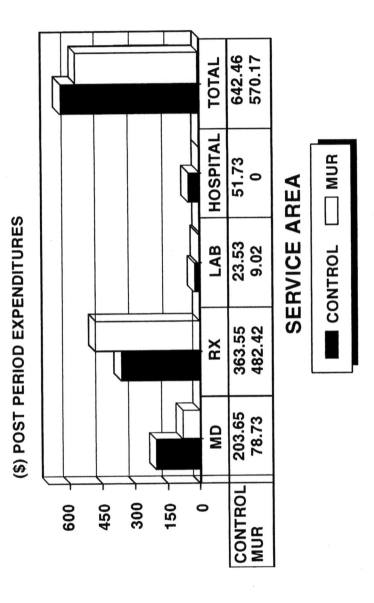

($) POST PERIOD EXPENDITURES

	MD	RX	LAB	HOSPITAL	TOTAL
CONTROL	203.65	363.55	23.53	51.73	642.46
MUR	78.73	482.42	9.02	0	570.17

SERVICE AREA

■ CONTROL   □ MUR

TABLE 9.3. Regimen Complexity: Number of Concomitant Maintenance Medications Per Patient During the One-Year Post Period

Number of Concomitant Medications	MUR Enrollees	Control Group
0	22 (21%)	227 (24%)
1	39 (38%)	435 (46%)
2	27 (26%)	198 (21%)
≥ 3	15 (15%)	86 (9%)

TABLE 9.4. Number of MUR Appointments Attended Per MUR Enrollee During the One-Year Post Period

Number of Appointments Attended	Number of Enrollees
1-3	12
4-6	8
7-9	19
10-12	64

CONCLUSION

At the managerial level, the findings indicate that enrollment of Medicaid recipients in an MUR program results in a significant increase in the level of authorized medication utilization and significant reductions in the use of physician, laboratory, and hospital services. These financial findings suggest an increased level of program efficiency and an enhanced quality of life for MUR participants. Moreover, achieved economies resulted in sufficient program savings to have facilitated reimbursement for the level of consultative services provided. At the policy level, these results argue for a systematic evaluation of community-based clinical pharmacy services and their potential to reduce aggregate health care expenditures.

LIMITATIONS

The results reported here represent the experience of a single study and as such may not be generalizable to other health care environments or to

TABLE 9.5. Multivariate Regression Analysis: Post Period Health Care Expenditures

Explanatory Variable	Regression Coefficient	t Statistic
Intercept	($) 183.74†	2.76
Age	3.14**	3.85
Gender	14.89†	2.49
MUR	−41.86**	−6.47
Physician (Prior)	0.63	0.76
Prescription (Prior)	0.69†	3.57
Laboratory (Prior)	−0.33	−0.34
Hospital (Prior)	0.94†	2.19
Complexity	29.64†	2.85
R^2	.2464	
F Statistic	30.739	
N	1,049	

†$p \leq 0.05$
**$p \leq 0.001$

the entire population of noninsulin-dependent diabetics. Further research is required before constructive policy decisions can be reached. Retrospective analyses using Medicaid paid claims data afford researchers an opportunity to examine financial issues with an enhanced sample size relative to that experienced in a clinical trial environment. However, there are distinct limitations in the use of financial data to address clinical outcomes. First and foremost, paid claims data does not include patient-level clinical information (i.e., history and physical); therefore, the use of prior period health care expenditures to approximate a patient's presentation represents an indirect measure of health status at best. Moreover, the statistical approach employed does not provide a longitudinal evaluation of the underlying comorbidities during the experimental period under examination. Second, reliance on aggregate (e.g., physician, hospital, laboratory) rather than specific health service expenditures associated with a given disease state portends significant threats to internal and external validity. Third, the technical difficulties of merging Medicare and Medicaid databases pose significant limitations for broad-based theoretical analyses. Thus the utility of a given retrospective comparison lies in its ability to stimulate prospective confirmation or rejection of that which has been previously modeled.

TABLE 9.6. Multivariate Regression Analysis: Post Period Health Care Expenditures by Service Area

Explanatory Variable	Regression Coefficient	
	Physician	Prescription
Intercept	($) 42.61	($) 38.74
Age	0.85	1.59†
Gender	6.33**	9.02†
MUR	−18.42**	27.69**
Physician (Prior)	0.17†	0.21*
Prescription (Prior)	0.08†	0.34†
Laboratory (Prior)	−0.11	0.13
Hospital (Prior)	0.01	0.47
Complexity	6.14	21.08**
R^2	.0792	5132
F Statistic	15.905	183.739
N̲	1,049	1,049

*p ≤ 0.10
†p ≤ 0.05
**p ≤ 0.001

TABLE 9.7. Multivariate Regression Analysis: Post Period Health Care Expenditures by Service Area

Explanatory Variable	Regression Coefficient	
	Laboratory	Hospital
Intercept	($) 6.51	($) 95.87†
Age	0.08	0.62*
Gender	1.94*	−2.40†
MUR	−1.19**	−49.94**
Physician (Prior)	0.03*	0.22†
Prescription (Prior)	0.11	0.16*
Laboratory (Prior)	−0.07**	−0.28
Hospital (Prior)	0.14	0.32†
Complexity	0.83*	1.59*
R^2	.0693	1156
F Statistic	13.910	23.663
N̲	1,049	1,049

*p ≤ 0.10
†p ≤ 0.05
**p ≤ 0.001

FIGURE 9.2. Influence of MUR on Health Care Services

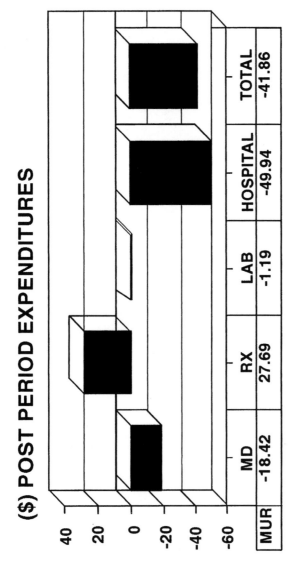

($) POST PERIOD EXPENDITURES

	MD	RX	LAB	HOSPITAL	TOTAL
MUR	-18.42	27.69	-1.19	-49.94	-41.86

SERVICE AREA

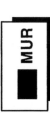

MUR

REFERENCES

1. Krowlewski AS et al. Onset, course, complications, and prognosis of diabetes mellitus. In: Marble A et al., eds. Joslin's diabetes mellitus. Philadelphia: Lea and Febiger, 1985.

2. Turner RC, Holman RR. Treatment of noninsulin-dependent diabetes mellitus with insulin. In: Skyler JS, ed. Insulin update: 1982. Princeton, NJ: Excerpta Medica, 1982;233-46.

3. Ward WK et al. Pathophysiology of insulin secretion in non-insulin-dependent diabetes mellitus. Diabetes Care 1984;7:491-502.

4. Olefsky JM. Pathogenesis of insulin resistance and hyperglycemia in non-insulin-dependent diabetes mellitus. Am J Med 1985;79(S3B):1.

5. Lebovitz HE. Clinical utility of oral hypoglycemic agents in the management of patients with noninsulin-dependent diabetes mellitus. Am J Med 1983; 75:94-9.

6. Carter Center of Emory University. Closing the gap: the problem of diabetes mellitus in the United States. 1985;8:391.

7. Clements RS, Bell DS. Complications of diabetes: prevalence, detection, current treatment, and prognosis. Am J Med 1985;79(S5A):2-7.

8. Nathan DM, Singer DE, Godine JE, Harrington CH, Perlmuter LC. Retinopathy in older type II diabetes: association with glucose control. Diabetes 1986;35:797-801.

9. Skyler JS. Non-insulin-dependent diabetes mellitus: a clinical strategy. Diabetes Care 1984;7(S1):118-29.

10. Prendergast BP. Glyburide and glipizide: second-generation oral sulfonylurea hypoglycemic agents. Clin Pharm 1984;3:473.

11. Lebovitz HE. Glipizide: a second-generation sulfonylurea hypoglycemic agent: pharmacology, pharmacokinetics and clinical use. Pharmacotherapy 1985;5:63-77.

12. Feldman JM. Glyburide: a second-generation sulfonylurea hypoglycemic agent. Pharmacotherapy 1985;5:43.

13. National Pharmaceutical Council. Pharmaceutical benefits under state medical assistance programs. Reston, VA: National Pharmaceutical Council, 1988.

Chapter 10

Impact of an Open Formulary System on the Utilization of Medical Services

Earle W. Lingle
C. Eugene Reeder
Christopher M. Kozma

INTRODUCTION

Formularies have been a part of medicine since the mid-fourteenth century, when they provided standards for medication formulations. Since that time, formularies have evolved from ingredient lists and compendia to guidelines for pharmaceutical therapy. Today, formularies are common provisions in public and private third-party prescription benefit programs.

Formularies are included in prescription benefit programs for two major reasons: to control utilization and to encourage rational or discourage irrational prescribing. Although formularies theoretically may be beneficial in achieving these goals, problems may arise when formularies are implemented as cost-containment devices without optimal patient care as their focus or when they are developed without sound clinical judgment. If cost control is the sole criterion, certain more costly pharmaceuticals may be excluded from a formulary on the basis of their unit costs without considering the alternative costs of excluding the product. The consequence of such action may be extended treatment with a less expensive agent or, more dramatically, substitution of more expensive modes of treatment, such as physician visits or institutional care.

As public and private third-party administrators are confronted with rising program expenditures and as the emphasis on cost containment continues, questions regarding the utility of formularies assume new im-

Previously published in *Journal of Research in Pharmaceutical Economics*, Vol. 2(3), 1990.

portance. This is particularly true in publicly funded prescription benefit programs such as Medicaid and Medicare, where administrators must allocate increasingly scarce resources among competing program priorities. Policy questions concerning the effects of a restrictive prescription formulary on the utilization of other medical services arise when the system impact is considered. Specifically, what are the effects of a restrictive formulary on the use of pharmaceuticals, physician services, outpatient hospital visits, and inpatient hospital admissions?

Literature Review

A review of the literature reveals numerous studies related to the development and evaluation of formulary systems. Most of these studies, however, focus on formularies in the hospital environment.[1-6] Very few studies focus on the effects of a restrictive formulary on utilization in outpatient prescription benefit programs. Attempts to assess the cost-effectiveness of restrictive formularies have been limited by problems of research design and scope.

In a study of state medical assistance programs, Hammel compared medical care expenditures for states with closed formularies to those without restrictions.[7] No relationship was apparent between the use of a prescription formulary and expenditures for medical services. In analyzing the data on a regional basis, Hammel reported that states in the South and West that used restrictive formularies experienced higher per capita expenditures for medical care than neighboring states without restrictive formularies. Unfortunately, results of this study were confounded by variations in pharmaceutical benefits and administrative costs among the programs.

The effects of restricting prescription medicine utilization through a formulary system have been studied in the Mississippi Medicaid Program.[8,9] Minor tranquilizers and nonnarcotic analgesics were removed from coverage when a formulary was implemented. Following these changes, substantial increases were observed in the frequency of prescribing of other psychotherapeutic agents and narcotic and nonnarcotic analgesics. These findings suggest that formularies may have the negative effect of encouraging physicians to prescribe more potent substances as substitutes for milder prescription medicines excluded from formulary coverage.

Hefner has studied the effects of eliminating certain categories of prescription medicines from the Louisiana Medicaid formulary on expenditures for pharmaceutical and nonpharmaceutical services and on the incidence of specific disease diagnoses.[10] Following the program change, prescription expenditures decreased by 11.4%, but total program expenditures increased by 7.3%. A high correlation between the classes of pharmaceuticals removed and an increase in the disease categories most affected by those agents was reported. Hefner concluded that formulary restrictions had an adverse impact on the health status of Medicaid recipients and increased total program costs. A follow-up study using a matched sample of Texas Medicaid recipients was conducted to ascertain if findings were unique to Louisiana or simply the reflection of a trend among all Medicaid eligibles. The large increases in total health expenditures and nonprescription services observed in the Louisiana program were not apparent in the Texas program.[11] Concerns about the generalizability as well as data reliability and causation have been expressed by Rucker and Morse in a critique of this research.[12]

Smith and Simmons compared prescription drug program expenditures across state Medicaid programs for the period 1973 through 1980.[13] Secondary data for the study were obtained from the National Pharmaceutical Council publication *Pharmaceutical Benefits Under State Medical Assistance Programs*. In addition to examining expenditures, Smith and Simmons also explored the effects of formulary exclusions on the participation rate in the program. Results of this analysis were mixed with therapeutic exclusions being associated with both higher and lower participation rates. Of particular note was their finding of no statistically significant relationship between expenditures or participation rates and formulary status. Patients in states with no formulary restrictions exhibited expenditure and participation patterns that were no different from those of their counterparts in states with restrictive formularies. Based on this finding, the authors question the wisdom of using formularies in Medicaid drug programs.

In a recent Pharmaceutical Manufacturers Association report, Moore and Newman concluded that Medicaid program expenditures may actually increase under a restrictive formulary when the substitution of other health services is considered.[14] This finding was based on the authors' comparison of secondary expenditure data for 47 state Medicaid programs. Specifically, use of a restrictive formulary was not related to a decrease in prescription expenditures. Moreover, states with restrictive drug formularies were shown to have significantly greater expenditures on physician and outpatient hospital services than states without restrictive formularies.

Although attempts have been made to assess the impact of formulary restrictions in public assistance programs, very few conclusions can be made about the consequences of such strategies. The preponderance of the evidence suggests that implementation of a restrictive formulary will, in the short-term, reduce prescription utilization and expenditures. However, results of research on the effects of formulary restrictions on utilization of nonpharmaceutical services are not as persuasive. In summary, it is apparent that precise estimates of the effects of formulary restrictions are not possible given the existing literature.

Objective

On October 1, 1984, the South Carolina Medicaid Drug Program implemented a relatively nonrestrictive formulary system for its prescription coverage. Prior to that time, the program provided pharmaceutical benefits under a restrictive, or closed, formulary that included pharmaceuticals from major therapeutic categories, but restricted payment to listed products only. The less restrictive system reimburses pharmacy providers for most prescription drugs and a minimal number of nonprescription products. Categories of pharmaceuticals excluded from coverage after the policy change include adult prescription vitamins, obesity control products, immunizing agents, and DESI products.

The objective of this study was to assess the impact of a relatively nonrestrictive formulary system on the utilization of medical services in the South Carolina Medicaid Program. Services of interest included pharmaceuticals, physician office visits, outpatient hospital visits, inpatient hospital admissions, and average length of stay.

METHODS

The study employed a one-group pretest-posttest quasi-experimental within subjects' repeated measures design. The pretest period consisted of the 12 months before implementation of the open formulary in the South Carolina Medicaid Program, October 1, 1983 through September 30, 1984. The 12 months from October 1, 1984 through September 30, 1985 comprised the posttest period.

The design employed was not truly experimental because random assignment of sample members to an experimental or control group was not possible. The before measure served as the control period to assess changes and trends in utilization of pharmaceuticals once the open formulary was implemented. The advantages of an external control group, such as another state's Medicaid population, were recognized. For the purposes of this project, such a control group was not feasible because during the study period the South Carolina Medicaid Program had, in effect, a limit of three prescriptions per month for each eligible person. Other states' programs had different cost-containment procedures, such as state MACs and formularies, during the study period; South Carolina's Medicaid population differed from those in other states regarding socioeconomic and demographic characteristics.

Implementation of the open formulary system was the only major change made in the South Carolina Medicaid Program during the two-year study period; thus, it serves as the experimental intervention. Furthermore, no remarkable events occurred that would jeopardize the study's internal validity; therefore, the study should not be seriously compromised by history or maturation effects. Although diagnosis related group (DRG) reimbursement for Medicare was being implemented during this period, its effects should be minimal for two reasons. First, only 25% of the DRG rates were based on the national averages at that time. Second, and more important, Medicare eligibles were excluded from the study. The only methodological problem that might have occurred as the result of DRGs was the extent to which physicians might have altered their treatment patterns of the general population to comply with DRG limitations. However, pretest results indicate this did not occur in the South Carolina Medicaid Program.

DATA COLLECTION

The sample was chosen from a Medicaid population that met two criteria. First, population members had to be continuously eligible for Medicaid benefits during the 30-month period from October 1, 1983 through March 31, 1986. This was necessary to ensure that the same persons were included in both the pretest and posttest periods. Although the study period was for the 24 months from October 1, 1983 through September 30, 1985, it was important that the subjects be eligible for an additional six months. Without this requirement, subjects may not have utilized medical care services in the earlier stages of the study, but may have died in October or November 1985 after experiencing substantial increases in medical care use during the terminal six months of life. Because subjects were required to be eligible for an additional six months after the study period, the health status of the subjects during the poststudy period, as related to mortality, should not be different from that of the previous three six-month periods. Second, population members could not be eligible for Medicare in addition to Medicaid at any time during the study. This criterion was invoked because the objective was to study the utilization for health care services for which Medicaid was the primary payer. Medicare eligibles were excluded from the sample because their Medicaid payments would represent only a minor portion of their total utilization. Exclusion of subjects eligible for both Medicare and Medicaid could affect the mean utilization patterns and hence limit the external validity of the study. The purpose of this study, however, was not to generalize to the population, but to assess the effect of a policy intervention. Including subjects who were eligible for both Medicaid and Medicare would have introduced error because utilization and expenditure data for Medicare eligibles were not available. From an internal validity perspective, it was assumed that a known bias (i.e., exclusion of individuals eligible for both programs) was preferable to an error in the dependent variable. The sample was selected by randomly choosing every seventh Medicaid eligible who met the criteria. Of the total 1984 South Carolina Medicaid population of 231,395 persons, 115,929 met the sampling criteria. Choosing every seventh eligible yielded a total sample of 16,561 persons.

Data for the study were taken from the South Carolina Department of Health and Human Services Finance Commission data files. Sample members' demographic and eligibility data were collected from respective recipient information records. Data on recipients' utilization of medical care services were retrieved from the claims files. Separate data files were created and maintained for each of the major service categories. All files were coded and merged by unique patient identification numbers.

A multivariate approach to the univariate analysis of repeated measures was used to analyze the data. The null hypotheses of equal population means for number of services or claims before and after implementation of the open formulary were tested at a probability level of .05. The multivariate approach to the univariate case was chosen because it permits unequal covariate weights over repeated measures. An approximation of the F-test, based on Pillai's trace, was used as the test statistic. This F approximation is one of the most robust statistics for a multivariate analysis and is sufficiently powerful to detect true differences when minor violations of the equal covariance assumption are encountered. If the overall F-test for unequal means was significant at the 0.05 level, post hoc comparisons of individual means were conducted to explain group differences in trends and level.

Utilization was computed as the average number of services or claims per period. Claims data were analyzed by the following groups:

1. Eligibles–All subjects who were eligible to receive services.
2. Recipients–A subset of eligibles who received at least one service during the two-year study period.
3. Frequent Users–A subset of recipients who received at least one service in each of the six-month periods.

The frequent users group was selected to associate the effects of an open formulary on frequent users of medical care services.

The effects of opening the formulary (on the level and trends of claims) were further investigated by using three post hoc contrasts of the means rather than simple comparisons of means. The three contrasts evaluated were: changes in level or location of means, changes in slope or trend, and presence or absence of a dominant trend.

A change in level can be thought of as an immediate shift in claims following the formulary change. A change in trend can be conceptualized as a change in the slope of the function after the formulary change. This change may be reflected as a greater upward slope or one opposite in direction. A third analysis was conducted to determine if a general, or dominant, trend existed over the entire study period. A dominant trend may occur in the presence of changes in level and slope and may override these other tendencies. All statistical analyses were conducted using the SAS statistical package General Linear Model.[15]

RESULTS

Of the individuals who satisfied the study criteria, 16,561 were randomly selected from the population of Medicaid eligibles. Characteristics of the sample and the population of South Carolina Medicaid eligibles are presented in Table 10.1. Sampling criteria resulted in a lower percentage of subjects in the 65-and-over age category than is prevalent in the population. The elderly were excluded from the sample because of confounding effects of reimbursement under Medicaid and Medicare. The sample included higher percentages of males and blacks than were found in the total South Carolina Medicaid population. The use of a systematic, simple random sampling strategy should have distributed other sources of error evenly among the groups.

The total sample of 16,561 subjects who were eligible for Medicaid benefits was analyzed and subdivided into two groups based on the utilization of prescriptions. A total of 12,139 subjects in the sample received at least one prescription during the two-year study period, and these subjects were considered "recipients" for the purpose of analysis. A second subgroup of 4,233 subjects included individuals who received at least one prescription per six-month period, and these were considered "frequent users" in the analyses. These groupings indicate that 4,422 eligibles did not have a prescription claim for prescription medicines during the study period.

TABLE 10.1. Characteristics of the Study Sample as Compared to the South Carolina Medicaid Population, 1984

	S. C. Medicaid Population		Study Sample	
	N	%	N	%
TOTAL	231,395	100.0	16,561	100.0
AGE (years)				
<6	38,826	16.8	4,064	24.5
6-20	61,022	26.4	6,064	36.6
21-64	74,204	32.1	6,375	38.5
>65	57,224	24.7	58	0.4
Unknown	119	0.0	0.0	0.0
GENDER				
Male	73,748	31.9	5,987	36.1
Female	157,228	67.9	10,542	63.7
Unknown	419	0.2	32	0.2
RACE				
White	61,821	26.7	2,617	15.8
Black	157,660	68.1	13,588	82.1
Indian	86	0.0	4	0.0
Asian	70	0.0	8	0.0
Hispanic	99	0.1	1	0.0
Unknown	11,659	5.1	343	2.1
ELIGIBILITY CATEGORY*				
Aged	46,397	15.5	22	0.1
Blind	1,833	0.6	146	0.9
Disabled	50,477	16.8	3,962	23.9
AFDC	201,455	67.1	12,429	75.1
Other	13	0.0	2	0.0

*Sum is greater than 231,395 due to some recipients eligible under multiple categories during the year.

Results are reported according to the specific medical care service studied. For analytical purposes, medical care services included outpatient pharmaceutical services, physician services, outpatient hospital services (e.g., emergency room, outpatient hospital clinic services), and inpatient hospital services. For each type of medical service, the dependent variable of interest was the average number of claims per period per person.

Formulary Restrictions

When a policy of fewer formulary restrictions is implemented, an increase in the number of different pharmaceutical entities prescribed and dispensed is expected. The extent of formulary restrictiveness can be inferred from the change in the number or percentage of different pharmaceuticals used. Table 10.2 shows the change in the number of different pharmaceutical entities used when the formulary moved from a closed to an open status, as well as the number of claims generated by these additional covered entities. For this comparison, a pharmaceutical entity was defined as a chemical entity that may be found in several different dosage forms. For example, promethazine tablets, syrup, suppositories, or injections would all constitute the same pharmaceutical entity, regardless of strength or manufacturer. While the number of different pharmaceutical entities used increased substantially (45.1%) for all categories, the number of claims for these products increased only marginally (8.0%). The greatest change in number of pharmaceutical entities prescribed was observed in the blood formation and coagulation agents category (69.3%). This increase can be explained in large part by the availability of numerous multivitamin products under the open formulary. A priori, one would not expect any dramatic therapeutic consequences from this change. Potentially important was the increase in pharmaceutical claims in the antibiotic, miscellaneous anti-infective, gastrointestinal, and hormone/enzyme categories.

A total of 329 pharmaceutical entities were prescribed in the open formulary period that were not covered under the restrictive formulary policy. An assessment of the clinical significance of these new entities was neither attempted nor desired.

Analysis of Outpatient Pharmaceutical Services

The average number of prescriptions per period per person for each group of subjects is presented in Table 10.3. The mean for each group increased significantly (p. < .05) in the year after the change in formulary policy. The effects of the formulary change on the level and trends of the data are presented in Table 10.4.

TABLE 10.2. Number of New Pharmaceutical Entities Available and Frequency of Use in the Open Formulary Period

Therapeutic Category	Change in Entities Used		Change in Claims Related to New Entities Used	
	N	%	N	%
Antibiotics	38	48.7%	922	6.5%
Central nervous system agents	61	31.6%	1,136	3.3%
Cardiovascular agents	11	14.1%	210	1.4%
Hormones and enzymes	61	50.4%	1,358	11.7%
Blood formation and coagulation agents	27	81.8%	756	69.3%
Gastrointestinal agents	10	31.3%	346	12.2%
Miscellaneous anti-infectives	28	54.9%	640	17.2%
Miscellaneous agents	93	64.6%	1,917	25.4%
TOTALS	329	45.1%	7,285	8.0%

TABLE 10.3. Average Number of Prescriptions per Period per Person by Group (with Standard Deviation)

Subject Group	Six-Month Study Period				F	PR>F
	I	II	III	IV		
All subjects n = 16,561	2.40 (3.99)	2.49 (4.35)	2.75 (4.49)	2.66 (4.51)	144.2	.0001
With at least one Rx during study n = 12,139	3.27 (4.34)	3.40 (4.76)	3.75 (4.88)	3.63 (4.93)	144.7	.0001
With at least one Rx per period n = 4,233	7.35 (4.83)	7.91 (5.34)	8.31 (5.35)	8.12 (5.45)	127.0	.0001

TABLE 10.4. Effects on Level and Trends of Average Total Number of Prescriptions per Period per Person by Group

Subject Group	F Values		
	Change in Level	Change in Trend	General Trend
All subjects (PR>F)	298.6 (.0001)	52.4 (.0001)	0.0 (.9546)
With at least one Rx during study (PR>F)	300.6 (.0001)	52.4 (.0001)	0.0 (.9546)
With at least one Rx per period (PR>F)	198.7 (.0001)	116.6 (.0001)	30.2 (.0001)

A significant increase in the average number of prescriptions can be explained by three independent sources. First, all three groups exhibited a significant increase in level or location of the means in the year following implementation of the open formulary. This shift is an indication of the immediate impact of the formulary change. Second, all three groups had a change in trend during the two years. Under the closed formulary, there was an upward trend in the average number of prescriptions per person; however, this trend reversed in the year following the formulary change. Hence, the rate of the average number of prescriptions per period per person decreased after implementation of the open formulary. The only group exhibiting a significant general trend was the frequent user group, which received at least one prescription during each period. Although this group also demonstrated a change in trend in the postperiod, the trend in the preperiod was sufficiently strong to dominate the overall trend in the data.

Analysis of Physician Services

Closely related to the utilization of prescription medicines is the utilization of physician services. To evaluate the effect of implementing an open formulary on the use of physician services, utilization patterns of the same cohort of patients were studied. The average number of physician visits per person per period was computed as the dependent variable for analysis. Again, the sample was subdivided into three groups: eligibles (N =

16,561); those who had used the service at least once during the study (recipient group, N = 13,291); and those who had used physician services at least once in each study period (frequent user group, N = 4,264). These groupings indicate that 3,270 eligibles did not have a Medicaid claim for physician services during the study period.

All three groups exhibited a change in the average number of physician visits per period per person following implementation of the open formulary. The greatest increases were seen in the eligible and recipient groups (Table 10.5). Although significant, the magnitude of the increase was not as large for the frequent user group. This is consistent with the findings for prescription utilization in this group. It is likely that members of the frequent user group have approached the maximum allowable routine physician office visits under Medicaid. The decreasing trend in physician visits that existed in the first year stabilized in the second year, accounting for significant changes in trend (Table 10.6). No trends were apparent for the high user group in this respect.

Analysis of Outpatient Hospital Services

Outpatient hospital services include emergency room and outpatient hospital clinic services. For the analyses of outpatient hospital services, the eligible group numbered 16,561 subjects, the recipient group consisted of 8,927 persons, and the frequent user group totaled 855 subjects. These groupings indicate that 7,634 eligibles did not have a Medicaid claim for outpatient hospital services during the study period.

Utilization of outpatient hospital services was measured by the average number of outpatient hospital visits per period per person by group and is presented in Table 10.7. The models for all three groups were significant and indicated an increase in the mean number of visits from the closed to the open formulary periods. These increases can be explained by significant changes in the levels and trends for each group during the two years under study (Table 10.8). The level change indicates that the mean number of visits was greater during the open formulary period than during the closed formulary period. However, the increasing trend that was evident during the closed formulary period was reversed during the open formulary period and actually showed a slight decline from Period III to Period IV.

Analysis of Inpatient Hospital Services

Analyses of inpatient hospital services were also performed for the three groups of sample members: eligibles, recipients, and frequent users.

TABLE 10.5. Average Number of Physician Visits per Period per Person by Group (with Standard Deviation)

Subject Group	Six-Month Study Period				F	PR>F
	I	II	III	IV		
All subjects n = 16,561	1.68 (2.58)	1.60 (2.65)	1.71 (2.66)	1.70 (2.77)	13.4	.0001
With at least one MD visit during study n = 13,291	2.09 (2.72)	2.00 (2.82)	2.13 (2.82)	2.12 (2.94)	13.4	.0001
With at least one MD visit per period n = 4,264	4.17 (3.33)	4.10 (3.46)	4.27 (3.47)	4.22 (3.65)	3.5	.0153

TABLE 10.6. Effects on Level and Trends of Average Number of Physician Visits per Period per Person by Group

Subject Group	F Values		
	Change in Level	Change in Trend	General Trend
All subjects (PR>F)	21.5 (.0001)	6.7 (.0098)	10.3 (.0013)
With at least one MD visit during study (PR>F)	21.5 (.0001)	6.7 (.0098)	10.3 (.0013)
With at least one MD visit per period (PR>F)	7.0 (.0083)	0.1 (.8015)	2.7 (.0977)

The eligible group consisted of the total sample of 16,561 subjects. Recipients (those having one inpatient hospital stay during the two-year study) numbered 3,197. The frequent user group was defined as subjects having one stay in each six-month period and totaled 28 individuals. As the size of the frequent user group was small and the models were not statistically significant, results are presented in the tables but will not be discussed. These groupings indicate that 13,364 eligibles did not have a Medicaid claim for an inpatient hospital stay during the study period.

Utilization of inpatient hospital services was measured as the average number of hospital admissions per period for each group and is presented in Table 10.9. The analyses indicated a significant decrease (p. < .05) in the number of admissions for the eligible and recipient groups in the year after the formulary was opened. Table 10.10 shows that the increase was due to a significant change in level or location of the means. A significant change in trend or a dominant trend was not evident in either group.

The average length of hospital stay per period for each group was used as a second measure of utilization. A significant decrease in the mean number of hospital days per stay was also found in the open formulary period (Table 10.11). This decrease was due to a significant change in level between the closed and open formulary periods (Table 10.12). The models did not exhibit a significant change in trend or a dominant trend.

TABLE 10.7. Average Number of Outpatient Hospital Visits per Period per Person by Group (with Standard Deviation)

Subject Group	Six-Month Study Period				F	PR>F
	I	II	III	IV		
All subjects n = 16,561	0.42 (1.66)	0.46 (1.71)	0.66 (2.97)	0.65 (2.40)	68.3	.0001
With at least one OP hopital visit during study n = 8,927	0.79 (2.19)	0.86 (2.25)	1.22 (3.96)	1.20 (3.17)	68.5	.0001
With at least one OP hospital visit per period n = 855	3.08 (5.83)	3.46 (5.75)	4.02 (6.55)	3.68 (4.48)	5.7	.0007

TABLE 10.8. Effects on Level and Trends of Average Number of Outpatient Hospital Visits per Period per Person by Group

Subject Group	F Values		
	Change in Level	Change in Trend	General Trend
All subjects (PR>F)	122.5 (.0001)	4.3 (.0388)	1.4 (.2341)
With at least one OP hospital visit during study (PR>F)	123.2 (.0001)	4.3 (.0386)	1.4 (.2351)
With at least one OP hospital visit per period (PR>F)	6.3 (.0124)	8.3 (.0040)	0.1 (.8499)

DISCUSSION

Results of this study are consistent with theoretical expectations about utilization under an open versus a closed formulary situation and offer support for the research hypotheses. Given the sample size used in this study, the results and the analyses are reliable. That is, if the study were to be repeated with a similar but separate group of South Carolina Medicaid eligibles, the results would, in all likelihood, remain the same. The study design and large sample size also render a very powerful statistical analysis and ensure that observed differences (or lack of differences) are true.

Pharmaceutical Services

Statistically significant increases were observed in the average number of prescriptions per period per person. Clearly, removal of formulary restrictions resulted in an immediate increase in the utilization of prescription medications. With the open formulary, physicians were free to prescribe most available medications for their Medicaid patients. It is reasonable to expect physicians to prescribe similarly for Medicaid and private-pay patients in this situation. Moreover, the freedom to prescribe

TABLE 10.9. Average Number of Hospital Admissions per Period per Person by Group (with Standard Deviation)

Subject Group	Six-Month Study Period				F	PR>F
	I	II	III	IV		
All subjects n = 16,561	0.08 (0.32)	0.08 (0.32)	0.07 (0.30)	0.07 (0.30)	8.1	.0001
With at least one admission during study n = 3,197	0.42 (0.63)	0.40 (0.63)	0.35 (0.60)	0.36 (0.61)	8.1	.0001
With at least one admission per period n = 28	1.61 (0.99)	1.43 (1.00)	1.39 (0.83)	1.25 (0.52)	1.1	.3408

TABLE 10.10. Effects on Level and Trends of Average Number of Hospital Admissions per Period per Person by Group

Subject Group	F Values		
	Change in Level	Change in Trend	General Trend
All subjects (PR>F)	21.8 (.0001)	1.7 (.1893)	0.24 (.6211)
With at least one admission during study (PR>F)	21.9 (.0001)	1.7 (.1893)	0.24 (.6211)
With at least one admission per period (PR>F)	MODEL NOT SIGNIFICANT		

was associated with a reduction in the rate at which prescription medications were being used. Under the open formulary, physicians prescribed a greater variety of products. A total of 329 pharmaceutical entities were prescribed during the open formulary that were not available under the restrictive formulary. This represents a 45.1% increase in the number of entities prescribed and accounts for an 8% increase in the number of prescription claims. An assessment of the impact of new drug availability on prescribing practices was not possible.

Further discussion of the three post hoc contrasts should be expository. All variables of interest exhibited statistically significant increases during the open formulary period. These changes could have been driven by three independent forces: a change in level, a change in trend, and/or a dominant trend in the data. With the exception of the frequent user category, all groups exhibited a significant increase in the level of all study variables. A change in level can be thought of as a "step up" in the function as a direct impact of the change in formulary policy.

Average utilization may also differ because of a change in trend or slope during a given period. All groups exhibited significant changes in trend; these changes were either a reversal of or a reduction in a positive trend that existed during the closed formulary period. Hence, utilization did not continue to grow at the same rate under the open formulary policy.

Finally, a general or dominant trend was apparent in all groups and variables except for the average number of prescriptions variable in the eligible and recipient groups. A general trend can be regarded as a dominant

TABLE 10.11. Average Inpatient Hospital Length of Stay in Days per Admission per Period per Person by Group (with Standard Deviation)

Subject Group	Six-Month Study Period				F	PR>F
	I	II	III	IV		
All subjects n = 16,561	0.285 (1.2736)	0.265 (1.2578)	0.241 (1.2039)	0.244 (1.2399)	5.2	.0014
With at least one hospital stay during study n = 3,197	1.48 (2.58)	1.37 (2.58)	1.25 (2.50)	1.26 (2.58)	5.2	.0014
With at least one hospital stay per period n = 28	4.26 (2.66)	4.07 (2.40)	4.42 (3.21)	4.90 (3.99)	0.5	.6270

TABLE 10.12. Effects on Level and Trends of Average Inpatient Hospital Length of Stay per Admission per Period per Person by Group

Subject Group	F Values		
	Change in Level	Change in Trend	General Trend
All subjects (PR>F)	7.8 (.0052)	0.78 (.3773)	0.13 (.7236)
With at least one admission during study (PR>F)	13.1 (.0003)	1.7 (.1952)	0.84 (.3600)
With at least one admission per period (PR>F)	MODEL NOT SIGNIFICANT		

force that existed in the utilization functions. That is, a series of observations is generally moving upward or downward with occasional increases or decreases in the trend. A very large change in one period will dominate a small change in another period and, hence, dictate the general trend. The general trend in the data also contributes to the observed increases in all three variables independent of the change in formulary status.

In summary, when only the medication portion of medical care costs is considered, implementation of an open or nonrestrictive formulary system is functionally related to an increase in the average number of prescriptions per person. This change may be explained not only by the direct impact of the formulary, but also by dominant trends and external forces.

Physician Services

As the number of entities available to the prescriber increases, it is reasonable to expect physicians to increase the number of entities prescribed. Availability of medications would seem to be related to the number of physician visits, as patients must visit the office to obtain new prescriptions or to receive refill authorizations. Results of this analysis suggest that a true increase in the average number of physician visits occurred for all three patient groups. This change was independent of an increasing trend in physician utilization. The frequent user group demonstrated greater stability in utilization than the other two groups, possibly reflecting the tendency of this group to approach program limits on utilization.

Outpatient Hospital Services

Utilization of outpatient hospital services increased significantly following implementation of the open formulary. This increase may be inversely related to the number of inpatient hospital admissions. Such a relationship would seem more logical than attributing the change to the formulary policy modification.

Inpatient Hospital Services

Proponents of an open formulary policy contend that the availability of appropriate pharmaceuticals ensures the greatest flexibility in outpatient treatment, resulting in improved patient care and fewer hospitalizations. Hence, the analysis of inpatient hospital services is central to any such argument. Findings of this study suggest that an open formulary may be functionally related to a decrease in the number of hospital admissions as well as a reduction in the average number of inpatient days per stay. This observation is strengthened by the findings of no significant change in trend and no dominant trend in hospital utilization. The data exhibited a sharp and immediate decrease following implementation of the open formulary.

Recipients of Pharmaceutical Services

During the data analysis phase of this study, a post hoc question was raised. Were the patterns of utilization different for subjects who actually received pharmaceutical services? Logically, subjects who utilized pharmaceutical benefits would more likely be affected by changes in the formulary than individuals who had not used prescription benefits.

As described earlier in this report, subjects who received at least one prescription claim during the study exhibited an increase in the average number of prescription claims. The rate of utilization of prescriptions was increasing in the periods prior to formulary repeal. In all cases, the utilization rates either stabilized or decreased during the open formulary period.

An exploratory analysis of changes in utilization of other services for subjects who actually used the prescription benefit was conducted. The level of utilization for physician visits increased for subjects who received at least one prescription during the two-year period. A dominant upward trend may explain a portion of this observed level change. The level of utilization for outpatient hospital visits exhibited similar increases. For the group who used prescription services, the effects on inpatient hospital services appear noteworthy. Both the number of inpatient hospital admissions and the average length of stay decreased.

These findings are observational, and the data need to be explored further before any conclusions can be drawn. Focusing future research on this cohort should prove enlightening.

LIMITATIONS

Use of secondary data may be a limiting factor in this type of research. The sample size and statistical analyses are appropriate and reliable, given the research design. Where differences are found, they are very likely to be true differences that can be extrapolated to the population of South Carolina Medicaid eligibles who met the study criteria. Other forces extraneous to the study, such as flu epidemics, were explored, but none was apparent. However, implementation of diagnosis related group (DRG) reimbursement began in the Medicare program at the onset of this study and was phased in over the study period. While the DRG reimbursement strategy did not apply to any subjects in this study, it is possible that a major Medicare policy change such as this might alter physician treatment behavior. Also, a DRG policy might have produced an increase in inpatient hospital utilization if administrators used non-Medicare patients to offset revenue effects of DRG reimbursement. Finally, formulary restrictiveness may also have an impact on study outcomes. If the closed formulary were, in fact, adequate to treat most conditions, then the effect of the change in formulary policy would be minimal. In this case, any significant findings would be a conservative estimate of the effects of a very restrictive formulary.

CONCLUSIONS

The findings of this study indicate that there were concurrent significant increases in utilization for prescription, physician, and outpatient hospital services. At the same time, inpatient hospital utilization significantly decreased. The value of this study lies in its contribution to a better understanding of the system impact of policy changes. Findings of this study are consistent with the earlier works that have raised the issue of the overall effectiveness of formularies within the context of total program expenditures. Studies that have focused solely on the effects of formularies on prescription expenditures have reported mixed results. In the short term, expenditures and utilization may decrease with a restrictive formulary. What is important is the further refining of the interrelationship of prescription drug availability and the use and cost of other services.

These changes in utilization for medical care services occurred simultaneously during the study period in a homogeneous group of Medicaid eligibles. The research design employed makes it possible to say that these events may be functionally related to the change in formulary policy. Results of this study have policy implications for Medicaid and other third-party program administrators. While a change from a restrictive, closed formulary to a nonrestrictive, open formulary was associated with an increase in pharmaceutical claims, these increases must be viewed in the context of total Medicaid utilization. A simultaneous reduction in hospital utilization possibly reflects the programmatic impact of the change in formulary policy. Medicaid agency directors must not view prescription benefits or any other service component of Medicaid coverage in isolation. All services are intricately interrelated, and total program utilization, cost, and quality of care should be the ultimate concerns.

REFERENCES

1. Muller C, Westheimer R. Formularies and drugs standards in metropolitan hospitals. J Am Hosp Assoc 1966; 40:97-102.

2. Muller C, Herbst M, Westheimer R. Use and cost of drugs for inpatients at four New York City hospitals. Med Care 1967; 5:294-312.

3. Muller C, Krasner M. Pharmacy purchasing, formularies and prices paid for drugs: a survey of hospitals in southern New York State. Am J Hosp Pharm 1973; 30:781-9.

4. Rosner MM. The financial effect of formularies in hospitals. Am J Hosp Pharm 1966; 23:673-5.

5. Swift RG, Ryan MR. Potential economic effects of a brand standardization policy in a 1000-bed hospital. Am J Hosp Pharm 1975; 32:1242-50.

6. Rucker TD, Visconti JA. A descriptive and normative study of drug formularies. College of Pharmacy, Ohio State University, June 1978.

7. Hammel RW. Insights into public assistance medical care expenditures. JAMA 1972; 219:1740-4.

8. Smith MC. Prescribing patterns, physician reactions, and economic effects of closed and open formularies. In: Proceedings of a symposium: revolution in health care. Columbia, SC: 1974; 1974; 41-5.

9. Smith MC, Maclayton DW. The effect of closing a Medicaid formulary on the prescription of analgesic drugs. Hosp Form 1977; 12:36-41.

10. Hefner DL. A study to determine the cost-effectiveness of a restrictive formulary: the Louisiana experience. Washington: National Pharmaceutical Council, 1979.

11. Hefner DL. Cost-effectiveness of a restrictive drug formulary. Washington: National Pharmaceutical Council, 1980.

12. Rucker TD, Morse ML. The Medicaid drug program in Louisiana: critique of the Hefner-Pracon study. Am J Hosp Pharm 1980; 37:1350-3.

13. Smith MC, Simmons SA. A study of the effects of formulary limitations in Medicaid drug programs. In: Proceedings of a symposium and workshop: the effectiveness of medicines in containing health care costs: impact of innovation, regulation and quality. Washington: National Pharmaceutical Council, 1982; 117-39.

14. Anon. Protecting Medicaid patients from restrictive formularies. Washington: Pharmaceutical Manufacturers Association, 1990.

15. SAS Institute, Inc. SAS user's guide: statistics version 5 edition. Cary, NC: SAS Institute, Inc., 1985.

PART III:
ANALYTICAL APPROACHES

Pharmaceutical economics is at once evolving and discovering useful tools from the past. This section begins with a proposed framework for research which combines the fields of economics and of epidemiology. This is followed by Luce and Elixhauser's brief premier on some techniques available to economics researchers.

Two specific research techniques, contingent valuation and repeated measures designs are described in chapters by Reardon and Pathak and by Kozma, Reeder, and Lingle. Einarson, Arikian and Shear then provide a three-phase economic analysis–drug cost analysis, drug regimen analysis, and expected cost analysis–as applied to a specific treatment area.

Finally, Pathob offers some incisive comments and poses hard questions about the use of quality adjusted life years (QALYs) in outcomes research.

Chapter 11

A Research Framework
for Economic Epidemiology

James A. Visconti
Mickey C. Smith

. . . thus illness creates poverty, which in time creates more illness.

–Henry Sigerist

INTRODUCTION

Discussions of the Catastrophic Coverage Act have again brought to the attention of health professionals the ineluctable interrelationship between the provision of health care services and the economic environment and characteristics of the patient. Greater recognition and attention should be given to a formal inclusion of economic consideration in all phases of health care, including that segment of health care study called epidemiology.

Although "economic epidemiology" is, as nearly as we can determine, a new term, its basic tenets are by no means new. However, the uses of economic studies in the field of health care have not been as broad as one would desire.

DEFINITIONS

There are a variety of definitions for epidemiology, but most are quite similar. A good one is provided by Morton and Huhn: "Epidemiology is the study of the distribution of a disease or condition in a population and of

Previously published in *Journal of Research in Pharmaceutical Economics*, Vol. 1(3), 1989.

factors that effect or are associated with the occurrence of cases."[1] Epidemiology has been divided into two classes–descriptive epidemiology and explanatory epidemiology–with the goals of discovering and describing variations in the occurrence of disease and of analyzing the reasons for differences in occurrence of disease among different subgroups of the population, respectively.[2] Other distinctions have been made in epidemiology, including the description of social epidemiology–defined as "the joining of *social* science focused on the definition and measurement of the independent variable (the social ideological factor) and *medical* science concerned with the identification and diagnosis of the disease state."[2] Although it was not considered separately in the above discussion of social epidemiology, economic epidemiology might, technically speaking, be considered part of social epidemiology, insofar as economics is considered a social science. In any case, we have defined economic epidemiology as "the study of factors and conditions that determine the occurrence and distribution of economic consequences of disease with the purpose of interrupting the natural history of these events."

This discussion is designed to acquaint those who provide medical services with basic principles for studying, preventing, and estimating the cost of diseases, and for points of interception, both economic and medical. Most medical care personnel are better oriented to treatment and, to a lesser extent, prevention than to economics and the cost of illness. A discussion of the need for application of the techniques of economic epidemiology is followed by a section on actual and theoretical use of such techniques.

NEED FOR ECONOMIC EPIDEMIOLOGIC STUDIES

What is the ultimate objective in studying the economics of a disease? In the broadest terms, the answer to this question is the same as the answer to a similar question concerning the pathology of a disease: to increase our understanding of the disease so that it can be prevented or treated more effectively. In stricter terms, we study the economic impact of disease to place the disease within a cost framework of all diseases so that we may determine priorities (i.e., which diseases are most costly in terms of direct and indirect expenditures) and, once priorities on particular disease states to be attacked are determined, to investigate the natural history of the disease with the hope of interjecting preventive barriers that are both logical and practical from a medical as well as an economic standpoint. We may think of this latter objective as a strategic decision about when and where action will be most effective. Economic epidemiology must go beyond incomplete evidence to fill gaps in knowledge for more effective resource allocation, prevention measures, and solutions to disease problems. Economic epidemiology is based upon existing bodies of knowledge that lead to a definition of the nature, extent, and significance of the problems and to the framing of questions for which answers are to be sought. The formulation of hypotheses follows a critical appraisal of existing disease information to disclose gaps in knowledge.

Insofar as the techniques of economic epidemiology are closely related to those of cost-benefit and cost-effectiveness analyses, the need for use of these techniques parallels its use in the latter types of applications. These techniques have been used for a variety of purposes, including the identification of the cost of illness for purposes of forecasting the economic responsibilities of the person contracting the disease; determining optimal allocations of biomedical research expenditures; selecting the most appropriate program for controlling diseases; and choosing from among research, education, and treatment as means of dealing with medical problems.

The health care industry consumes resources that have alternate uses and are scarce. This operation, therefore, has the economic opportunity to be suboptimal. It can be too large or too small. From the textbook viewpoint, the optimal scale of the health care industry and its many components is that in which marginal costs and marginal revenue are equal. Not enough is known about either the cost or the revenue, with the revenue (derived from the "product," as not yet defined clearly) area still lacking precise delineation. Health care has traditionally concerned itself with either prevention or therapy, whereas epidemiology has focused on the prevention activities, and economic epidemiology should be no exception. Prevention involves studying the succession of events that cause the exposure of certain types of individuals to specific types of environment leading to or aggravating bodily changes in those individuals. These environments will have economic elements, and bodily changes may be accompanied by changes in the economic status of the individual and the society of which he or she is a part.

An epidemic has been defined as "the occurrence in a community . . . of a group of illnesses of similar nature, clearly in excess of normal expectation."[3] Under this definition, one is tempted to describe the current rate of increases in most health care costs, particularly hospital costs, as a form of "economic epidemic." Carrying the simile further, we might point out that costs are also communicable. For example, an economically debilitating illness may make a family a medical ward of the community. Thus, the costs are transmissible. It is also worth noting that both chronic and acute costs exist and that they parallel the medical characteristics of disease in both the nature of their severity and the effective term.

It is in the area of prevention that the economic epidemiologist may make his greatest contribution. Indeed, the most challenging purpose of economic epidemiology is that of identifying those economic components of causal (or contributory) mechanisms that enable the formulation of effective preventive measures with the ultimate goal of either reducing costs or increasing the effectiveness of health care investments.

Economic epidemiology should provide a strategy for action. Just as in clinical medicine, where physical, social, psychological, and laboratory information is gathered to establish certain facts for treatment and prevention, in economic epidemiology data are collected to establish facts for preventing economic problems.

Major aims and purposes of economic epidemiology include:

1. Analyzing the interactions of agent, host, and environmental factors in the natural history of disease in order to discover gaps in knowledge and to contribute to preventing economic consequences of disease.
2. Describing and analyzing disease economics (costs) and their distribution according to such variables as age, race, sex, occupation, economic status, and payment mechanism.
3. Filling gaps in knowledge about the costs of disease processes by observing illness and its economic consequences in populations.
4. Studying immediate and special problems in the field of health economics, including the cost of new diseases (e.g., drug-induced disease) and administrative problems (e.g., cost-benefit and cost-effective analysis of preventive health programs, cost and benefits of monitoring drug use and drug reactions).
5. Stimulating and using an orderly approach to scientific research in the costs of illness.

In the discussion that follows, the details of agent, host, and environmental factors are presented to show how epidemiology approaches an analysis of disease causation. This presentation involves a logical procedure similar to that used by the clinician in thoroughly examining the patient.

STEPS IN THE ECONOMIC EPIDEMIOLOGY METHOD

Economic epidemiology may be thought of as an orderly sequential procedure used in the solution of economic problems related to disease. This epidemiologic approach is based on five steps used to study disease in groups of individuals on a mass basis.

Step 1

Step 1 involves definition of the problem and clarification of objectives including:

A. Nature, extent, and significance of the problems
B. Preliminary questions for which answers are sought
C. Statement of ultimate and immediate objectives of the study
D. Explanation of terms
E. Statistical planning

Illustration of Step 1
(Adverse Drug Reaction Economics)

A. The nature of the problem relates to methods of adverse drug reaction case finding. Very few cases are reported, even in control environments (i.e., hospitals), and so far no good method that is both economically and medically feasible has been developed for better case reporting.

The extent of the problem can be visualized from several studies of hospitalized patients and from estimates made by the U.S. Public Health Service. A very conservative estimate of 1% of all patients hospitalized are admitted to hospitals because of untoward drug complications. Very little data describing drug reactions taking place outside of the hospital environment is available.

The significance of the problem lies in the fact that there has been general disregard of the economic consequences of drug reactions, although it is generally agreed that many take place.

B. A few of the preliminary questions for which answers are sought include:

1. Will investigation lead to successful monitoring systems, and what will these systems cost?
2. How effective will the system be in relation to the cost? What alternate systems are available, and how effective are they in relation to cost?
3. Which reactions are most important economically?

C. The immediate objectives are to find cases of drug reactions and to investigate the economic implication of these cases. The ultimate objective is to construct barriers to prevent drug reactions from becoming economically or medically important to the patient.

D. Explanation of terms. *Adverse drug reaction:* any response in a patient to a drug properly administered in the accepted dose range that is unintended and undesired by the prescribing physician, necessitating a reduction in drug dose, discontinuation of the drug, administration of an antidotal drug, hospitalization, or prolonged hospital stay.

Step 2

Step 2 involves appraisal for existing medical and economic information. The literature must not only be reviewed, but must also be critically evaluated so that the investigator is aware of errors in published reports. Step 2 includes:

A. Search of the literature
B. Classification, organization, and evaluation of existing information to reinforce or to invalidate the conclusions made in published reports
C. Finding gaps in knowledge (This is a logical step following Part B, designed to disclose what facts are really known, what is speculation on the part of investigators, and what needs to be known about the economics of disease.)

Illustration of Step 2

A. One of the purposes of the literature search is to get information on the merits of different methods of reporting adverse drug reactions and the cost-effectiveness of alternative methods of reporting.

B. Information is classified and organized into inpatient studies, outpatient studies, and economics of illness studies.

C. There has been no good evaluation of various monitoring systems and their costs and no agreement on definition of the problem.

D. Despite the considerable accumulation of information on adverse drug reactions, there has been no complete evaluation of all of the economic implications of these reactions. One study only discusses particular economic consequences of drug-induced diseases that took place in the medical service of a university teaching hospital.

Step 3

Step 3 involves formulation of hypotheses and includes:

A. Statement of important questions needing study and formulation of hypotheses (All questions that need study are considered so that hypotheses can be formulated and the most important can be chosen for testing.)

B. Consideration of needs, interests, and resources (The needs that stimulated the original problems are important in selecting hypotheses for testing. The needs are related to the significance of the problems. The investigator must have an interest in the work as well as available resources to conduct the study.)

C. Selection of hypotheses to be tested

Illustration of Step 3

A. Important questions needing study include: What are the incidence rates of adverse drug reactions? Do rates differ in institutional versus outpatient settings? How useful as a method of identification is a pharmacistmonitor? Can a pharmacist monitor help prevent reactions?

B. Besides cooperation of the medical staff, the use of a computer that can act as a data bank is necessary to obtain information that could not otherwise be processed.

C. There is almost an endless number of hypotheses relating to adverse drug reaction epidemiology that could be tested. One hypothesis central to our study was that drug reactions caused economic consequences for patients, the hospital, and the community.

Step 4

Testing hypotheses includes planning and executing the study:

A. Design of an experiment (includes definition of units of observation, e.g., individuals with and without adverse drug reactions)

   1. Definition of units of observation (Precise definition of specific characteristics of the units to be observed in the study is necessary. The units may be individuals from specific populations [e.g., patients in a hospital, patients with ulcerative colitis]. Characteristics of the units of observation must be defined carefully so that patients exhibiting such characteristics will be included in the study.)

   2. Frequency, method, and type of observation

   3. Location and time factors

   4. Design of record and observation forms

B. Collection of data

C. Classification, organization, and data tabulation

D. Analysis of collected data

Illustration of Step 4

A. A study could consist mainly of a community-wide survey of drug reactions with subsequent calculation of the costs of such reactions to patients, third parties, hospitals, and the community.

1. The unit of observation would be each patient treated by a physician in the community.
2. The study would include the reactions of all treated patients to drugs and the presence or absence of economic complications due to reactions in these patients.
3. The circumstances under which the observations will be made are not unique. They could, however, represent a typical community. Each MD, DO, DDS, and RPh will be asked to complete a drug identification and patient profile form providing data on the patient, drugs, etc. Each patient exhibiting some untoward drug complication will be followed until any reaction sequelae are resolved. The study area could include one city or a metropolitan area. The time of the study could be one year.
4. A special record form designed so that it can be easily placed on punch cards would be constructed. The form will include all pertinent information on every patient seeking medical care, whether he or she experiences a drug reaction or not.

Step 5

Conclusions and practice application include:

A. Evaluation of results
B. Conclusions
C. Presentation of results
D. Practical applications of results

Illustration of Step 5

Results of a study with 685 hospital patients in the general medical service of a university teaching hospital have provided specific information about the economics of drug reactions, the incidence of drug-induced disease, and the usefulness of a pharmacist-monitor in drug reaction case reporting.

The results of this study left little doubt that adverse drug reactions are expensive to the nation. The investigation indicated that adverse drug reactions causing hospitalization were the most expensive for patients, the hospital, and the community.

SUMMARY

This chapter has described our concept of economic epidemiology. From the standpoint of economic epidemiology and preventive medicine, it is not enough to be aware of the definite association between disease and economic consequence. The manner in which disease factors influence departure from health and contribute to economic disability also deserves attention. Equally important is the identification of points of intervention to reduce or to prevent economic disability from disease. These concepts provide the basic framework for economic epidemiology. By applying these economic principles, researchers can make progress in preventive medicine and reduce the cost of disease.

REFERENCES

1. Morton WE, Huhn LA. Epidemiology of genital health disease. JAMA 1966;195(13):129.

2. Suchman EA. Sociology in the field of public health. New York: Russell-Sage Foundation, 1963;53.

3. Anonymous. The control of communicable diseases in man. 9th ed. New York: American Public Health Association, 1960.

Chapter 12

Socioeconomic Evaluation and the Health Care Industry

Bryan R. Luce
Anne Elixhauser

INTRODUCTION

In the past, decisions about the use of health care technologies have been based solely on the clinical safety and efficacy of the technology. Upwardly spiraling medical costs, as well as the unique burden associated with managing chronic disease, have sensitized health care decision makers to the problems of scarce resources and multiple competing interventions. These problems have encouraged decision makers to examine additional criteria before deciding whether and when to use and to pay for a particular technology.

Socioeconomic evaluations have emerged as tools that enable decision makers to systematically compare health care technologies, such as medications and medical devices, to assess the personal, social, and economic effects of those technologies. Although numerous evaluations of technologies have been reported, the quality of the research has been inconsistent. Consequently, there is a perceived need among decision makers for guidance in interpreting these studies, in judging their quality, and in determining their applicability to particular settings.

DEFINITION OF SOCIOECONOMIC EVALUATIONS

Socioeconomic evaluations are research methods based on the social sciences, primarily economics and psychology. They are methods that

This work was supported in part by CIBA-Geigy, Ltd.

Previously published in *Journal of Research in Pharmaceutical Economics*, Vol. 2(4), 1990.

enumerate the costs and consequences of medical products and services. Costs are the monetary valuations of resource inputs required to produce a health outcome. Consequences are the monetary and nonmonetary results of applying a particular intervention. It is vital to recognize that socioeconomic evaluations are grounded in the clinical efficacy of the interventions they evaluate; the clinical effects of a medication must be clearly understood before the relevant socioeconomic hypotheses can be generated.

It is helpful to visualize two streams of events pertaining to each medical intervention. The first is the medical stream. In this stream, a patient arrives at a physician's office, receives treatment, and is cured or not cured. Paralleling this stream is the socioeconomic stream of events. Each activity in the medical stream is associated with a particular socioeconomic result—medical services and other resources are used; the patient's level of social, personal, or employment functioning is altered, etc. The task of a socioeconomic evaluation is to delineate this latter stream of events.

Through socioeconomic evaluations, it is possible to make more informed decisions regarding the use, distribution, and financing of health care services and technologies. Although socioeconomic evaluations are not a panacea for rising health care costs, they provide information that health care decision makers can use to optimize their resource allocation decisions.

TYPES OF SOCIOECONOMIC EVALUATIONS

There are a number of evaluations that can estimate the socioeconomic effects of medical technologies. They are distinguished primarily by whether and how costs and consequences are measured. Three types of studies assess both the costs and the consequences of medical interventions: cost-benefit, cost-effectiveness, and cost-utility analyses.

In cost-benefit analysis (CBA), the costs and the consequences of a technology are expressed in monetary terms. This often means placing a dollar value on health outcomes. Because all consequences are valued in the same metric, cost-benefit analyses allow comparisons of disparate types of interventions having widely divergent outcomes. Theoretically, one could compare the construction of a hospital to the construction of a dam. One drawback of CBA, however, is that not all consequences are easily estimated in monetary terms, and placing dollar values on human lives can be problematic. Furthermore, consequences that are not easily expressed in monetary terms may be ignored in a CBA, thus allowing for miscalculation of an intervention's true consequences.

Cost-effectiveness analysis (CEA) was developed to address this limitation of CBA, and it has been used extensively in medical care. In CEA, input costs are measured in monetary units, but health outcomes or consequences are measured in their natural units, such as number of lives saved, years of life saved, cases diagnosed, or cases prevented. The strength of CEA lies in the fact that no dollar value is placed on human life or health outcomes. It is assumed that economic costs are not valid representations of the entire effects of a treatment and that decisions should not be based solely on economic effects. Although CEA allows researchers to examine the costs per unit of health outcomes, only interventions whose outcomes are measured in equivalent units can be compared. For example, in a CEA, it is assumed that all years of life are equivalent: adding ten years to one person's life has the same value as adding one year to the lives of ten people. A year in the life of a debilitated cancer victim is considered the same as a year in the life of a patient with high blood pressure.

Cost-utility analysis (CUA) addresses this limitation of CEA by measuring the utility or value of years of life rather than just enumerating them. Outcomes are measured in terms of their quality or states of consumer preference. One drawback of this method is that the field of utility analysis is relatively new, and the methodology is still developing. Another drawback is that, unlike CEA, which can examine a number of intermediate health outcomes such as cases found or cases prevented, CUA has only one outcome measure: quality-adjusted life years (QALYs).

Another type of socioeconomic evaluation that can be helpful in assessing health care technologies is the cost-of-illness (COI) study. Cost-of-illness studies are the precursors of other socioeconomic evaluations. Rather than looking at the impact of treatments, cost-of-illness studies focus on the economic consequences of the medical conditions themselves. In essence, cost-of-illness studies illustrate the socioeconomic relevance of the condition or disease. No comparison of treatment modalities is involved.

The choice of which socioeconomic evaluation to perform is guided by the interventions, the clinical problem, the data available, and how outcomes can be valued (monetarily, in natural units, or in terms of patient preferences). These socioeconomic evaluations attempt to measure the social and economic effects of diseases or their treatments. They step beyond an assessment of the clinical efficacy of a treatment or intervention and attempt to reveal the effects of medical technologies in a much broader sense. One type of socioeconomic evaluation is not inherently better or worse than another; however, in any particular case, one method is likely to be more appropriate than another based on the types of questions asked and the types of data available.

THE RESEARCH QUESTION

A socioeconomic evaluation begins with a clinically based hypothesis and a research question that states the objective of the study. The research question outlines the alternatives that will be examined, the perspective that will be taken, and the pathway of clinical management that will be considered.

The Socioeconomic Hypothesis

To develop relevant socioeconomic hypotheses, socioeconomic analysts must first understand the clinical effects of the technology. For example, hypotheses that are designed to test the costs and consequences of a medication are derived from clinical information on the quality, efficacy, and safety of the drug. The clinical efficacy of a drug is the basis for any socioeconomic advantages, and a drug with socioeconomic advantages may lead to lower outpatient costs (fewer concomitant medications, fewer outpatient visits), lower inpatient costs (fewer hospitalizations, shorter stays), lower costs in the nonmedical sector of the economy (fewer days absent from work, longer productive life), and greater quality of life (improved social and emotional functioning, greater sense of well-being).

Alternatives

Most socioeconomic evaluations compare one treatment alternative with another, even if the comparison is no treatment. Ideally, socioeconomic evaluations should examine those alternatives that are actually available or that would be realistic options in the clinical setting, even though the alternatives may represent completely different classes of interventions. It is important that the choice of alternatives not be too narrow. For example, there may be a tendency to compare one drug against another drug when a feasible—and possibly illustrative—option is to compare the drug to a nondrug therapy, such as surgery or behavioral and educational approaches.

The selection of alternatives can introduce unanticipated biases into the study. The cost-effectiveness of a particular intervention depends to a large extent on the alternative analyzed. Thus, the report should justify the selection of specific alternatives and the omission of others.

Perspective

Perspective is the viewpoint from which the study is performed; in other words, whose interests are considered in the evaluation? Perspective largely defines the costs and consequences that will be assessed and is also a powerful determinant of the conclusions that will be drawn from the study results. The perspectives of society, the third-party payer (insurance companies or national sickness funds), and the health care provider are the most common in socioeconomic evaluations. Studies are rarely performed from the perspective of patients alone. Generally, the societal perspective is preferred because it considers the welfare of society in general rather than the well-being of a specific player in the health care arena. Because studies conducted from the viewpoints of specific players will tend to examine only those costs and consequences that are relevant to the players' budgets, the solutions from these narrower perspectives are almost always suboptimal and may lead to wasteful decisions when examined in the context of the general social welfare.

For example, a government agency in charge of decisions about reimbursement for a particular medication may wish to examine the impact of that drug on its own health care expenditures. Such a narrow analysis would ignore a vast array of costs and consequences that should be considered in the adoption of medications. Such costs might include nonreimbursed costs borne by the patient, costs covered by other third-party payers, and costs absorbed by health care providers. Inclusion of these costs and consequences provides a much richer base of information for decision makers, allowing them to understand the varied effects of an intervention, including those costs that are often hidden and those consequences that fall outside the limited scope of the agency's perspective. Ignoring these costs and consequences can result in decisions that are not optimal for society in general. The budget of one sector of the economy may benefit, but overall costs may increase.

Clinical Management Pathways

The research question sets the parameters for the pathways of clinical management that will be assessed in the evaluation. These pathways define the clinical stream of events that forms the basis for estimating the socioeconomic stream. At this point, the potential areas of resource use are defined. The results of the study can be altered considerably by the addition or deletion of a particular category of costs or consequences, that is, by including one pathway of clinical management rather than another. Clinical knowledge is absolutely vital at this stage of describing the pathways of clinical management because without clinical knowledge, important inputs and outcomes may be neglected. Enough information should be provided in the research report to allow the reader to identify those significant costs and consequences that were *not* assessed.

FUNDAMENTAL CONCEPTS OF ECONOMIC ANALYSIS

Two fundamental concepts lie at the heart of all economic analyses: opportunity cost and marginal analysis.

Opportunity Cost

The true economic cost of an intervention is the value of the benefits that would be derived from using the resources required for that intervention in their next best use. This is called the opportunity cost. The concept of opportunity cost is the basis of the monetary valuation of medical resource use.

In a truly competitive market, prices will equal economic or opportunity costs. The medical care market, however, is not a truly competitive one because of influences such as lack of consumer sensitivity to prices (due to health insurance coverage) and providers' control of demand for services. As a result, the prices or charges affixed to goods and services do not generally reflect their true economic value. Nonetheless, because of the difficulty of estimating the opportunity cost, most socioeconomic evaluations use prices or charges as a proxy for costs. To the extent that the purpose of the analysis is to assist in making choices between alternatives rather than to determine true societal value, prices and charges may be an acceptable proxy for costs. This decision depends on the perspective of the study.

Marginal Analysis

The second fundamental concept of economic analysis is marginal analysis. Generally, the basic question assessed in socioeconomic evaluations is not whether to employ a particular intervention, but when to employ it, how often, under what clinical conditions, and in what specific circumstances. The researcher asks: What is the additional cost of producing one more unit of that good or service, and how much additional benefit will be derived from that level of investment? This question deals with the marginal or incremental costs of an intervention and the marginal benefits expected.

Although socioeconomic evaluations ideally should examine marginal costs and consequences, a major limitation faced by these studies is that, generally, only data on average costs and consequences are available. Using average rather than marginal costs and consequences makes determination of the optimal use of a technology, such as medications, much more difficult.

MEASURING COSTS AND CONSEQUENCES

Ideally, socioeconomic evaluations should include all potentially relevant costs and consequences over all time. However, practical compromises must inevitably be made. Because of limitations in money, time, and data availability, many studies examine only those particular costs and consequences that are expected to be most salient. Researchers must use judgment in simplifying a broadly stated research question into a workable study plan.

Costs

There are two general categories of costs: direct costs and indirect costs. Direct costs include actual changes in resource use that are attributable to the intervention. It is important not only to examine those direct medical costs associated with the intervention, but also to look beyond these costs to other sectors of the health care market. Direct nonmedical costs include resource expenditures outside the medical care market, such as costs borne by patients in seeking care. Most studies do a good job of including direct medical costs; however, direct nonmedical costs, such as patient transportation, out-of-pocket costs, and child care expenses, are often ignored.

Direct costs are subdivided into fixed and variable costs. Variable costs fluctuate with the volume of services rendered while fixed costs remain constant across the entire range of service volumes. By definition, variable costs, such as medical supplies or medications, are gained or lost depending on whether they are used and in what volumes. On the other hand, fixed costs are stationary; that is, they cannot be saved, at least in the short run, regardless of whether or not they are used. From a decision maker's standpoint, it is critical that costs be examined carefully to estimate which are truly variable to the program that is affected by the medical technology under study.

Less obvious, but important to many comprehensive economic evaluations, are indirect costs. Indirect costs reflect the value of changes in health status and productivity that results from the health care intervention. These costs are termed indirect because they are not directly expended in the production of health care services or products. These changes in health status may be valued in monetary or nonmonetary terms.

There are two main approaches to reaching the monetary value of indirect costs. In the human capital approach to measuring indirect costs, changes in productivity are measured as the average earnings of persons in the labor force that will be lost or gained as a result of using an intervention. The human capital approach is most commonly used in health care evaluations. Another approach to placing a monetary value on health and life is the willingness-to-pay method; it is preferred conceptually by many economists because, theoretically, it takes into account a broader array of costs than the human capital approach. The willingness-to-pay method elicits values that individuals would spend to stay healthy. Indirect costs are important in many socioeconomic evaluations because the economic impact of interventions is not limited to the health care arena.

Three major considerations dictate the type of resource changes that are valued in monetary terms in a socioeconomic evaluation. These include the type of analysis to be performed (cost-benefit, cost-effectiveness, or cost-utility), the perspective taken in the study, and the alternatives to which the technology in question will be compared.

Consequences

The consequences of medical interventions are the clinical, psychosocial, and economic outcomes of employing that intervention. Clinical consequences include measures of death, disability, and illness. Psychosocial consequences include personal outcomes, such as pain and anxiety, and social effects, such as work days lost and job changes resulting from illness. Many of these outcomes were considered intangible until methodological advancements like utility analysis and quality of life assessment were made. Economic consequences are health outcomes that have been valued in monetary terms. Of course, very important economic consequences of a medical intervention are the changes in health care costs themselves, the savings or additional expenditures that result from the use of particular interventions. Although the goal of socioeconomic evaluation is to assess the full range of consequences that result from the use of a medication, this is often not feasible, practical, or sometimes even necessary.

Measuring consequences is a challenging task for the researcher. Many important outcomes are not quantifiable in monetary terms, and thus cost-benefit analysis is not always possible. Clinical consequences, such as morbidity and mortality, may be appropriate for a given research question;

however, these measures often do not capture the full range of outcomes that results from treatment. Utility analysis is a means of measuring those effects that have previously been considered intangible. Utility analysis seeks to compress a wide array of psychological and functional effects into one summary measure to compare vastly divergent outcomes in terms of a common metric, usually expressed on a scale that ranges from 1 (perfect health) to 0 (death). Life years weighted by utility values form the denominator of a cost-utility ratio, a measure that is easily grasped and effectively summarizes health effects information.

In general, researchers should begin a study by enumerating the full range of consequences that is based on the clinical evidence available. They should evaluate which consequences are most relevant and which are most likely to differ among the alternatives compared. They should examine these consequences to appraise which are measurable in monetary terms, which are measurable in natural units, and which can be valued using quality of life or utility measures. Finally, in reporting results, researchers should clearly state which potentially important outcomes are not included in the final results and what the impact of these omissions might be on the interpretation of results. A qualitative description of the consequences that have been excluded from the analysis is often helpful. Readers of socioeconomic studies can go through the same type of analytic process to determine whether all relevant consequences were included and adequately expressed.

Sensitivity Analysis

Researchers face significant challenges in accurately estimating the impact of interventions on costs and on patients' well-being. These challenges often mean that relatively gross estimates must be made and that these estimates are subject to considerable uncertainty. Assumptions must often be made regarding resource use, the costs of resources, or the health effects of an intervention. When such assumptions are made, researchers cannot be certain that their conclusions are tenable; that is, whether the conclusions are sensitive to changes in these assumptions. Sensitivity analysis is an important analytical tool that can be used to test whether the conclusions of a study change as assumptions are altered. It should be performed whenever there is uncertainty about key variables.

When faced with uncertainty about the true value of some costs or consequences, researchers will generally begin by choosing a value that is a best estimate. They will then vary that estimate, usually suggesting a high value and a low value, and then repeat the calculations to see whether their results change under the high and low assumptions. If the conclusions drawn from the study do not change as these values are altered, the results of the analysis are insensitive to changes in this variable. We can accept the conclusions of the study if the sensitivity analysis encompasses the true range of possible values for that variable. If the conclusions change with sensitivity analysis, then our faith in the analysis is less certain.

Discounting

When costs or consequences do not occur within a relatively short time frame or when costs and consequences do not occur at the same time, the results of the socioeconomic evaluation should be adjusted to reflect the positive value of time preference. This means that costs and consequences incurred in the present have greater value than those that will occur in the future. Discounting reduces future costs and consequences to their present value by a discount rate (usually between 3% and 5% annually).

OTHER STUDY DESIGN ISSUES

Socioeconomic evaluations can be conducted by using prospective or, more commonly, retrospective data. Prospective data might be collected in conjunction with a randomized controlled trial (RCT) of a device, medication, or other intervention, whereas a retrospective study uses data from existing sources, such as the clinical and economic literature or a claims database from a third- party payer.

Inclusion of economic measures and quality of life surveys within a clinical trial is a relatively recent phenomenon, but this practice can be expected to increase in the future. Such prospective studies can supply highly valid information because of the strength of the RCT design. However, there may be problems in generalizing the results to other patient groups. Because RCTs are expensive, they are often performed on relatively small and specialized groups of patients; therefore, it is not clear that the results can be generalized to other populations.

On the other hand, retrospective studies often make use of large population-based data sets, or they use best estimate values in conjunction with analytic modeling techniques to simulate general population values. These studies suffer from a different kind of uncertainty. Because the data are seldom derived from well-controlled studies, the precision of values may suffer. Sensitivity analysis, as discussed above, is particularly helpful in analyzing the results and improving the credibility of retrospective studies.

CONCLUSION

Although researchers conducting socioeconomic evaluations attempt to measure and evaluate the costs and consequences of a medical treatment as accurately as possible, they face the restrictions of having to gather data in the real world and having to draw conclusions on the basis of incomplete information. As a result, the costs measured in economic analyses are not true opportunity costs; rather, they represent a proxy such as an imperfect price set in a noncompetitive marketplace or an arbitrary price set by a government commission. And even though marginal analysis is a critical goal of an economic evaluation for optimal decision making, average costs and consequences are usually the only costs available. Furthermore, researchers conducting socioeconomic evaluations generally collect data on only the most salient costs and consequences on a few alternatives, and they do so over a relatively restricted time frame. As a result, some important costs and consequences may be neglected, and some important alternatives may be ignored. In assessing a research report, it is important to evaluate whether significant changes might be anticipated if other costs and consequences had been incorporated and if other alternatives had been compared. The perspective of the analysis also determines, to a large extent, the outcome of a study. Studies conducted from the perspective of society take into account costs and consequences regardless of those to whom the costs and consequences accrue. Therefore, these studies are least likely to result in a shifting of costs from one segment of society to another.

Socioeconomic evaluations are important tools for decision makers in the health care field. These decision makers face increasingly difficult choices between competing alternatives, such as choices between medications with apparently equivalent efficacy. If these choices are based simply on a comparison of the monetary costs per dose of the drugs, other important costs and consequences may be disregarded, including costs such as those associated with the utilization of medical resources to treat significant adverse reactions and consequences such as differences in quality of life. Socioeconomic evaluations can provide balanced and impartial appraisals of the relative costs and efficacy of interventions and are becoming essential tools for decision making.

REFERENCES FOR FURTHER READING

General Overviews of Socioeconomic Evaluation

Dao TD. Cost-benefit and cost-effectiveness analysis of drug therapy. Am J Hosp Pharm 1985;42:791-802.

Drummond MF, Stoddart GL, Torrance GW. Methods for the economic evaluation of health care programmes. Oxford: Oxford Medical Publications, 1987.

Warner KE, Luce BR. Cost-benefit and cost-effectiveness analysis in health care. Ann Arbor, MI: Health Administration Press, 1982.

Cost-Benefit Analysis Studies

Geweke J, Weisbrod BA. Clinical evaluation vs. economic evaluation: the case of a new drug. Med Care 1982;20:821-30.

Koplan JP, Schoenbaum SC, Weinstein MC, Fraser DW. Pertussis vaccine–an analysis of benefits, risks, and costs. N Engl J Med 1979;301: 906-11.

Weinstein MC. Estrogen use in postmenopausal women–costs, risks, and benefits. N Engl J Med 1980;303:308-16.

Cost-Effectiveness Analysis Studies

Henriksson R, Edhag O. Cost-effectiveness comparison of estrogen therapy and orchidectomy in patients with prostatic cancer. Int J Tech Assess Health Care 1987;3:523-9.

Oster G, Epstein AM. Cost-effectiveness of antihyperlipemic therapy in the prevention of coronary heart disease. JAMA 1987;258:2381-7.

Cost-Utility Analysis Studies

Willems JS, Sanders CR, Riddiough MA, Bell JC. Cost-effectiveness of vaccination against pneumococcal pneumonia. N Engl J Med 1980;303: 553-9.

Thompson MS, Read JL, Hutchings HC, Paterson M, Harris ED. Cost-effectiveness of auranofin: results of a randomized clinical trial. J Rheumatol 1988;15:35-42.

Cost-of-Illness Studies

Eisenberg JM, Koffer H, Glick HA, Connel ML, Loss LE, Talbot GH, Shusterman NH, Strom BI. What is the cost of nephrotoxicity associated with aminoglycosides? Ann Intern Med 1987;107:900-9.

Oster G, Colditz GA, Kelly NL. The economic costs of smoking and benefits of quitting for individual smokers. Prev Med 1984;13:377-89.

Hartunian NS, Smart CN, Thompson MS. The incidence and economic costs of cancer, motor vehicle injuries, coronary heart disease, and stroke: a comparative analysis. Am J Public Health 1980;70:1249-60.

Chapter 13

Assessment of a Contingent Valuation Technique with Utility Estimation Models

Gregory Reardon
Dev S. Pathak

Responses to a mail questionnaire were obtained from 143 allergic rhinitis sufferers with a history of antihistamine use. For each subject, scores for the five utility estimation models were compared with contingent valuation measures for sixteen orthogonal and three holdout antihistamine product profiles. The results support the hypothesis that Huber-hybrid models provide better prediction of subjects' contingent valuations for full profile descriptions of antihistamine products than self-explicated models. Further, the results provided support for the use of open-ended questions in mail surveys as an alternative to measurement of contingent valuation by traditional direct interview methods.

INTRODUCTION

During the last two decades there has been a steady growth in the literature in formalized economic evaluation of health care programs. Two of the most commonly used techniques for such evaluation are cost-benefit analysis (CBA) and cost-effectiveness analysis (CEA).[1] The application of these techniques to pharmaceutical programs, however, has been limited to the measurement of benefits of important and successful new drugs and a few path-breaking drugs, such as antiulcer agents, vaccines,

---

Previously published in *Journal of Research in Pharmaceutical Economics*, Vol. 1(3), 1989.

antipsychotics and antituberculins. Ordinarily, close substitutes for these drugs have not been available. This presents a potential bias in which the selection of a drug for CBA/CEA evaluation is based upon expected or observed dramatic benefits. Unfortunately, the need for formalized economic review is often less for such drugs because the answer to the CBA/CEA analysis of these drugs is usually obvious.

As Wagner indicates, most cost-benefit analyses of pharmaceuticals have concentrated on:

> ... direct and indirect costs, leaving psychosocial costs to be considered in some other way. The benefits of a strategy are generally measured as reductions in the direct and indirect costs of illness resulting from the outlay of direct program costs. This approach represents a step back from the attempt to measure "willingness-to-pay" for a given consequence in favor of a "human capital" approach in which the value of a consequence is determined by its effect on an individual's ability to produce goods and services.[2]

Because the productivity, or human capital, method represents the norm in cost-benefit analysis of pharmaceuticals, these studies value costs and benefits of the use of pharmaceuticals in terms of calculable production gains and losses to society. However, many, if not most, pharmaceuticals may lack a *readily measurable* effect on productivity.

Productivity loss is typically measured in hours of missed work time.[*] If a drug affects quality of work performed rather than the quantity of hours worked, the productivity measure would need to be refined to include qualitative aspects. Further, "psychosocial costs" may account for a greater proportion of the total benefit value for those pharmaceuticals without dramatic, life-altering properties. For these drugs, the value of the health consequences cannot be assumed to be the same as the direct or derived market value of human productivity.[3] Fortunately, innovative valuation methods, including contingent valuation and the health status index, have been proposed in the health care literature as alternatives to be employed in cases where assessment of quality in equivalent quantitative terms (monetary in the former and scaled value in the latter) is desired.

The terms *willingness-to-pay* (WTP) and *contingent valuation* (CV) have often been used interchangeably in the literature. However, CV refers to a

---

[*]Recent research using the human capital approach has begun to place a greater emphasis upon a more general operational definition of opportunity costs. For example, some studies have used equivalent market labor costs as measures of the value of homemaker services.

hypothetical market scenario in which individuals are asked to trade money for an economic good or related goods, whereas the term WTP has been used more loosely to describe a number of valuation techniques from both individual and societal perspectives. The CV approach is founded on basic economic utility theory.[4] For example, in his ground-breaking work in consumer theory, Lancaster suggested that it is the properties or characteristics of a good and not the good itself from which consumer utility is derived. Thus, consumer preference for a good occurs only indirectly as a result of the values that the consumer assigns to the characteristics that the good possesses.*[5]

ANTIHISTAMINES AND ALLERGIC RHINITIS

The goal of the current study was to assess the validity of a contingent valuation technique to measure the value of antihistamine drug therapy for the treatment of allergic rhinitis. In a condition like allergic rhinitis, one would expect that psychosocial costs would be more important than direct productivity costs although this would not be the case with more serious diseases.

Because application of formalized contingent valuation techniques to specific pharmaceutical products is lacking, it was necessary to develop methodology that could be used as a model. Contingent valuation methodologies used in both health- and nonhealth-related studies have employed a number of techniques to value a good or service. However, few contingent valuation studies have made use of demographic, disease severity, or other postdictive or concurrent criteria to support claims that the obtained contingent valuation estimates are indeed reasonable. Such comparisons within a well-established theoretical framework, such as economic utility theory, are scarce.

To address this shortcoming, this study examined the association between expressed monetary (dollar) and utility valuations that are linked to the features of antihistamine pharmaceutical products used in the treatment of allergic rhinitis. Because the foundations of contingent valuation are based in

---

*In his model, Lancaster assumes that the characteristics possessed by a good area "objective"; hence, ". . . the consumer choice arises in the choice between collection of characteristics only, not in the allocation of characteristics to the good." Unlike Lancaster's model, however, the CV approach does not assume that product attributes are perceived to be the same by all consumers. The CV approach proposes that an individual's willingness to trade money (i.e., willingness to pay or accept) for a product resource or health status is the individual's net resolution of the attributes perceived to be possessed by the product, resource, or health status.

economic utility theory, previously tested utility measures for multiattribute alternatives were used as a basis of comparison with contingent valuation measures.[6] Validity of the proposed contingent valuation measure was tested by examination of correlation with these utility measures. Although many different utility measurement techniques have been studied, two major techniques were examined: the *self-explicated utility measurement* and the *Huber-hybrid utility measurement*.

ATTITUDINAL-UTILITY MODELS

The first approach, known as the compositional or self-explicated approach, computes the overall utility for a given multiattribute alternative (which may be a good or service) as the sum of a subject's ratings for each attribute component of that alternative.

There are two basic types of self-explicated models: *unweighted* and *weighted*. In the unweighted self-explicated model, the overall utility is derived through use of the following equation: [7]

$$U_{(h)} = \sum_{i=1}^{n} u_{ik(h)}$$

where $U_{(h)}$ is the overall utility of alternative h with attribute categories, i, of 1 through n, each having a specific attribute level for each category, identified by k. The expression on the right side of the equation, then, is simply the sum of the "desirability" or utility ratings, u_{ik}, for each attribute level that is characteristic of the alternative, h.[8]

The *weighted self-explicated* (two-stage) model adds the dimension of attribute "importance" to overall utility. This is represented by the following equation:[9]

$$U_{(h)} = \sum_{i=1}^{n} w_i u_{ik(h)}$$

where the equation is the same as for the unweighted type, except that an "importance" rating, w_i, has been assigned by the subject for each attribute category.[8]

The second approach to utility measurement is known as the Huber-hybrid model. Originally proposed by Huber and his colleagues, this model is an extension of the self-explicated approach.[10] In the Huber-hybrid model, subjects are asked to rate individual attribute levels of an alternative in terms of desirability, as in the unweighted self-explicated approach. The same individuals assign global value ratings of desirability for alternatives that are described as a "package" of various attribute levels. There are three types of Huger-hybrid models. The first type is the *additive hybrid*, and it is represented as:[5]

$$V_{(h)} \approx \alpha + \sum_{i=1}^{n} \beta_i \, u_{ik(h)}$$

where $V_{(h)}$ is the overall desirability rating assigned by the subject to the entire product profile, h, for a given alternative.[8,10,11] On the right side of the expression, β_i is the coefficient that has been derived to reflect the relative contribution of attribute i to $V_{(h)}$, α is an intercept term, and $u_{ik(h)}$ is the same "desirability" rating for each level, k, of attribute, i, as used in the unweighted self-explicated model. Ordinary least squares can be used to derive the beta and alpha coefficient terms by using self-explicated measures as independent variables and ratings of selected product profiles as the dependent variable. The predicted overall utility, $V_{(h)}$, is the stochastic analog of the deterministically derived overall utility, $U_{(h)}$.

The second type of Huber-hybrid model is the *addilog hybrid*. This model is represented as:[12]

$$V_{(h)} \approx \alpha + \sum_{i=1}^{n} \beta_i \, \log u_{ik(h)}$$

and is the same as the additive model, with the exception that the attribute "desirability" ratings are transformed logarithmically. Huber, Sahney, and Ford proposed this model, hypothesizing that a person's perception of differences in stimuli may be proportional to the logarithm of the actual difference.[10] In other words, an individual's true perception of desirability increases, but at a logarithmically decreasing rate, for each additional interval scale unit of desirability that the individual assigns to an attribute.

A third type of Huber-hybrid model has been advocated as one possibly superior to the first two.[10,13] This is the *multiplicative hybrid*, and it is described as follows:[14]

$$V_{(h)} \approx \prod_{i=1}^{n} \alpha_{u\,ik\,(h)}{}^{\beta_i}$$

This model would be especially useful in adjusting for interactions that may occur among attributes.* Further, this model has been suggested as especially useful where some stimulus variables act as screening variables.[10]

METHODOLOGY

The major objective of this study was to use overall utility scores for antihistamine product profiles, derived from each of the five functional equation forms shown above, as comparative criteria for a contingent valuation measure for each individual subject. The study design consisted of the following steps: design of a self-administered survey instrument, development of 16 orthogonally coded product profiles of hypothetical antihistamine products and profiles for three holdout or market basket products for validation, sample selection from a target population, and calculation of utility scores based on five utility models as comparative criteria for contingent valuation estimates obtained from respondents.

Subsequent to a review of antihistamine literature and discussion with a panel of pharmacists, a list of 47 potentially relevant antihistamine product features was developed. A panel of ten allergic rhinitis sufferers was then asked to rate the importance of each product feature. Analysis of allergy sufferer responses yielded seven categories of features for inclusion in the final study questionnaire. For each category, two to four levels were assigned to describe the range of features associated with antihistamine products. A description of the categories and levels chosen for the study is shown in Table 13.1. The instrument was designed so that subjects could rate the desirability of each of the 18 feature levels on a nine-point bipolar scale of desirability. In addition, a seven-point unipolar scale provided subjects with the opportunity to evaluate the importance of each of the seven feature categories.

Full product profiles of hypothetical antihistamine products were then constructed by selecting single levels from each of the seven categories. An asymmetrical orthogonal array of antihistamine products (the type dis-

---

*Taking the log of the left side of the addilog hybrid equation and keeping the right side as it is produces an expression equivalent to the multiplicative hybrid equation.

cussed by Green) was selected according to a factorial design suggested by Addelman.[9,15] The total number of product profiles constructed consisted of 16 orthogonally coded profiles and three holdout, or market based, products. The holdout profiles were used as a check on the reliability of the utility model and were designed to be similar in appearance to commonly used antihistamine products in the marketplace.

TABLE 13.1. Antihistamine Categories and Levels Used in the Study

Category	Levels
Onset of Action	1. 30 minutes. 2. 90 minutes.
Dryness	1. YES, the product causes some dryness of the mouth, nose, and eyes. 2. NO, the product has no dryness effect.
Prescription Status	1. YES, one needs a prescription to buy product. 2. NO, one can buy product without prescription.
Interaction	1. YES, the product worsens intoxication for one who has taken alcohol or tranquilizers. 2. NO, the product has no effect on intoxication for one who has taken alcohol or tranquilizers.
Effectiveness of Relief	1. 4 persons in 10 reported "good to excellent" relief of allergic rhinitis symptoms (similar to placebo). 2. 6 persons in 10 reported "good to excellent" relief. 3. 7 persons in 10 reported "good to excellent" relief.
Duration	1. Product is taken two times daily. 2. Product is taken three times daily. 3. Product is taken four times daily.
Drowsiness	1. 1 person in 10 reported some drowsiness after taking product (similar to placebo). 2. 3 persons in 10 reported drowsiness. 3. 4 persons in 10 reported drowsiness. 4. 6 persons in 10 reported drowsiness.

The target population was a full-time faculty and staff members employed at a large Midwestern university who were recent allergic rhinitis sufferers with a history of antihistamine use. Questionnaires were mailed during November 1986 to 2,000 employees who were randomly selected from a computerized employee roster. Nine hundred and fifteen respondents returned completed questionnaires, yielding a response rate of 45.8%. As a check on potential nonreturn bias, respondents were evenly split into "early" and "late" respondent categories. Comparisons using T-tests, or chi-square where appropriate, revealed no significant differences between early and late respondents (p < .05) for any of the demographic or health status related variables. Two hundred and forty-nine respondents (27.2%) claimed to have had some symptoms of allergic rhinitis during the six months prior to the study; 168 of these allergic rhinitis sufferers had revealed a history of antihistamine use during the six-month period and were eligible for analysis in this study. However, only 143 (85%) of these were usable.

Applying each of the five utility models, utility scores were calculated by individual subject for each of the 16 orthogonal product profiles.* Five sets of sixteen utility scores were thus obtained for each subject. These are represented in Table 13.2 as Matrix U.

Contingent valuation estimates were obtained from each subject for each of the orthogonal and holdout product profiles. Subjects were asked in an open-ended format to indicate their contingent valuation amount for six months' use of each of the products.** For orthogonal product profiles, the set of data available for each of the subjects is represented in Table 13.2 as

---

*For the two self-explicated models, the utility scores, $U_{(h)}$, were calculated deterministically. For the three Huber-hybrid models, utility scores were calculated from an ordinary least square function; predicted utility scores, $V_{(h)}$, from the three stochastic functions were used as the basis for subsequent analyses.

**In practice CV estimates can be obtained with questions using an open-ended, closed-ended, or iterative bidding format. In this study, subjects were first asked to estimate the total amount spent by them for treating allergic rhinitis for six months by specific cost categories: physician fees, prescription medications, non-prescription medication, air-conditioning and purification costs, travel costs to health professionals' offices to treat allergic rhinitis, and other costs. Subjects were also asked to estimate the percentage of each cost category paid by the insurer and that paid by the subject. The subjects were then asked to identify a global amount they would pay for total relief from allergic rhinitis with the instruction to imagine that they have no health insurance and were asked to keep in mind the estimated total cost of treating allergic rhinitis for six months calculated earlier. Finally, subjects were asked to refer back to the contingent valuation amount immediately prior to indicating their contingent valuation for each of the antihistamine products.

Vector C. Five sample linear regression models were analyzed for each subject as represented:[16]

$$C = \beta U_{.y} + \alpha$$

where C is the contingent valuation and U is the desirability score from utility model y (y = 1, . . . ,5), for each of the sixteen orthogonal product profiles. Thus, from Table 13.2 the Vector C was regressed onto each of the five columns of Matrix U, yielding a set of five correlation coefficients for each subject.

To avoid potential skewness problems with correlations, each subject set of correlation coefficients was transformed to Fisher's Z values, producing a mean vector, μ_z, for testing significance. For reporting purposes, though, a mean vector, μ_p, was also calculated for the entire sample as a retransformation of μ_z. The Bonferroni test for simultaneous comparison of means was used to test the significance of the differences (two-tailed) between the ten pair-wise combinations of values from μ_z, as well as the significance of the positive relationship (one-tailed) of each of the five values in μ_z. Thus, the Bonferroni test held the total number of comparisons made to m = 15 and experiment-wise error to < .05.

RESULTS

The results of the Bonferroni test are shown in Table 13.3. The mean correlations ranged from .59, with the self-explicated model, to .79, with the additive Huber-hybrid model. Each of the correlations is significantly greater

TABLE 13.2. Data Matrixes for Orthogonal Design

$$U = \begin{bmatrix} U_{11} & U_{12} & V_{13} & V_{14} & V_{15} \\ U_{21} & U_{22} & V_{23} & V_{24} & V_{25} \\ U_{31} & U_{32} & V_{33} & V_{34} & V_{35} \\ U_{41} & U_{42} & V_{43} & V_{44} & V_{45} \\ U_{51} & U_{52} & V_{53} & V_{54} & V_{55} \\ \cdot & \cdot & \cdot & \cdot & \cdot \\ \cdot & \cdot & \cdot & \cdot & \cdot \\ \cdot & \cdot & \cdot & \cdot & \cdot \\ U_{x1} & U_{x2} & V_{x3} & V_{x4} & V_{x5} \end{bmatrix} \quad C = \begin{bmatrix} C_1 \\ C_2 \\ C_3 \\ C_4 \\ C_5 \\ \cdot \\ \cdot \\ \cdot \\ C_x \end{bmatrix}$$

U_{xy} = utility score for product x, model y; C_x = contingent valuation for product x; (x = 1, . . .,16; y = 1, . . .,5).

than zero. Table 13.3 shows that all of the pair-wise differences for means of correlation coefficients are significantly different from zero, with the exception of unweighted/weighted self-explicated model and additive/addilog Huber-hybrid model comparisons. The self-explicated models, while not statistically different from each other, were outperformed by each of the Huber-hybrid models. Although mean correlation values obtained for the additive and addilog Huber-hybrid models are not statistically different, both models had significantly higher mean correlations than the multiplicative Huber-hybrid model.

The reliability of the utility models was checked by a comparison of predicted contingent valuations from the data with actual contingent valuations of the three holdout products, which were not used in the derivation of functional values.[†] Desirability ratings of individual feature attributes (and importance ratings for the weighted model) were input into the equational forms of the five utility models previously derived for each subject. Utility scores were thus calculated for the three holdout product profiles for each subject. Predicted contingent valuations were then obtained for the three holdout products by using the beta values obtained from the individual subject models of regression of orthogonal product contingent values from the contingent valuation equation e. The correlations, across all individuals, between actual and predicted contingent valuations for holdout products are

TABLE 13.3. Bonferroni Test of Mean Correlation Coefficients–Orthogonal Profiles

Models	UNWTD Self	WTD Self	Additive HH	Addilog HH	Multipl HH
Mean r	.5890	.6088	.7899	.7838	.7594
UNWTD Self	*	NS	*	*	*
WTD Self		*	*	*	*
Additive HH			*	NS	*
Addilog HH				*	*
Multipl HH					*

* = Significant, NS = Not Significant, at 95% Level of Confidence for simultaneous intervals. Diagonal entries are one-tailed comparisons with zero, off-diagonal entries are two-tailed pairwise comparisons between models.

[†]One of the three holdout products is available as Rx-only. The other two are over-the-counter drug products.

shown in Table 13.4. Means of actual and predicted contingent values are shown in Table 13.5. The range of correlation coefficients across the models and holdout products was from .79 to .94. Using Fisher's Z-test and holding experiment-wise error to < .05, by product, each of the correlations was significantly greater than zero. For Seldane 60 mg. and Benadryl 25 mg., the Huber-hybrid correlation coefficients tended to be higher than the self-explicated ones. However, the opposite relationship was seen in the case of Chlorpheniramine 8 mg.

An open-ended question asked subjects to state their maximum CVs for avoidance of allergic symptoms like those they had experienced during the previous six months. Of the 249 subjects identified as allergic rhinitis sufferers, 228 (91.6%) had responded to the question. The mean bid for six

TABLE 13.4. Correlation Coefficients–Holdout Products

Holdout Product B: "Chlorpheniramine 8 mg."

N = 141

Predicted CV

	UNWTD Self	WTD Self	Additive HH	Addilog HH	Multipl HH
Actual CV	.9010	.8908	.8432	.8440	.8189

Holdout Product I: "Seldane 60 mg."

N = 143

Predicted CV

	UNWTD Self	WTD Self	Additive HH	Addilog HH	Multipl HH
Actual CV	.8729	.8499	.9397	.9369	.9233

Holdout Product O: "Benadryl 25 mg."

N = 142

Predicted CV

	UNWTD Self	WTD Self	Additive HH	Addilog HH	Multipl HH
Actual CV	.7949	.8030	.8782	.8904	.8679

TABLE 13.5. Mean Contingent Valuations for Holdout Products–Models vs. Actual

Holdout Product B: "Chlorpheniramine 8 mg."

	N	Mean $	STD DEV
Predicted:			
UNWTD SE	141	47.76	70.36
WTD SE	141	42.82	62.69
Additive HH	141	38.21	59.77
Addilog HH	141	38.29	58.31
Multiplic HH	141	37.52	55.36
Actual	141	61.81	95.03

Holdout Product I: "Seldane 60 mg."

	N	Mean $	STD DEV
Predicted:			
UNWTD SE	143	56.83	88.68
WTD SE	143	57.72	92.05
Additive HH	143	60.16	92.92
Addilog HH	143	59.92	90.88
Multiplic HH	143	57.30	87.11
Actual	143	70.50	122.45

Holdout Product O: "Benadryl 25 mg."

	N	Mean $	STD DEV
Predicted:			
UNWTD SE	142	33.08	54.17
WTD SE	142	36.05	52.44
Additive HH	142	37.13	73.94
Addilog HH	142	33.47	71.89
Multiplic HH	142	36.50	76.16
Actual	142	31.61	59.63

months' avoidance was $223.32; however, the distribution was highly skewed to the right. Contingent valuations ranged from $0.00 to $5,000. Several demographic and health-related variables were studied as correlates of the contingent valuation for six months of allergic rhinitis avoidance. The results of simple linear regression models are presented in Table 13.6. For those health-related and demographic variables measured on a noncontinuous scale, the independent variable was dummy coded. These results are presented in Table 13.7.

Of the health-related variables listed in these tables, allergy severity (both types), perceived cost-of-illness, maximum CV for an antihistamine product,

TABLE 13.6. Simple Linear Regression

Allergy Severity

"During the time of the year when my allergy is worst"

Model: CV = 104.387 (Allergy severity rating) + 467.118

N = 214   R-Square = .0765
F = 17.552   Prob > F = .0001

Allergy Severity

"During the entire year"

Model: CV = 139.316 (Allergy severity rating) + 677.024

N = 211   R-Square =. 0969
F = 22.418   Prob > F = .0001

Cost of Illness

Model: CV = .92574 (Amount spent on allergic rhinitis) + 84.496991

N= 199   R-Square = .3029
F = 85.615   Prob > F = .0001

Age

Model: CV = 4.860561 (Age in years) + 17.221297

N = 218   R-Square = .0130
F = 2.838   Prob > F = .0935

Maximum CV for an Antihistamine Product

Model: CV = 1.099344 (Maximum CV) + 114.763

N = 141   R-Square = .1278
F = 20.376   Prob > F = .0001

TABLE 13.7. Regression of Dummy Coded Variables

Cyclicality of Symptoms

	n	Mean CV	Mean CV - b_0
"Allergy comes and goes"	128	130.789	0
"Allergy all/nearly all of year"	89	292.472	161.683

F = 8.32   R-Square = .03725
Prob > F = .0043

Sex

	n	Mean CV	Mean CV - b_0
Female	129	168.287	0
Male	90	235.133	66.847

F = 1.40   R-Square = .006421
Prob > F = .2376

Asthma

	n	Mean CV	Mean CV - b_0
Yes	30	228.833	0
No	188	190.989	−37.844

F = .22   R-Square = .001005
Prob > F = .6417

Income

Gross Family Income (1985)	n	Mean CV	Mean CV - b_0
Less than $5,000	2	25.000	0
$5,000 to $9,999	8	125.250	100.250
$10,000 to $17,499	27	85.926	60.926
$17,500 to $24,999	28	185.250	160.250
$25,000 to $34,999	42	143.929	118.929
$35,000 to $49,999	48	282.083	257.083
$50,000 to $69,999	44	205.341	180.341
$70,000 to $100,000	18	309.278	284.278
Over $100,000	2	62.500	37.500

F = .86   R-Square = .03168
Prob> F = .5521

TABLE 13.7 (continued)

Education

Highest Educational Level Completed	n	Mean CV	Mean CV - b_0
Some High School	2	45.000	0
High School Graduation	12	95.417	50.417
Some College	42	314.881	269.881
College Graduation	43	148.721	103.721
Postgraduate College	120	183.467	138.467

F = 130   R-Square = .02373
Prob > F = .2709

and cyclicality of symptoms were significantly (p < .05) correlated with CV for six months' avoidance; only asthma was not significantly correlated. No significant relationship was found for any of the demographic variables listed in these tables (p < .05).

DISCUSSION

Missing Data

For allergic rhinitis sufferers, the response rate to open-ended CV questions for six months' avoidance of the disease symptoms was 91.6%. For allergic rhinitis sufferers with a history of antihistamine use, 85% of the responses for contingent valuation of the orthogonal and holdout product profiles were usable. These response rates are less than ideal and introduce the possibility of nonresponse bias into the results. However, the response rate was higher than anticipated. The response rate for an open-ended WTP question for complete relief of chronic arthritis was only 27% in Thompson, Read, and Liang's work.[17] The higher response rate in the current study is encouraging, but it may well be the product of differences between study samples.

Thompson, Read, and Liang's sample consisted of a large number of unemployed subjects, ". . . a significantly higher proportion (71%) of those with paid employment responded suggest[ing] that WTP methods will have greater applicability among such populations" (p. 209). Further, these researchers noted greater response rates with more highly educated subjects.

Because the sample in the current study was much higher in terms of both education and employment status, the relationships found by these researchers appear to be supported.

Additional reasons for CV item nonresponse are not clear, but the length of the questionnaire was likely to have been a major factor. Several subjects complained that the number of product profiles was too great. A few individuals stated that it was extremely difficult to answer the contingent valuation questions; they did not know what they would be willing to pay for the products. This may be a function of the hypothetical market or the open-ended CV question format. Many of these same individuals responded to the desirability/importance measures while leaving the contingent valuation questions blank.

Contingent Valuation of Orthogonal Products

Analysis of the mean correlation coefficients for the individualized utility function/CV measures of orthogonal product profiles revealed very high correlations, particularly for the Huber-hybrid models. The multiplicative, addilog, and additive Huber-hybrid models explained 58%, 61%, and 62% of the variance (on average) of the dependent antihistamine product contingent valuations, respectively. Although the correlation coefficients were high for the unweighted and weighted self-explicated models, the percentage of variance explained for these models was 35% and 37%, respectively. Thus, it seems that the additional information provided by the inclusion of utility measures for the full product profiles contributes significantly to the explanatory power of the model. Several possible explanations can be suggested.

First, self-explicated ratings might seem less realistic to the respondent than would full product profile descriptions. Responses to these items may, therefore, have less reliability because of the subject's difficulty in conceptualizing isolated individual attributes. A second explanation of these results could be that the subject perceives the product attributes as related; hence, there may be considerable interaction between perceptions of attributes. The Huber-hybrid models may have reduced the effect of attribute interaction by readjusting the beta weights of individual attributes to reflect these interattribute relationships.

An interesting point is the somewhat lower performance of the multiplicative Huber-hybrid model in comparison to the additive and addilog models. Although the practical significance of this difference is not great (explanation drop of 4%), this finding is contrary to prior expectations. Akaah and Korgaonkar found a slightly better explanation for the multiplicative model.[8] The findings of the present study give no evidence that one or more product categories act as "screening" variables.

Contingent Valuation of Holdout Products

Probably the most encouraging finding of this study was seen in the analysis of holdout products. Although the correlation analysis was made across individuals for each holdout product, it was believed that such an analysis was appropriate because predicted contingent values were based upon individual utility/CV functions. For Chlorpheniramine 8 mg., the contingent valuations predicted by the unweighted self-explicated model explained 81% of the variance of the actual contingent valuations assigned by subjects to the product description. For Seldane 60 mg., 88% of the variance was explained by the additive Huber-hybrid model. For Benadryl 25 mg., the addilog and additive Huber-hybrid models explained 79% and 77% of the variance, respectively. Although, in line with the findings of the orthogonal products, the additive and addilog Huber-hybrid models showed superior performance for two of the holdout products, it is uncertain why the self-explicated models outperformed each of the Huber-hybrid ones for Chlorpheniramine.

Subject Demographic and Health-Related Variables

A study of the linear association between characteristic variables of respondents (demographic and allergic rhinitis disease state) revealed some interesting findings. Of the four demographic variables examined (sex, age, income, and education), none showed a significant (alpha = .05) linear relationship with contingent valuation to avoid allergic rhinitis for six months. Thompson, Read, and Liang had used CV for relief of arthritis, as a percentage of income, as the dependent variable in their study.[17] Thus, it is difficult to make comparisons. However, as in the present study, no significant linear relationships were found with nearly all demographic variables reported in Thompson, Read, and Liang's work.*

Interpretation of the findings for disease-related attribute variables are stated as follows (alpha = .05):

1. Allergy severity, for both "the entire year" and "the time of the year when my allergy is worst," was positively associated with CV for

---

*Education was found to be positively associated with contingent valuation in the Thompson, Read, and Liang study.

allergic rhinitis avoidance. However, this relationship was not very strong: less than 10% of the variance was explained for each type of allergy severity.

2. As expected, perceived cost of illness was significantly related to CV to avoid allergic rhinitis. In this case, 30% of the variance was explained by the regression equation.

3. Maximum CV from the set of antihistamine product profiles was also significant, but in this case only 13% of the variance was explained.

4. Cyclicality of symptoms was significantly related to CV. For this health state variable, individuals indicating perennial-type allergies had contingent valuations more than twice as great as seasonal sufferers. This was expected. However, the percentage of variance explained by this relationship is small; only 4% of the variance in the CV measure is explained.

5. Asthma was not significantly related to CV for six months' allergic rhinitis avoidance. This is surprising because it was posited prior to analysis that asthmatics would be willing to pay more for relief of allergy conditions that presumably aggravate their asthma than allergy sufferers without this concurrent respiratory disease.

RECOMMENDATIONS FOR FUTURE RESEARCH

Recommendations for future studies of contingent valuation research in health care are as follows:

1. Randall, Hoehn, and Brookshire have suggested the importance of sociopsychological research into the decision-making processes involved in contingent valuation research.[18] This need cannot be overemphasized. Much of previous CV research focused upon obtained CV bids and their applications to public policy decisions. Unfortunately, the validity of many of these valuations was not assessed, and one may question the utility of these previous study results for public policy.[19] It is recommended that more basic research in theory development of contingent valuation methodology be undertaken.

2. The schools of contingent valuation research and explicit utility assessment have made significant advancements in recent years. However, the present study is one of the few that attempts to bridge theoretical concepts from both schools. Contingent valuation research may provide a means of overcoming some of the practical limitations of the explicit utility school (e.g., aggregation of data),

while explicit utility research can provide some of the needed theoretical foundations for contingent valuation assessment. The potential for major research in bridging this gap is unlimited.

3. Many potential applications of contingent valuation to health care are evident. The results of the present study are encouraging and suggest that future health research in this area, particularly for applications of CV to low mortality disease conditions, may be quite fruitful.

4. Although not studied here, the dilemma of willingness to pay or willingness to accept continues to pose a problem for both health care and nonhealth care research. Research in this area has led many to conclude that the answer to the choice of compensatory or equivalent measures is far from simple. Traditional hypothetical explanations for differences between the two measures are not validated in practice. Applications of psychometric theory to consumer decision-making processes may provide some insight into the problem.

5. The interaction of product or service attributes in an area worthy of further investigation. Explicit utility theory has explored some of the effects of various assumptions of attribute independence, but strong empirical research is lacking. The results of this study suggest that such assumptions should not be taken lightly. More work can be done to develop empirically tested models that control for possible interactive attribute effects.

6. The statistical strategy used in this study was adapted from marketing and behavioral literature.* The objective of this study was to use full profile utility scores derived from previously tested models as comparative criteria for the contingent valuation estimates for the antihistamine products. Five functional forms (two deterministic and three stochastic) were chosen *a priori* from the same literature to produce these full profile utility scores. In reality, however, any of an infinite number of functional forms (stochastically or deterministically based) may be tested. An a posteriori approach has been used in econometrics, which, through maximum likelihood estimation, applies a test of functional specification devised by Box and Cox to identify an "optimal" transformation from a range of possible logarithmic linear models.[14,20] This approach may be quite useful in selecting an optimal stochastic model, as suggested by the data, for explaining the importance and contribution of the desirability rating

---

*Thanks are extended to an anonymous reviewer for suggesting this and the following recommendation.

of each product feature to the overall desirability rating for the product profile.

7. Finally, once the contingent valuation estimates can be validated using the economic utility theory framework, additional tests may be conducted by correlating the CV approach results with real market behavior. For example, when there is more than one alternative available to satisfy the same basic health need, it can be hypothesized that consumers will select the products with highest consumer surplus or highest net-benefit-to-cost ratio. Actual purchases by consumers and market share data could then be used to provide further evidence for the validity of using the CV approach from a realistic market behavior perspective.

REFERENCES

1. Larson LN, Bootman JL, McGhan WF. Demystifying cost-benefit/cost-effectiveness analysis. Pharm Exec 1985; 595:64-7.

2. Wagner JL. Economic evaluations of medicines: a review of the literature. Washington: Pharmaceutical Manufacturers Association, 1982:7.

3. Hansen RW. New pharmaceuticals reduce cost of illness. Can Pharm J 1985; 119:318-25.

4. Roberts KJ, Thompson ME, Pawlyk PW. Contingent valuation of recreational diving at petroleum rigs, Gulf of Mexico, Trans Amer Fisheries Soc 1985; 114:214-19.

5. Lancaster KJ. A new approach to consumer theory. J Polit Econ 1966; 74:132-52.

6. Keeney RL, Raiffa H. Decisions with multiple objectives: preferences and value tradeoffs. New York: Wiley, 1976.

7. Acton JP. Evaluating public programs to save lives: the case of heart attacks. Santa Monica, CA: Rand Corp., 1973; Report R95ORC.

8. Akaah, IP, Korgaonkar PK. An empirical comparison of the predictive validity of self-explicated, Huber-hybrid, traditional conjoint, and hybrid conjoint models. J Market Res 1983; 20:187-97.

9. Addelman S. orthogonal main effect plans for asymmetrical factorial experiments. Technometrics 1962; 4(1):21-46.

10. Huber GP, Sahney VK, Ford DL. A study of subjective evaluation models. Behav Sci 1969; 14:483-89.

11. Huber GP, Daneshgar R, Ford DL. An empirical comparison of five utility models for predicting job preferences. Organiz Behav Human Perform 1971; 6:267-82.

12. Bishop, RC, Heberlein TA, Kealy MJ. Contingent valuation of environmental assets: comparisons with a simulated market. Nat Resources J 1983; 23:619-33.

13. Einhorn HJ. The use of non-linear, non-compensatory models in decision making. Psychol Bull 1970; 73:221-30.

14. Box GEP, Cox DR. An analysis of transformations. J Royal Statis Soc 1964; 26(Ser. B.):211-43.

15. Green PE. On the design of choice experiments involving multifactor alternatives. J Consumer Res 1974; 1:61-8.

16. Boyle KJ, Bishop RC, Welsh MP. Starting pint bias in contingent valuation bidding games. Land Econ 1985; 61:188-94.

17. Thompson MS, Read JL. Liang M. Feasibility of willingness-to-pay measurement in chronic arthritis. Med Decision Making 1984; 4:195-215.

18. Randall A, Hoehn JP, Brookshire DS. Contingent valuation surveys for evaluating environmental assets. Nat Resources J 1983; 23:635-48.

19. Keeler E. Models of disease costs and their use in medical research resource allocations. Santa Monica, CA: Rand Corp., 1970; P-4537.

20. Ehrlich I. Capital punishment and deterrence: some further thoughts and additional evidence. J Polit Econ 1977; 85:741-87.

Chapter 14

Using Repeated Measures Designs to Evaluate Interventions: A Multivariate Approach

Christopher M. Kozma
C. Eugene Reeder
Earle W. Lingle

INTRODUCTION

The purpose of this chapter is to describe and demonstrate a multivariate approach to a univariate analysis for interpreting changes in response variable means accompanied by an intervention. Issues related to experimental design, statistical design, and analysis will be discussed and illustrated with a study that used this methodology. The intervention could be a compliance treatment or a prescription copayment, as well as implementation or removal of a formulary. In any case, the question of interest is the effect of the intervention. With large data sets, this question may be answered efficiently using a repeated measures design and a multivariate procedure. This methodology may be applied in many types of economic, social, and administrative research involving large data sets when the treatment of interest is an intervention. The intent of this paper is to offer researchers an alternative to the traditional approach to analysis of an intervention. Those who are evaluating intervention may find this approach more efficient, given a specific research question; however, the effectiveness and efficiency of all statistical methods are situation-dependent.

The removal of a drug formulary from a state Medicaid program will be the example used to demonstrate this methodology. Although the scope of

Previously published in *Journal of Research in Pharmaceutical Economics*, Vol. 2(1), 1990.

the overall project was much broader, only a portion of the analysis will be used for illustration. In this example the primary question is, "What was the effect on utilization of prescription services when the formulary was removed?" In this type of analysis, researchers frequently stop with the question, "Did the number of claims change?" When dealing with interventions, however, it is helpful to have a methodology that goes further than just addressing questions about changes in means or level. A methodology that also addresses the effect of the change in the slope of the utilization curve is needed. An example of this would be questioning whether utilization was increasing before the intervention and then decreasing after the intervention. The effects of time will also be taken into consideration with this methodology. This allows partial development of a moving picture of change over time.

SAMPLE

To use this methodology, it is necessary to have data from the same subjects that can be divided into time periods or that are collected in time series. To illustrate one approach to establishing repeated measures with a large sample, a brief discussion of the data used in the example study will be given. The sampling frame consisted of 115,929 subjects who were continuously eligible for Medicaid benefits for a two-year period. The study sample was chosen by randomly selecting every seventh Medicaid patient in the sampling frame, yielding 16,561 subjects who were continuously enrolled in Medicaid for the entire two-year study period. Because patients were continually enrolled, it is possible to divide the data into time periods to obtain repeated measures.

A large sample size is important because it has an effect on the power of statistical tests. As sample size increases, the ability of statistical tests to detect true differences increases.[1] With a sample size of 16,561 subjects, it is possible that trivial differences will be found statistically significant. Evaluation of results must also include the use of tools such as the percentage of explained variance to account for the effect of large sample sizes. Large sample sizes will also affect the choice of statistical analysis methods.

DESIGN

Two facets of research design will be discussed: experimental design and statistical design. There are a myriad of possible approaches; however, attention is focused on a situation that may be encountered by researchers in the economic, social, or administrative fields. This example is only one possible case, and the methodology is adaptable to many other problems.

Experimental Design

The optimum approach to evaluate the effects of formulary removal would be to use a true experimental design. In a true experimental design, two randomized samples of Medicaid patients would be selected. The experimental group would be treated with a closed formulary, and the control group would be treated with an open formulary. In this true experimental design, most threats to the internal and external validity would be controlled.[2] This ideal will not typically be possible in practice situations because Medicaid programs will not normally treat groups of patients differently.

Given this constraint, two other choices merit consideration. The first is use of an equivalent control group. In this case the state with the closed formulary would be the experimental state, and a second, similar state with no formulary or an open formulary would serve as the control. An equivalent group serves to control for threats to validity only in as much as the two groups are similar. In Medicaid programs there may be large differences in the characteristics of state programs.[3] Frequently, very different methods of expenditure control are used in each program service area, and patient characteristics may also differ.[4] In reality, truly equivalent state Medicaid programs do not exist.

A second possible design is preexperimental. In a preexperimental design, the effects of external factors are ruled out qualitatively. While this approach is not as desirable as a true experimental design, it can be as effective. Its effectiveness is dependent on identification of external factors that may be responsible for results. This preexperimental design is the approach that will be used for this demonstration. The basic methodology, however, could be adapted to many experimental designs.

Statistical Design

A traditional approach to evaluation of the effects of an intervention may only compare one mean before and one mean after the intervention (Figure 14.1). These means could then be statistically evaluated with a t-test or an analysis of covariance. Analysis of covariance (ANCOVA) would be used to control for differences that are known to exist between subjects, such as age, sex, or diagnoses.

This chapter proposes an alternative statistical design. Data in this case are available on Medicaid subjects over a two-year period. This design involves segmenting the data into four six-month periods, yielding four repeated measures on each subject (Figure 14.1). This approach allows detection of a change in level and trend (slope) over the short run (Figure 14.2). The primary advantage of a repeated measures design is the ability to better partition the total variance[5] (Figure 14.3). It is known that patients differ from one another. The repeated measures design allows filtering of variance due to differences between subjects. The differences being evaluated are aggregate effects of the way the intervention changed individual use patterns.

This methodology can be viewed as a precursor to time series analysis. Frequently, available data are not amenable to time series analysis because at least 60 months of data would be needed.[6] This method permits description of changes in trend in the near term. If the changes are significant, the need for a more complete time series analysis is indicated. If the trend changes are not significant, an expensive and resource consuming time series analysis can be avoided.

STATISTICAL ANALYSIS

With a repeated measures design, there is a choice of specific statistical analysis procedures. An analysis of variance (ANOVA) procedure or a multivariate analysis of variance (MANOVA) may be used. If an ANOVA procedure is used, the statistical design would be a randomized block design

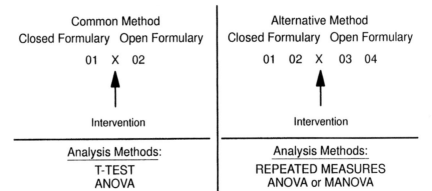

FIGURE 14.1. Research Design

Common Method	Alternative Method
Closed Formulary Open Formulary	Closed Formulary Open Formulary
01 X 02	01 02 X 03 04
↑	↑
Intervention	Intervention
Analysis Methods:	Analysis Methods:
T-TEST	REPEATED MEASURES
ANOVA	ANOVA or MANOVA

FIGURE 14.2. Level and Slope Changes, Conceptual View

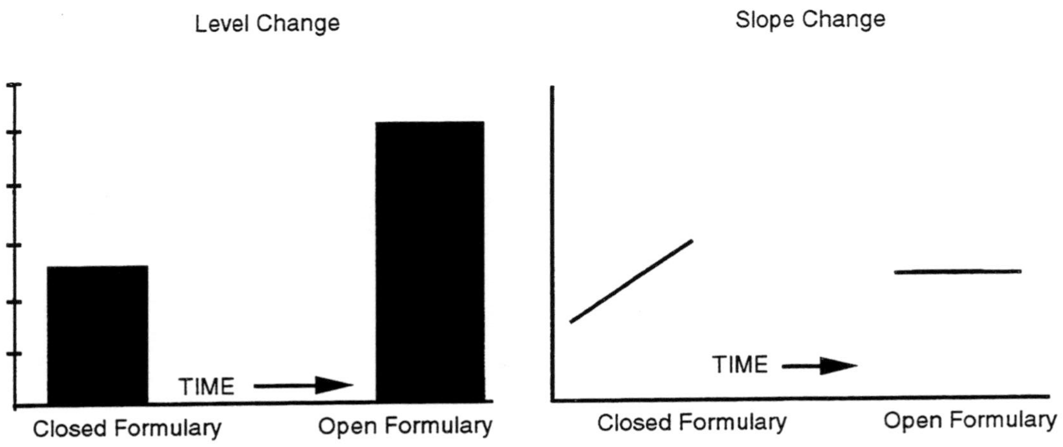

Level Change

Slope Change

Closed Formulary   Open Formulary

Closed Formulary   Open Formulary

TIME

TIME

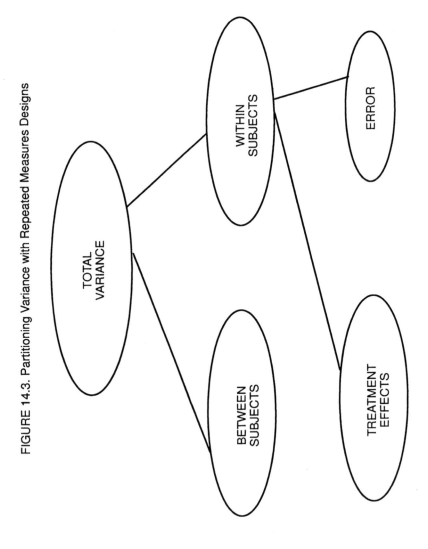

FIGURE 14.3. Partitioning Variance with Repeated Measures Designs

with subjects as the blocking factor and the four time periods as treatment levels.[7] Observations of utilization are made on each subject for each time period, and the treatment is the removal of the formulary at the midpoint of the study.

If repeated measures are used in a univariate analysis, there are several assumptions that must be satisfied.[8] The first assumption is that the population covariances between pairs of treatment levels are constant. In this example, the assumption would hold that covariances between the six-month time periods be equal. The second assumption of the univariate analysis is that population variances for the treatment levels are homogeneous. This would mean that the population variances for the six-month periods are equal. If these assumptions are violated, it is necessary to adjust the degrees of freedom for the omnibus f-test to make the test more conservative.[9] Several techniques, such as the Geisser-Greenhouse or the Huynh-Feldt methods, may be used to make such adjustments.[9,10] Fleiss has criticized the use of ANOVA for the analysis of repeated measures designs when time effects are being investigated on the basis that many of the above assumptions may not be satisfied.[11]

In this study the assumption of sphericity is not made. One form of sphericity, compound symmetry, requires that all variances of the repeated measures be equal and that all correlations between pairs of repeated measures be equal.[8] This is a difficult assumption to meet in studies involving medical care utilization. The best predictor of the next period's use of medical care is likely to be use in the previous period. Also, as periods diverge, the correlation will likely decrease. Given these circumstances the multivariate approach is more appropriate.* A multivariate test, such as the Hotelling-Lawley trace or the Pillai trace, can be used to test the null hypotheses of no differences between means.[12]

When the statistical design is a mixed effect model, a generalized error term is used to perform significance tests. If the assumption of sphericity is violated, this generalized error term is distorted. The recommendation has been made to use specific error terms generated by a multivariate analysis to test contrasts between means. Multivariate analysis of variance will also circumvent the assumption of sphericity.[13]

The use of computer resources also presents a problem when the ANOVA procedure is used with large data sets. In the commonly used statistics package, Statistical Analysis System (SAS), it is necessary to produce a

---

*Readers who desire more background on multivariate methods for analyzing repeated measures design are referred to Reference 13.

design matrix of observations that is four times the size of the data set.[14] For this example (16,561 subjects), this would be 66,244 observations.

There is controversy over which method is best. Several studies have compared traditional methods with the MANOVA approach.[15,16] There is no one procedure that is uniformly more powerful. Power differences depend on sample size and technical relationships about which researchers have little knowledge.[13] With a large sample, power is not as great a concern, and the MANOVA procedure is more efficient. The best strategy is to use a method that is statistically efficient and explainable.

DEPENDENT MEASURES

In the example study, utilization and expenditure data for pharmaceutical, physician, and inpatient and outpatient hospital services are the dependent measures. The multiple dependent measures are means for the number of claims per person, total expenditures per person, and mean expenditures per person for each of the four six-month time periods during the study. The analysis is repeated independently for each measure of expenditure and utilization and for each service area. For this demonstration, only the utilization (number of claims) measure for pharmaceutical services will be included in the discussion. An example of how the utilization measure was calculated is shown in Table 14.1.

CONTRASTS OF MEANS

If an overall multivariate test such as the Pillai trace is significant, the next step is to perform a priori contrasts among the means to determine how the means differ. In actuality, the omnibus test need not be performed if the desired contrasts are postulated in advance. Contrasts can be conceptualized as comparisons between means or sets of means for the purpose of detecting differences.

It is possible to contrive a set of orthogonal contrasts that allow the total sums of squares to be completely partitioned. Orthogonality plays an important role in determining the importance of each contrast. The maximum number of orthogonal contrasts is equal to the number of groups minus one $(k - 1)$. In this case there are four repeated measures; therefore, it is possible to have three orthogonal contrasts $(4 - 1 = 3)$. In some cases a larger number of contrasts may be desirable, depending on the conditions the researcher is attempting to explain. In this case three contrasts were

TABLE 14.1. Sample Calculation of Dependent Measures

DATA

Subject 1		Subject 2	
Date	Amount Reimbursed	Date	Amount Reimbursed
10/02/83	6.43	10/15/83	56.88
10/24/83	10.89	11/22/83	56.88
10/24/83	8.23		
11/01/83	29.56		

COMPUTATIONS

1. Number of Claims (Subject 1)
   $1 + 1 + 1 + 1 = \underline{4}$

1. Number of Claims (Subject 2)
   $1 + 1 = \underline{2}$

AVERAGES PER PERSON

1. Average Number of Claims per Person = 6/2 = 3*
*This same procedure is repeated within each time period for each subject.

DEPENDENT MEASURES

Subject	Repeated Measures Time Period			
	10/1/83 - 4/1/84	4/1/84 - 10/1/84	10/1/84 - 4/1/85	4/1/85 - 10/1/85
S1	4	3	4	6
S2	2	2	6	2
.	.	.	.	.
.	.	.	.	.
.	.	.	.	.
S_n	n_1	n_2	n_3	n_4
Dependent Measures	Mean 1	Mean 2	Mean 3	Mean 4

chosen to explain changes in level and slope and to detect general tendencies in the data. The means being evaluated for this demonstration are shown in Table 14.2.

Again, it should be emphasized that the large sample size increases the probability that trivial differences may be statistically significant. In addition to testing the means, it is also necessary to evaluate the magnitude of the differences between means. Even if statistically significant, the difference should be sufficient to be of practical significance. To evaluate this,

TABLE 14.2. Utilization of Prescription Services per Person per Period Sample Means

Dates	Repeated Measures Time Period			
	10/1/83 - 4/1/84	4/1/84 - 10/1/84	10/1/84 - 4/1/85	4/1/85 - 10/1/85
MEAN	3.27	3.40	3.75	3.63
Standard Deviation	4.34	4.76	4.88	4.93

the Omega-squared statistic should be used with the percentage of sums-of-squares explained by each contrast.

First Contrast

The first contrast is used to determine whether a change in level has occurred. This test is analogous to a t-test between before and after periods and is computed with the following formula:

$$\frac{\text{Mean 1} + \text{Mean 2}}{2} - \frac{\text{Mean 3} + \text{Mean 4}}{2}$$

This represents the difference between the mean of the first and second period and the mean of the third and fourth period. If the means are equal, the sum of squares for the contrast will be equal to zero (Figure 14.4). The differences in prescription utilization were statistically significant, with an f-value of 300.6 and a probability of a greater f-value of 0.0001.

Second Contrast

The second contrast focuses on a change in trend. It compares similarity in the slope of the line before the formulary was removed and the slope of the line after the formulary was removed. The formula for this contrast is:

$$(\text{Mean 1} - \text{Mean 2}) - (\text{Mean 3} - \text{Mean 4})$$

FIGURE 14.4. Average Number of Prescriptions per Person, Level Contrast

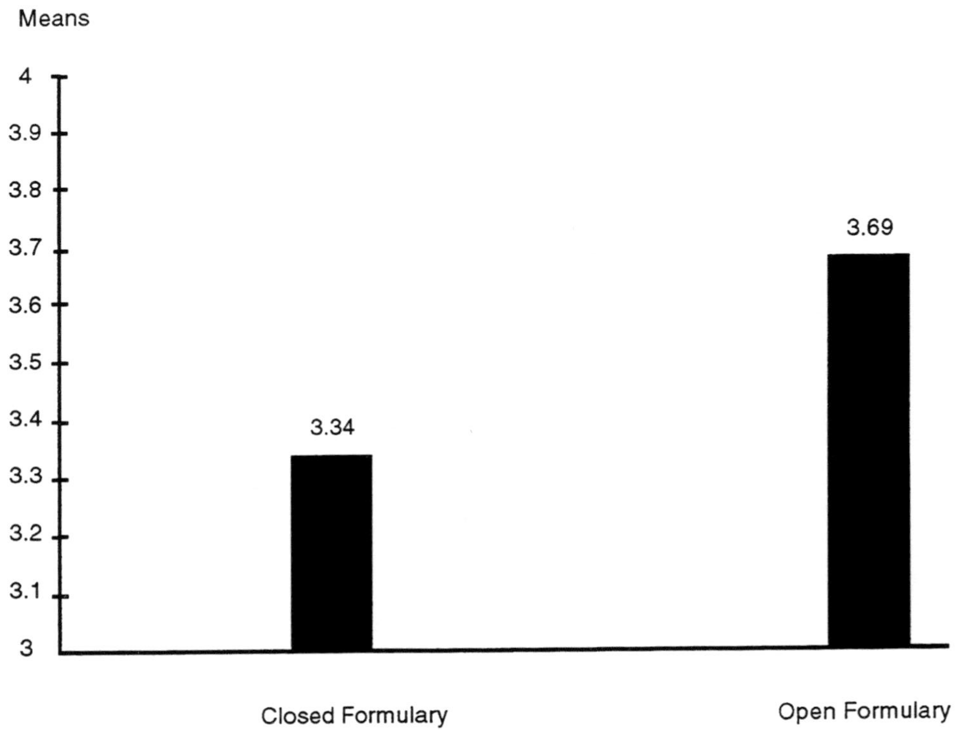

This contrast asks whether the difference between means from periods one and two is greater or less than the difference between means three and four. If the slopes of the two lines are equal, regardless of the level, the contrasts will not be significant (Figure 14.5). The second contrast indicated a significant change in slope ($F = 52.4$, $p = 0.0001$).

Third Contrast

The final contrast is more subtle. If a change in level is found, a question may be raised about why the change occurred. It may be possible that the change in level was due to an existing trend in utilization or expenditures. The third contrast addresses that question. If there is a dominant upward or downward trend in the data, this contrast will be significant. The formula for the contrast is as follows:

$$(\text{Mean } 1 - \text{Mean } 2) \ + \ (\text{Mean } 3 - \text{Mean } 4)$$

If the differences offset each other, the contrast will not be significant. If the differences are moving in the same direction, the contrast will be significant. Care must be taken in the design of the project because this contrast may also detect seasonality in the data. Referring again to Figure 14.5, there was not a constant effect either upward or downward. The f-test was not significant.

INTERPRETATION OF RESULTS

In the demonstration case, an increase in level of utilization of prescription services occurred at the midpoint of the study when the formulary was removed. A change in slope also occurred, indicating that prescription use peaked and then stabilized upon removal of the formulary, or that an increasing trend reversed after formulary removal. The third contrast was not significant for this sample; if it had been significant, the interpretation would change.

If there had been a general increasing trend in prescription utilization, it may have been possible to explain a portion of the variance associated with the level change. In other words, a portion of the increase in level of prescription use may have been due to an increase in prescription use independent of the formulary change. In fact, this may occur frequently with expenditure data in service areas that are difficult to control for inflation. There are many possibilities for interpretation that are dependent on the

FIGURE 14.5. Average Number of Prescriptions per Person, Slope and General Trend Contrasts

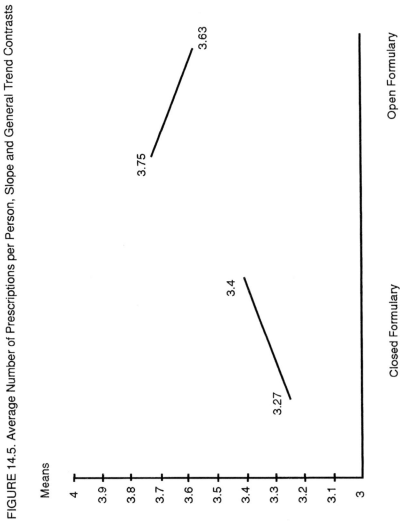

combination of significant contrasts and the direction of movement of the means. A visual inspection of the means should be conducted to reveal the direction of the change if significant differences in slope, level, or trend are detected.

MAGNITUDE OF EFFECTS

Once it has been determined that differences in means exist, attention should be shifted toward the significance of the effects. Because of the large sample size, it is possible that the effects are significant but trivial from a practical perspective. It is reasonable to ask how much the formulary affected prescription utilization. Second, if there was an overall effect, which contrast accounted for the largest percentage of variance. For example, if the model accounts for a significant amount of variance and a change in level, slope, or trend is detected, it is important to know which contrast effect was most important. These two measures of magnitude of the effect will be addressed by the use of omega-squared and the percentage of variance accounted for by each of the orthogonal contrasts.

Strength of Association

A significant omnibus f-test indicates an association between independent and dependent variables. It has been noted that a trivial association may achieve statistical significance if the sample size is large. Hayes has described a parameter, omega-squared, that indicates the magnitude of a population effect.[17] The omega-squared statistic is given by:

$$w^2 = \frac{SS_B - (k-1)\, MS_{RES}}{SS_{TOTAL} + MS_{RES}}$$

SS_B = Sum of squares between groups
k = Number of treatment levels
MS_{RES} = Mean squared residual
SS_{TOTAL} = Sum of squares total

Calculations using this formula will yield a number between zero and one. This number indicates the strength of association between independent and dependent variables. Omega-squared is conceptually analogous to r-squared in regression.

When applying this formula to the model for utilization of prescription services, the omega-squared calculation yields a value of 0.006 or 0.6%.

This indicates that the strength-of-association between the removal of the formulary and the time periods is small. Only 0.6% of the variance in the number of claims per person per period is related to the change in formulary status at the midpoint of the study. In this case, however, even a small change in the number of prescriptions per person may lead to a significant dollar expenditure because of the large number of recipients. If the differences between means are large enough to produce costs savings when extrapolated to a Medicaid program, this is also an indication of practical significance.

Percentage of Explained Variance

Once the issue of significance of the overall model has been put into perspective, attention can be concentrated on methods for determining whether one of the contrast effects dominated. Does the level change, the slope change, or the general trend explain the highest proportion of the total variance? To determine this, the percentage of the total sums of squares accounted for by each contrast can be computed. In the demonstration case the results were as follows:

Average Number of Prescription Claims	Percentage
Level contrast	89.5
Slope contrast	10.5
General trend contrast	0.0

In this case the largest amount of variance is explained by the change in level. Both level and slope contrasts are significant. Observing the direction of movement of the means over time indicates utilization of prescription services went up sharply upon removal of the formulary, then began to stabilize. Because the slope contrast was significant, the need for a more complete time series analysis may be warranted. This would allow more exact determination of the shape of the utilization curve. The dominant effect, however, was the increase in level of utilization. Although the design was nonexperimental, the increase in level is strong enough to argue that it is formulary related. If it were not formulary related, the likelihood is that the general trend contrast would have explained a larger portion of the total variance.

USING THE METHODOLOGY

Finally, the following is given as an example of the Statistical Analysis System (SAS) commands used to perform this analysis for the basic case.

Other statements may be needed for full analysis of means. For example, polynomial contrasts, univariate statistics, and correlation analysis should also be incorporated. This is the basic model for a repeated measures design in which differences between the means for each time period are detected using the three contrasts described.

PROC ANOVA;

Model Mean 1 Mean 2 Mean 3 Mean 4 – /int;

(Mean 1 to Mean 4 are the means from the repeated measures)

Manova M =   Mean 1 – Mean 2 – Mean 3 – Mean 4,
Mean 1 – Mean 2 – Mean 3 + Mean 4,
Mean 1 – Mean 2 + Mean 3 – Mean 4
H = _All_ /ORTH SUMMARY; [14]

SUMMARY

The intent of this chapter was to provide a description of a methodology that may be useful for researchers evaluating economic, social, and administrative interventions. Although a specific example was described, this methodology is adaptable to many experimental designs where repeated measures are available or can be collected. The availability of sophisticated data analysis packages makes the use of multivariate techniques easier, and multivariate techniques are frequently more efficient when the analysis involves large data sets. This type of evaluation may be advantageous for many types of pharmaceutical research.

REFERENCES

1. Cohen J. Statistical power analysis for the behavioral sciences. New York and London: Academic Press, 1969.

2. Campbell DT, Stanley JC. Experimental and quasi-experimental designs for research. Boston: Houghton Mifflin Company, 1966.

3. U.S. Department of Health and Human Services, Health Care Financing Administration. Program statistics: analysis of state Medicaid program characteristics, 1984. Baltimore, MD, August 1985.

4. Nelson AA, Reeder CE, Dickson WM. The effect of a Medicaid drug co-payment program on the utilization and cost of prescription services. Med Care 1984;22(5):727.

5. Neter J, Wasserman W, Kutner MH. Applied linear statistical models. Homewood, IL: Richard D. Irwin, 1985.

6. McCleary R, Hay Jr RA. Applied time series analysis for the social sciences. Beverly Hills, CA: Sage Publications, 1980.

7. Kirk RE. Experimental design: procedures for the behavioral sciences. Belmont, CA: Brooks/Cole Publishing Company, 1968.

8. Rogan JC, Keselman HJ, Mendoza JL. Analysis of repeated measures. Br J Math Stat Psychol 1979;32:269-86.

9. Huynh H, Feldt LS. Conditions under which mean square ratios in repeated measurement designs have exact F-distributions. J Am Stat Assoc 1970;65:1582-9.

10. Geisser S, Greenhouse SW. An extension of Box's results on the use of the F- distribution in multivariate analysis. Ann Math Stat 1958;29:885-91.

11. Fleiss JL. The design and analysis of clinical experiments. New York: John Wiley and Sons, 1986.

12. Sall JP. SAS regression applications. Revised ed. SAS Technical Report A-102. Cary, NC: SAS Institute, 1981.

13. O'Brien RG, Kaiser MK. MANOVA method for analyzing repeated measures designs: an extensive primer. Psychol Bull 1985;97(2):316-33.

14. SAS Institute, Inc. SAS user's guide: statistics. Cary, NC: SAS Institute, 1985.

15. Davidson ML. Univariate versus multivariate tests in repeated measures experiments. Psychol Bull 1972;77:446-52.

16. Huynh H. Some approximate tests in repeated measures designs. Psychometrika 1978;43:1582-9.

17. Hays WL. Statistics for psychologists. New York: Holt, Rinehart and Winston, Inc., 1963.

Chapter 15

Pharmacoeconomic Analysis of Oral Treatments for Onychomycosis: A Canadian Study

Thomas R. Einarson
Steven R. Arikian
Neil H. Shear

INTRODUCTION

According to Balfour and Faulds, fungal infections represent a major form of infection throughout the world.[1] Onychomycosis is the infection of the nail by fungus.[2] More than 90% of nail infections in Canada are due to dermatophytes, with yeasts (primarily *Candida* species and molds) comprising the remainder.[3] The primary pathogenic organisms in onychomycosis are dermatophytes of the *Trichophyton, Microsporum,* and *Epidermophyton* species. Four types of onychomycosis are generally recognized: (1) distal subungual (most commonly involving distal nail bed and hyponychium, with secondary involvement of the underside of the nail plate); (2) white superficial (invading the toenail plate on the nail surface); (3) proximal subungual; and (4) *Candida* (whole nail). Moisture and heat foster the growth of those infections. Immune defects play a role.[4] Unlike other dermatophytoses, onychomycoses are all noninflammatory.[5] Positive diagnosis is made using potassium hydroxide microscopy and/or mycological cultures.[6]

Onychomycosis represents about 30% of all superficial fungal infections and 1.5% of all new visits to dermatology centers.[4] This disease is

The authors thank Jacki Gordon, PhD, and Fred Robin for their help in the preparation of this chapter.

Previously published in *Journal of Research in Pharmaceutical Economics,* Vol. 6(1), 1995.

more common in adults than in children, affecting males and females with equal frequency. The toenails are affected more often (80%) than the fingernails (20%), with the great toenail being affected most often. Fingernail infections are treated more easily than those of the toenails since toenails grow very slowly. Goldfarb and Sulzberger reported a cure rate of 41% in fingernails versus only 3.5% (2 of 58) in toenails.[7]

Drug treatment includes oral administration of griseofulvin (GRI), ketoconazole (KET), and more recently terbinafine (TER). Griseofulvin was the first effective drug used to treat onychomycosis because it penetrates well into skin and achieves therapeutic concentrations after oral administration. However, it is fungistatic, must be taken over very long periods of time (months for fingernails, years for toenails), and relapses are common. Ketoconazole, an imidazole antifungal drug related to miconazole and econazole, is also effective orally, but is mainly fungistatic. The occurrence of unacceptable side effects has curtailed its use significantly. Terbinafine, a recently developed drug of the alkylamine class, is effective orally against a wide variety of dermatophytes. It is particularly effective against onychomycosis because of its excellent penetration into the nail plate. Terbinafine is fungicidal, whereas other oral agents are fungistatic. The few alternate treatments include avulsion (revmoval) of the nail by physical or chemical means and mechanical debridement.[8]

The purpose of the research reported here was to evaluate the economics of oral antifungal therapies available in Canada for treatment of onychomycosis of the fingernail and toenail.

METHODS

Research Plan

This research was carried out by an independent group of university-based investigators. Health Economics Research (HER) of Secaucus, New Jersey, served as a consultant to Sandoz Canada, Inc. HER provided an unrestricted grant to the University of Toronto for this research. The pharmaceutical sponsor was not involved in any phase of the study. This approach has been suggested by Laupacis and coworkers and Hillman and colleagues as being the preferred method for minimizing bias.[9,10]

A separate independent panel of clinical experts was assembled from across Canada to guide and critique all aspects of the project. These experts are renowned dermatologists in active practice who are affiliated with teaching institutions in different geographical areas of the country.

By using a nationwide expert panel, we attempted to minimize bias due to regional differences in perspective.

Pharmacoeconomic Model

A three-phase model was used to guide the research. Phase I consisted of problem definition, Phase II was a meta-analysis designed to provide estimates of clinical outcomes, and Phase III comprised the pharmacoeconomic analysis.

Phase I: Problem Definition. During this phase, the purpose of the project was defined, as were the scope and perspectives of analysis. The purpose of this research was to perform an economic analysis of oral drug therapies for treatment of onychomycosis in Canada. Three sets of data were evaluated: drug cost analysis, cost of regimen analysis, and expected cost analysis (a form of cost-effectiveness analysis). The scope was limited to treatment of infections that require using the oral drugs GRI, KET, and TER. GRI and KET are currently the only oral drugs approved for treating onychomycosis in Canada. At this writing, TER, which belongs to a new class of antifungals, has just recently received its Notice of Compliance after review by the Health Protection Branch in Canada.

Separate analyses were required for onychomycosis of the toenail and fingernail. The perspectives identified were those of the government payer and the patient payer. The analytic time frame was one year or a maximum of three courses of treatment, making the economic end point of this analysis cost per patient per year.

Phase II: Meta-Analysis of Clinical Outcomes. Phase II consisted of quantification of clinical outcomes using meta-analysis of published clinical trials. The outcomes of interest were clinical success rates, relapse rates, and side-effect profiles. Clinical success was defined as the complete clinical cure of the infection or microbiological cure plus significant clinical improvement with only residual signs of the infection.

A stepwise meta-analytic approach was adopted, as described by Einarson, Leeder, and Kohen.[11] The literature was searched for all clinical trials that examined the use of oral GRI, KET, or TER in treating dermatophyte onychomycosis of the fingernail or toenail. Databases searched included Medline, Embase, and International Pharmaceutical Abstracts. In addition, all references from retrieved articles and review papers identified in the search were examined. Data were retrieved from accepted articles by two data extractors and differences were reconciled by a third reviewer. Rates were combined using a technique described by Velanovich for combining Bayesian probabilities; this technique was based on a modification of the method presented by DerSimonian and Laird.[12,13]

This method provides a point estimate and standard error (SE) for such data.[12] The resultant estimate is superior to that of other methods in that it incorporates between-study variance as well as within-study variance into its estimates. It also provides 95% confidence intervals to allow for statistical assessment of the findings. A 95% confidence interval may be calculated simply, as its limits are 1.96 SEs above and below the calculated average value.

In the model reported here, separate analyses were done for each indication (i.e., fingernail onychomycosis, toenail onychomycosis). Relapse rates and side-effect rates were calculated. The results from Phase II provided relatively robust quantitative point estimates of clinical outcomes that served as inputs into the economic analysis.

Phase III: Economic Analysis. Phase III comprised the actual pharmacoeconomic analysis. The main focus was on cost minimization among the three alternative drug regimens. Decision analytic principles formed the underlying methodological structure. The process involved calculating and summing expected utilities for each drug. All patient outcomes were identified, valued, and classified for relevance to each analytic perspective.

First, drug regimens were defined. The expert panel was consulted to determine, by means of consensus, what is considered to be standard therapy. Included were drug quantity, frequency of administration, and treatment duration; workup required; administration; and routine monitoring.

Next, patient outcomes were identified. Successes, relapses, and failures constituted patient outcomes. Clinical outcomes from the meta-analysis in Phase II were used as inputs. Success rates are listed in Table 15.1. The expert panel recommended that when a primary treatment failed, a secondary treatment be delivered, with another drug. KET was selected by the panel as the secondary (failure) drug for TER, and TER was the secondary drug for the other two.

Since the analysis spanned a time frame of one year, therapeutic relapses were a consideration. Clinical outcomes from the Phase II meta-analysis were employed. Patients were retreated with the primary therapy in each case of relapse. It was assumed that the success rate for retreatment would be very high, with at least 90% responding. That assumption was based on clinical experience and the fact that patients had already responded to one treatment regimen, although the beneficial effects had subsided. Also, those patients who had failed first course of primary

TABLE 15.1. Clinical Success Rates Derived from the Meta-Analysis

		Comparator		
		TER	GRI	KET
Fingernail Infection	Patients (Studies)	*N* = 172 (5)	*N* = 143 (6)	*N* = 106 (3)
	Primary success rate, % (SE)	95.0 (3.0)	59.6 (11.6)	80.9 (12.4)
	Primary relapse rate, %	6.6	40.0	33.0
	Primary retreatment success, %	90.0	90.0	90.0
Toenail Infection	Patients (Studies)	*N* = 84 (4)	*N* = 191 (5)	*N* = 20 (4)
	Primary success rate, % (SE)	78.3 (2.8)	17.5 (6.6)	40.8 (11.5)
	Primary relapse rate, %	6.6	40.0	38.0
	Primary retreatment success rate, %	90.0	90.0	90.0

therapy were switched to the secondary therapy, which was likely to elevate the success rate in the re-treated group.

In addition to successes and failures, it was necessary to consider the impact of adverse effects. As above, results from the Phase II meta-analysis were used. A dermatologist with expertise in assessing and treating adverse drug reactions (ADRs) was consulted to evaluate the ADRs reported. For each drug, the summary list of adverse events was presented. The average cost of treating each ADR was determined, as was the usual method of treatment. When necessary, medical specialists were consulted for their particular expertise. For minor, self-limiting (but annoying) complaints such as headache, diarrhea, or gastrointestinal upset, it was assumed that patients had consulted with their pharmacist and followed recommendations. Information on pharmacist recommendations for common complaints was extracted from the current Maclean Hunter Survey.[14] All results were presented to the expert panel for evaluation.

COST DATA

After verification of all clinical data by the expert panel, costs for each patient outcome were determined. The acquisition cost of each comparator included both the drug cost and administration costs. Drug costs were determined from the current edition of the Ontario Drug Benefit Formulary.[15] The cost was considered to be the number of total units for treatment (tablets or capsules) multiplied by the cost per unit plus the average dispensing fee. Prescription fees were those derived from the latest Maclean Hunter Survey of Canadian pharmacies.[14] One dispensing fee was added for each 100 days' supply of medication, as per the standard practice in Canada, where the analysis was conducted.

Cost of drugs prescribed to treat side effects was also estimated using the current Ontario database price list.[15] For those drugs not on the list, and for the purchase of nonprescription items, pharmacies in Ontario were contacted to establish the price for a standard package of the item in question. Costs of side effects treated by a physician, including referral to specialists and surgery, were calculated using the current Schedule of Benefits for Physicians' Services of the Ministry of Health for Ontario.[16] Costs of medical care were calculated by multiplying the number of incidents (e.g., consults) by the unit cost for that incident, as indicated in the Schedule of Benefits. Cost of hospitalization due to side effects was obtained by contacting the Ontario Hospital Association. Calculation of costs was done by multiplying the incidence of adverse events by the proportion of those ADRs that were treated, then multiplying by the cost of the treatment regimen. To determine the costs of laboratory tests, a testing laboratory was contacted. Costs extracted were those paid by the Ontario Ministry of Health.

Indirect costs were those associated with receiving therapy, including assessments and follow-up visits for monitoring or for treatment of ADRs. Costs included such expenses as transportation and lost wages due to time away from work. Canadian statistical data for wages were derived from Facts Canada and projected to the present using the Consumer Prince Index as an inflator.[17]

OUTCOMES
OF PHARMACOECONOMIC ANALYSIS

Three main analyses were performed for each perspective. They included drug cost analysis, cost of regimen analysis, and expected cost analysis. The drug cost analysis involves calculation of the acquisition costs plus administration costs for each drug regimen, ignoring clinical parameters and indirect costs. The cost of regimen analysis considers all direct and indirect costs of therapy with a drug, including costs of its side effects. This analysis also ignores clinical outcomes. Included in the cost of therapy are costs of drug acquisition and administration, routine medical care, adverse effect management, laboratory tests, and indirect costs. The expected cost analysis is a full economic analysis that considers therapeutic outcomes.

A clinical decision tree was constructed to model therapy for each drug (Figure 15.1). Branches of the tree represent treatments and their outcomes. Probabilities for branches are represented by clinical success rates for each drug and its relapse rates. Costs are the total expected cost for each regimen used on a particular branch of the tree. Table 15.2 presents the formulas for each branch of the tree. When probabilities are multiplied by the costs for their respective branches and summed for all branches, we arrive at the total expected cost for each drug. The drug having the lowest total expected cost is the preferred choice. In addition, one may calculate ratios between the expected cost for each comparator and the lowest comparator.

PERSPECTIVE ANALYSIS

Two perspectives were considered: that of the patient payer and that of the government payer. The former is essentially that of society in that it includes those indirect costs associated with treatment that must be paid by the patient, but that would not be a factor for the government payer. Indirect costs include time away from work for physician visits or for treatment of adverse events. In Ontario, the government pays for all costs of physician visits and procedures performed, consultations with specialists, laboratory tests, and hospitalization. All service providers must accept the government payment and cannot charge the patient any additional fees for these services.

For the government perspective, we first calculated overall cost-effectiveness by assuming that the government would pay for all prescription drugs for all people, as in a socialized health care system. However, in many jurisdictions, the government pays for drugs for only a proportion of its citizens. For example, in Ontario (where this analysis was conducted), the government pays for about 40% of all of the drugs purchased in the province. In other provinces, the rates vary from 30% (Manitoba) to

FIGURE 15.1. Diagram of Decision Tree for Calculating Outcomes, Probability of Success, and Overall Costs of Therapy

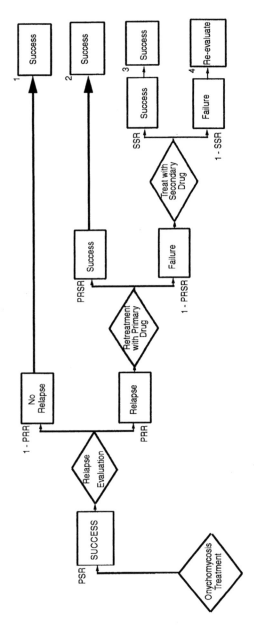

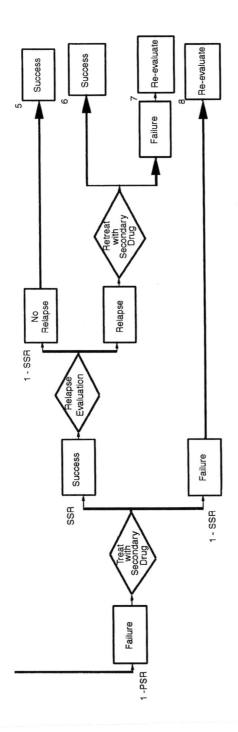

TABLE 15.2. Formulas for Probabilities and Costs

Branch	Probability	Cost
1	PSR*(1-PRR)	PTC
2	PSR*PRR*PRSR	2*PTC
3	PSR*PRR*(1-PRSR)*SSR	2*PTC + STC
4	PSR*PRR*(1-PRSR)*(1-SSR)	2*PTC + STC
5	(1-PSR)*SSR*(1-SRR)	PTC + STC
6	(1-PSR)*SSR*SRR*SRSR	PTC + 2*STC
7	(1-PSR)*SSR*SRR*(1-SRSR	PTC + 2*STC
8	(1-PSR)*(1-SSR)	PTC + STC

PTC = primary treatment cost, STC = secondary treatment cost, PSR = primary treatment success rate, PRR = primary treatment relapse rate, PRSR = primary retreatment success rate, SSR = secondary treatment success rate, SRR = secondary treatment relapse rate, and SRSR = secondary retreatment success rate.

100% (Saskatchewan). Therefore, the analysis was recalculated, varying the drug cost as a sensitivity analysis.

For the patient perspective, the patient payer would bear all costs of treatment. In effect, this perspective provides the "real" data for cost of care because all costs are paid by some payer within the system (e.g., government, insurance, out-of-pocket). Indirect costs would include loss of revenue due to time lost for treatments and medical consultations, as well as for transportation. A conservative estimate of $25 was used for transportation and meal costs for each day.

RESULTS

Only two comparative trials for onychomycosis were found; therefore, we were obliged to use open trials for determination of success rates.[18,19] A problem with open trials is the potential for bias. However, that caveat would hold for all drugs, and since every comparator had open trials, it was considered that there would be minimal bias against any individual comparator. Nonetheless, the results could be higher than those encountered in clinical practice. Thirteen studies of oral drugs in onychomycosis were found, 12 of which reported results for fingernails. Results appear in Table 15.1.[18-29]

Economic Analysis 1: Onychomycosis of the Fingernail

Terbinafine had the highest success rate of the three comparators (Table 15.1). It should be noted that, for all studies of this drug, the definition of success included both clinical and mycological cure. Clinical evaluations of the other two drugs, particularly GRI, were done many years ago and often included only clinical success. Thus, rates for TER could be underestimated with respect to the comparators.

The cost per tablet (Table 15.3) of TER that was selected for this analysis is greater than the unit cost of either of the comparators. However, because the length of treatment is much shorter with TER, it is not the most expensive choice for a treatment course; it falls between the two comparators. TER is fungicidal, whereas the other two drugs are fungistatic. This accounts for the longer treatment regimens for GRI and KET.

TABLE 15.3. Drug Cost Analysis of Oral Drugs for Onychomycosis

Infection	Component	Drug		
		TER	**GRI**	**KET**
Fingernail	Days of therapy	90	180	180
	Dosage in mg/day	250	500	200
	Total doses	90	180	180
	Cost per dose	$3.50*	$0.53	$2.07
	Drug cost	$315.00	$95.40	$372.60
	Dispensing fee**	10.00	20.00	20.00
	Total	325.00	115.40	392.60
Toenail	Days of therapy	120***	365	365
	Dosage (mg/day)	250	500	200
	Total doses	120	365	365
	Cost per dose	$3.50*	$0.53	$2.07
	Drug cost	$420.00	$193.45	$755.55
	Dispensing fee**	20.00	40.00	40.00
	Total	440.00	233.45	795.55

*   Cost data provided by Sandoz Canada, Inc.
** Per Canadian pharmacy survey.
*** 120 Days is the mean for terbinafine.

Thus, the drug cost analysis would identify GRI as the best alternative; however, decisions based only on those figures are often not valid since they do not project the true cost picture.

In the cost of regimen analysis (Table 15.4), TER emerges as the least costly alterative due to less medical care required and substantially lower indirect costs for the patient. The other two comparators require close monitoring to avoid toxicity and undesirable side effects such as hepatotoxicity.

In the expected cost analysis (Table 15.5), TER emerges as the most cost-effective alternative because of the short duration of treatment, higher clinical success rates, and lower relapse rates. This analysis considered complete costs of treatment. The cost-effectiveness analysis was based on using TER for 90 days, but more recent literature, as well as the expert panel suggests that this drug may be efficacious after only two months of treatment. A sensitivity analysis using a 60-day course of therapy would result in cost-effectiveness values of $431 for TER, $747 for GRI, and $1,034 for KET.

The government normally pays about 40% of all prescriptions in Ontario, where this analysis was undertaken. However, this year the proportion rose to 50%. Other provinces pay as little as 30% while Saskatchewan pays a full 100%. Thus, we performed a sensitivity analysis to evaluate cost-effectiveness based on drug reimbursement share. This analysis showed TER to be the most cost-effective alternative for the government in all drug reimbursement scenarios. For fingernail onychomycosis, the government would pay $334 and $259 for TER with a 50% and 30% cost reimbursement share, respectively. For GRIs, costs would be $650 and $592, respectively, while KET would cost $772 and $658.

Economic Analysis 2: Onychomycosis of the Toenail

Clinical results, presented in Table 15.1, show TER to be superior to the other two agents in all respects. Table 15.3 identifies the costs involved in prescriptions for the three antifungal agents. Griseofulvin has the lowest unit acquisition cost. However, it must be administered for an entire year to achieve clinical efficacy. Terbinafine has the highest unit cost, but it is administered over a shorter period of time, as described above. Ketoconazole is intermediate in cost but, like GRI, it must be taken for one year to elicit its maximal effect. This, it becomes the most expensive drug based on acquisition cost for a treatment regimen.

For the patient payer (Table 15.6), cost of regimen was lowest with TER, second with GRI, and highest with KET. This type of analysis does not consider clinical success rates and therefore does not reflect the total

TABLE 15.4. Cost of Regimen Analysis of Oral Drugs for Onychomycosis of the Fingernail

Perspective	Cost	Comparator		
		TER	GRI	KET
Patient payer	Drug acquisition	325.00	115.40	392.60
	Routine medical care	86.20	262.70	262.70
	Laboratory tests	28.30	99.05	99.05
	Adverse effect management	0.33	3.65	1.11
	Indirect costs	186.20	651.41	651.75
	Total	626.03	1132.21	1407.21
Government (100%)	Total*	439.83	480.80	755.46

*Excludes indirect costs, which are paid by the patient. All other cost components are the same as for the patient payer.

TABLE 15.5. Expected Cost Analysis for Onychomycosis of the Fingernail

Branch	TER	GRI	KET
Patient Payer			
Total Therapy	763	1686	1927
CE Ratio	1	2.21	2.52
% Savings	–	54.7	60.3
Government Payer (100%)			
Total Therapy	520	795	1058
CE Ratio	1	1.53	2.03
% Savings	–	34.6	50.9

cost of treatment for the disease. Table 15.7 presents the expected cost analysis, which considers clinical success rates, as determined in the Phase II meta-analysis. As in the other analyses, TER emerges as the most cost-effective drug, with a total cost substantially below the others.

For each drug in a cost-effectiveness analysis, the major cost factor is not primary success, but primary failure because of the necessity of using two treatment regimens. TER also has the lowest relapse costs due to a very low rate of relapse.

As with the fingernail onychomycosis data, we used a longer time period for treatment than may be necessary in clinical practice. Using a 90-day treatment regimen produced similar results, with TER emerging as the most cost-effective alternative. We also performed a sensitivity analysis using different payment shares for the government. When the government's share

TABLE 15.6. Cost of Regimen Analysis of Oral Drugs for Onychomycosis of the Toenail

Perspective	Cost	Comparator		
		TER	GRI	KET
Patient payer	Drug acquisition	440.00	233.45	795.55
	Routine medical care	156.80	333.30	333.30
	Laboratory tests	84.90	169.80	169.80
	Adverse effect management	0.33	3.65	1.11
	Indirect costs	372.20	837.41	837.76
	Total	1054.23	1577.61	2137.52
Government (100%)	Total*	682.03	740.20	1299.76

*Excludes indirect costs, which are paid by the patient. All other cost components are the same as for the patient payer.

TABLE 15.7. Expected Cost Analysis for Onychomycosis of the Fingernail

Branch	TER	GRI	KET
Patient Payer			
Total Therapy	1656	2610	3142
CE Ratio	1	1.58	1.90
% Savings	–	36.6	47.3
Government Payer			
(100%)			
Total Therapy	1050	1389	1936
CE Ratio	1	1.32	1.84
% Savings	–	24.4	45.8

of the drug cost was 50%, the overall cost of TER was $717, a 30% share cost was %583. For GRI, costs were $1,071 and $944, respectively, and for KET, they were $1,337 and $1,097, respectively.

From the perspective of both the patient payer and the government payer, TER has the preferred cost profile among the three drugs. It should be noted that its higher acquisition cost did not result in a higher overall cost. Pharmacoeconomic evaluation has thus demonstrated that a more expensive per unit drug can be the most cost-effective therapeutic alternative.

CONCLUSIONS

This comprehensive research is the first study of its type to focus on oral antifungals in onychomycosis. The nature of the model was such that all precautions were taken to avoid analytic bias. Using an expert panel of dermatologists provided excellent input and necessary clinical guidance. Maintaining independence from the funding source supported academic neutrality essential to pharmacoeconomic research. The sensitivity analyses that were performed, beyond those reported, all confirm the findings of the main analyses. Thus, we are confident that the findings in this study are genuine and not inflated. If anything, the analysis was somewhat biased in favor of GRI and KET regarding several issues. For example, the definition of successful therapy may have been more stringent for TER than for the two comparators.

This pharmacoeconomic analysis has demonstrated that TER is associated with a higher success rate, a shorter treatment time, and a lower relapse rate than GRI or KET in the treatment of onychomycosis of the fingernail or toenail. Terbinafine has the lowest expected cost compared with the other two agents from the patient payer and government payer perspectives in the Canadian health care system.

ACKNOWLEDGEMENTS

The authors thank the following Canadian dermatologists for their expert guidance and critique of the clinical parameters and results of this study:

G. Daniel Schachter, MD, FRCPC
Women's College Hospital
University of Toronto
Toronto, Ontario

Jay Taradash, MD, FRCPC
Diplomate of American Academy of Dermatology
Women's College Hospital
Toronto, Ontario

Wayne Gulliver, MD FRCPC
Clinical Assistant Professor of Medicine (Dermatology)
Director of Dermatology
Grace General Hospital
St. John's, Newfoundland

Robin C. Billick, MSc, MDCM, FRCPC
Chief of Dermatology
Jewish General Hospital
Montreal, Quebec

Sylvia Garnis-Jones, MSc, MDCM, FRCPC
Determatology
Ottawa Civic Hospital
Royal Ottawa Hospital
Ottawa, Ontario

REFERENCES

1. Balfour JA, Faulds D. Terbinafine: a review of its pharmacodynamic and pharmacokinetic properties, and therapeutic potential in superficial mycoses. Drugs 1992;43:259-84.
2. Zaias N. Onychomycosis. Arch Dermatol 1972;105:263-74.

3. Summerbell RC, Kane J, Krajden S. Onychomycosis, tinea pedis and tinea manuum caused by non-dermatophytic filamentous fungi. Mycoses 1989;32:609-19.

4. Andre J, Achten G. Onychomycosis. Int J Dermatol 1987;26:481-90.

5. Jones HE. Consensus of the role and positioning of the imidazoles in the treatment of dermatophytosis. Acta Derm Venereol Suppl (Stockh) 1986;121 (Suppl):139-46.

6. Daniel CR, Lawson LA. Tinea unguium. Cutis 1987;40:326-7.

7. Goldfarb NJ, Sulzberger MB. Experiences in 137 patients treated with oral griseofulvin. ARch Dermatol 1960;81:859-62.

8. White MI, Clayton YM. The treatment of fungus and yeast infections of nails by the method of "chemical removal." Clin Exp Dermatol 1982;7:273-6.

9. Laupacis A, Feeny D, Detsky AS, Tugwell PX. How attractive does a new technology have to be to warrant adoption and utilization? Tentative guidelines for using clinical and economic evaluations. Can Med Assoc J 1992;146:473-81.

10. Hillman AL, Eisenberg JM, Pauly MV, Bloom BS, Glick H, Kinosian B, Schwartz JS. Avoiding bias in the conduct and reporting of cost-effectiveness research sponsored by pharmaceutical companies. N Engl J Med 1991;324:1362-5.

11. Einarson TR, Leeder JS, Koren G. A method for meta-analysis of epidemiologic studies. Drug Intell Clin Pharm 1988;22:813-24

12. Velanovich V. Meta-analysis for combining Bayesian probabilities. Med Hyoptheses 1991;35:192-5.

13. DerSimonian R, Laird N. Meta-analysis in clinical trials. Control Clin Trials 1986;7:177-88.

14. Maclean Hunter. A survey of drug store trends 1991 survey of findings. Toronto, Canada: Drug Merchandising/Le Pharmacien, 1992.

15. Ontario Drug Benefit Formulary/Comparative Drug Index No. 32. Toronto, Canada: Ontario Ministry of Health, July 1992.

16. Schedule of benefits: physician services under the Health Insurance Act. Toronto, Canada: Ministry of Health, April 1, 1991.

17. Facts Canada 1990: an international business comparison. Ottawa, Canada: Prospectus Publications Ltd., 1991.

18. Baudraz-Rosselet F, Rakosi T, Wili PB, Kenzelmann R. Treatment of onychomycosis with terbinafine. Br J Dermatol 1992;126(Suppl 39):40-6.

19. Goodfield MJD. Short-duration therapy with terbinafine for dermatophyte onychomycosis: a multicentre trial. Br J Dermatol 1992;126(Suppl 39):33-5.

20. Rakosi T. Terbinafine and onychomycosis. Dermatologica 1990;181:174.

21. van der Schroeff JG, Cirkel PK, Crijns MB, Van-Dijk TJ, Govaert FJ, Groeneweg DA, Tazelaar DJ, De-Wit RF, Wuite J. A randomized treatment duration-finding study of terbinafine in onychomycosis. Br J Dermatol 1992;126 (Suppl39):36-9.

22. Zaias N, Serrano L. The successful treatment of fingernail *Trichophyton rubrum* onychomycosis with oral terbinafine. Clin Exp Dermatol 1989;12:120-3.

23. Hay RJ, Clayton YM, Griffiths WA, Dowd PM. A comparative double blind study of ketoconazole and griseofulvin in dermatophytosis. Br J Dermatol 1985;112:691-6.

24. Robertson MN, Hanifin JM, Parker F. Oral therapy for dermatophyte infections unresponsive to griseofulvin. Rev Infect Dis 1980;2:578-81.

25. Svejgaard E. Oral ketoconazole as an alternative to griseofulvin in recalcitrant dermatophyte infections and onychomycosis. Acta Derm Venereol Suppl (Stockh) 1985;65:143-9.

26. Davies RR, Everall JD, Hamilton E. Mycological and clinical evaluation of griseofulvin for chronic onychomycosis. Br Med J 1967;3:464-8.

27. Kaminsky A. Comparative effects of griseofulvin on onychomycosis and on psoriasis unguium. Arch Dermatol 1960;81:838-40.

28. Maibach HI, Kligman AM. Short-term treatment of onychomycosis with griseofulvin. Arch Dermatol 1960;18:733-4.

29. Galimberti R, Negroni R, da Ellas MRI, Robles AM, Arechauala A, Tuculet MA. The activity of ketoconazole in the treatment of onychomycosis. Rev Infect Dis 1980;2:596-8.

Chapter 16

QALYs in Health Outcomes Research: Representation of Real Preferences or Another Numerical Abstraction?

Dev S. Pathak

INTRODUCTION

Health care spending as a percentage of gross domestic product (GDP) has continued to rise in the western hemisphere in recent years. Although there is a great deal of concern about the rising level of health care expenditure, the more urgent question is: What is the worth or, more precisely, the efficiency of the resources utilized in the health care sector? Unfortunately, an answer to this question has remained elusive because of the frustrations associated with the identification of an appropriate output measure for health care interventions.[1] While early years of economic evaluation of health care programs and services concentrated on the cost-benefit analysis using the human capital approach, this approach has received less attention in recent years because it equates value of livelihood with value of life.[2,3] The problems associated with the applications of cost-benefit analysis in the health care sector have convinced many researchers to concentrate on cost-effectiveness analysis where outputs (or benefits) are measured only in terms of physical units such as life years gained, number of lives saved, and reduction in the number of hospitalization days.[4] One major problem with studies using cost-effectiveness analysis is that these studies, although easy to understand and conduct, do not

---

This chapter was originally prepared during the author's sabbatical at the Glaxo Research Institute during 1993. The author thanks Zafar Hakim for his comments and suggestions in the preparation of this manuscript.

Previously published in *Journal of Research in Pharmaceutical Economics*, Vol. 6(4), 1996.

have a common unit of output for all health care programs that combines both quality and quantity of healthy life. Hence, results of these studies do not allow decision makers to compare the efficiency of varying health care programs. In addition, many physical output measures do not represent patients' preferences. As a solution to these problems, a new analytical technique, called cost-utility analysis (CUA), was devised. CUA uses a new measure of output for health care programs–quality adjusted life years (QALYs).[5,6] This measure, proposed in the 1970s, accounts for the effects of health care programs on both the quantity and quality of patients' lives.[6]

Early researchers used many variants of the term QALY: quality adjusted years of life, function years, value adjusted years, and well years.[7-10] However, the 1977 article by Weinstein and Stason can be credited with the first operationalization of the term "quality adjusted life years" (QALYs).[6] Since then, many articles related to various aspects of QALY have been published. However, during the 1990s, the interest in this concept of common unit of output for health care programs has intensified because of the introduction of at least one competing measure, the healthy years equivalent (HYE) and because of growing interest among public policymakers in this concept in countries such as Australia, Canada, and the U.S.[11-15]

The objectives of this chapter are to review briefly the concept and the components of QALY, to outline the approaches used in the measurement of each component of QALY in the literature, to discuss the issues involved in the measurement of each component at the individual level, and to outline a few emerging measures of health care output combining quality and quantity of life. This chapter does not address the issues involved in the aggregation of preferences, nor does it discuss the ethical implications of the use of QALY in clinical or societal resource allocation decisions. Also, the chapter is restricted to the use of QALY as an output measure in CUA and does not address the issues involved in the measurement of cost in any CUA analysis. Finally, it is assumed that the reader is familiar with and understands the axioms underlying von Neumann and Morgenstern's approach to deriving the utility function and the differences between terms such as utility vs. value, cardinal vs. ordinal, risky vs. riskless decisions, and judgment vs. choice.[16-17]

QALY:
IN THEORY AND IN PRACTICE

The measurement of QALY consists of three major components: life years (Y), quality of life (QOL or Q) weights, and QALY which is multi-

FIGURE 16.1 QALY: In Theory and Practice

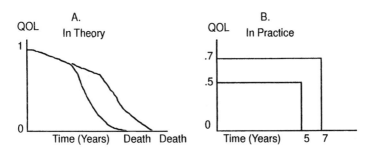

plication of Q and Y. In 1977, Weinstein and Stason defined QALY as follows:

> The general approach that has been used is to derive some measure like "quality adjusted life years" to express the total health effects in common units. The first approaches to this problem fall under the rubric of "health-status indexes." A health-status index is essentially a weighting scheme: each definable health status, ranging from death to coma to varying degrees of disability and discomfort to full health, and accounting for age differences, is assigned a weight from zero to one, and the number of years spent at a given health status, Y_s, is multiplied by the corresponding weight, λ_s, to yield a number $\lambda_s Y_s$, that might be thought of as an equivalent number of years with full health–a number of quality adjusted life years (QALYs). The source of these weights is ultimately subjective . . . .[6]

Based on Weinstein and Stason's definition, QALY, in theory, requires generation of utility function over life years *and* health states for an individual that can be used in evaluating the outcomes of different interventions. This characterization of QALY is presented in Part A of Figure 16.1. However, in practice, for chronic health states, QALY is measured as a multiplication of utility of health states times life years for the rest of a subject's life (see Part B of Figure 16.1). Although this discussion of QALY measurement has focused on chronic health states for the sake of simplicity, it should not be interpreted to mean that QALYs cannot be calculated for temporary health states.

A question is frequently raised as to why QALY should be used as a measure of output when measures of utility could suffice as a denominator in any CUA analysis. A major reason for using a numeric measure of

QALY, and not of utility, in the denominator of CUA calculations is simply the understandability of these two concepts by decision makers. In other words, the major benefit of QALY as a measure of output of any health program is that it seems to have significant intuitive appeal to decision makers in the pubic policy arena.[18]

Although advocates of the QALY concept have not justified the measurement of QALY on the basis of its relationship with the theory underlying the willingness to pay (WTP) or the contingent valuation (CV) measures, there is a striking similarity between the rationale underlying these two measurements.[19-21] Assume, for example, that an individual had ten years to live in a chronic disease state. If this individual assigns a utility score of .7 to this state, then QALY is 7 years (0.7 × 10 years) in perfect health. In other words, this individual is willing to trade off (pay) three years of his disease-based life for living in perfect health. Thus, in this case, the measurement unit is life years as opposed to money, as used in the contingent valuation approach.

MEASUREMENT OF Y
(QUANTITY OF LIFE)

Although the term QALY implies that the quantity of life (Y) should be measured in years, the measurement unit could be years, days, or even hours. Frequently, the Y component of the term QALY is operationalized by asking the respondent to consider terms such as "rest of your life," "specified number of years," or "specified number of days." In fact, the Y component of QALY can be measured in terms of any unit of time to reflect the life expectancy of the respondent. Hence, the term quality adjusted life years (QALY) can be defined as quality adjusted life expectancy (QALE). Regardless of the unit of time used, the emphasis in the measurement of Y for the purposes of calculating QALYs is on longevity as a substitute for the meaning of life years in survival.

MEASUREMENT OF Q
(QUALITY OF LIFE WEIGHTS)

Various approaches are used in the measurement of Q, i.e., the quality of life weights. The intent behind these approaches is to obtain the weights that capture the true preferences of respondents since "ignoring these preferences in the process of decision making can result in choosing the wrong (i.e., less preferred) service" and, ultimately, in lower individual and societal welfare.[18]

One approach commonly used to accomplish this goal of capturing preferences of patients and/or decision makers is to derive utility functions over life years and health states of the respondents based upon a set of axioms proposed by von Neumann and Morgenstern (vNM) to evaluate the outcomes of different health care programs.[16] vNM's axiomatization of utility theory consists of three axioms: complete ordering (including transitivity), continuity, and substitutability (also referred to as independence or IIA, i.e., independent of irrelevant alternatives). Based on these three axioms, vNM theory proposes that an individual who follows the axioms underlying the theory should, when faced with different lotteries (gambles or bets) consisting of risky outcomes, choose the lottery with the highest expected utility. In other words, vNM theory outlines how an individual should make decisions under conditions of risk and how to measure numerically the strength of preferences (i.e., utilities) of an individual among risky outcomes. Because the outcomes of health care programs are risky, vNM theory is viewed as directly relevant to decision making in health care and, in fact, is viewed as a gold standard for rational decision making under risk at an individual level. The method most commonly used to measure individual preferences under risk is the standard gamble (SG) technique using the probability equivalence approach.[18] A simplified interpretation of how the SG technique is used to arrive at the utility weights to be used in the QALY calculations for any chronic health state is presented in Figure 16.2. For the sake of simplicity, let us assume that healthy life and death represent all or nothing in the health domain and serve as reference states, i.e., the utility weights for a healthy life and death

FIGURE 16.2. The Standard Gamble Method for Obtaining Utility Weights for the Measurement of QALY for a Chronic Health State for the Rest of Life (Y)

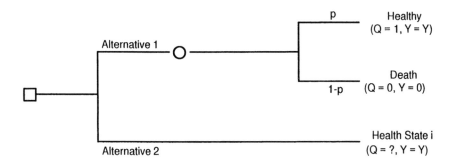

are set equal to 1 and 0, respectively. This representation also assumes that, within the health domain, all people are equal. Hence, the utility of a full healthy life from birth to death is set equal for each individual.

Figure 16.2 shows that a subject in a chronic health state is offered two alternatives. Alternative 1 is a health care program (intervention, treatment) that has two outcomes: the patient is cured and returns to being healthy (the most preferred outcome) and lives the rest of life (Y) without disease (a probability of p) or the patient dies immediately (the least preferred outcome) (a probability of $1-p$). Alternative 2 has the certain outcome of chronic health state i for the rest of life (Y years). To obtain the utility weight for living in the chronic health state for Y years, the probability p is varied until the patient or the respondent is indifferent between the two alternatives. The obtained indifference $p*$ value is the utility weight for the health state i.

The above holistic approach of using the SG technique to measure the strength of individual preferences via the vNM utility theory is not the only approach used in the literature for measuring Q. Techniques such as time trade-off (TTO), magnitude estimation (ME), and visual analogue scale (VAS) have also been used to arrive at the Q values of outcomes of various programs. The difference between the Q values obtained through the use of the SG technique and those obtained through the other techniques has been explained in terms of the underlying assumption of the nature of risk associated with the decision. The Q scores obtained through the SG technique are assumed to be for "risky" decisions, and these scores are referred to as "utilities," whereas the numbers obtained with the use of TTO, ME, or VAS are called "values" obtained from "riskless" decisions.

Since health state preferences are multiattribute decisions, the holistic approach could become quite cumbersome, time consuming, and cognitively burdensome to the respondents. Hence, many studies use a decomposed approach that allows the researcher to obtain values from the patient or decision maker for all health states without requiring the subject to assign values to each and every possible combination of multiattribute health states. A variety of strategies can be used to apply the decomposed approach to the measurement of health state preferences. A detailed account of these strategies is provided by Fisher; Veit, Rose, and Ware; and Froberg and Kane.[22-24] Some of the instruments used to measure the values assigned to health outcomes of various programs are the Quality of Well-Being Scale (QWB), the Crichton Royal Behavioral Rating Scale (CRBRS), the Life Satisfaction Index (LSI), the Index of Health-Related Quality of Life (IHQL), the European Quality of Life Instrument (EuroQol), and the Health Utilities Indexes (HUI).[25-30] Instead of explaining the assumptions underlying each of these instruments and the strengths and weaknesses of each instrument, this paper is limited to addressing the issues involved in obtaining Q values through the SG technique because some health care researchers consider this technique to be a "gold standard."[5,31]

MEASUREMENT OF QALY

Let us assume that the chronic health state presented in Figure 16.1 is mild angina, the rest of life consisted of 20 years for a subject, and the indifference probability (i.e., the utility score) was .6. Then, in this case, it can be stated that the QALY value assigned to the health state of mild angina is 12 years for this individual. In other words, although QALY is a bivariate utility function $\{QALY = U(Q \cdot Y)\}$, QALY is currently measured in practice by the following formula: $QALY = U(Q) \cdot Y$. This approach to the measurement of QALY as a bivariate function is true only under certain restrictive conditions beyond those prescribed by the vNM utility theory. These conditions are: (A) utility (as well as mutual utility) independence; (B) constant proportional trade-off property; and (C) linearity (or risk neutrality) with respect to time. The technical explanation of these conditions is provided by Pliskin, Shepard, and Weinstein.[32] However, an attempt is made below, following Kamlet, to provide a nontechnical description of these conditions.[15]

A. The attributes of quality and quantity must be utility independent as well as mutual utility independent (i.e., preference for gambles on one attribute should be independent of the other attributes). For example, consider an individual who is indifferent between living 17 years in mild pain and a lottery where he has a probability of .5 of living 24 years in mild pain or a .5 chance of living 6 years in mild pain (Figure 16.3). In this case, the trade-off involved is for quantity of life and not quality of life because the health outcomes involved in both alternatives are identical, i.e., mild pain. If the utility independence assumption holds for this individual, then replacing the outcome of mild pain with severe pain should result in the same preference

FIGURE 16.3. Assumption of Utility Independence

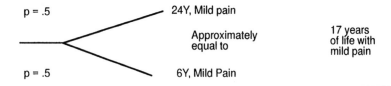

for the length of life. Similar scenarios could be created for showing that the trade-off between levels of pain should not change if the length of life involved is held constant.

B. The trade-off of quantity with quality must exhibit the constant proportional trade-off property (i.e., the proportion of the remaining life that one would trade off for a specific quality improvement should be independent of the amount of remaining life). For example, assume that a patient reported being indifferent between 24 years of healthy life and 32 years of life with migraine. The same patient should be indifferent between 15 years of healthy life and 20 years of life with migraine. This is because the patient is willing to trade off one-fourth of disease-based life for disease-free life.

C. The single attribute utility function for additional healthy life years must be linear with time (i.e., for a fixed quality level, one's utility should be directly proportional to longevity, a property also referred to as risk neutrality with respect to time). If this assumption holds, an individual should be indifferent between seven years of disease-free life and a gamble with a .5 chance of immediate pain-free death (0 years of life) and a .5 chance of 14 years of healthy life. In other words, the expected value of the gamble is equal to the certainty equivalence value (Figure 16.3).

Based on these assumptions, Pliskin and colleagues point out that "multiattribute function can be written as a function of life years times the value function for health status, i.e., $Y \bullet U_r(Q)$, in one of the following forms, indexed by the risk parameter r:

$$U(Y,Q) = 1/r \: \{[Y \bullet U_r(Q)]^r - 1\} + r \qquad \text{(for } r \neq 0)$$

or

$$U(Y,Q) = \log [Y \bullet U_r(Q)] \qquad \text{(for } r = 0).\text{''}\,[32]$$

$U_r(Q)$ can be interpreted as the proportion of any given remaining life span at full quality that has the same utility as the entire remaining life span at quality Q. In fact, if $r = 1$ (i.e., risk neutrality where the utility function on longevity is linear), then $U_r(Q)$ becomes a linear function and can be written as:

$$U(Y,Q) = Y \bullet U_1(Q).$$

This is the QALY function identified at the beginning of this section and is used in the literature.

ISSUES IN THE MEASUREMENT OF Y

If QALY is to represent a bivariate utility function for quantity and quality of life, then the *utility of life years (or expectancy) in survival* could be interpreted as the meaning of life years in survival. The measurement of Y (quantity of life) as some unit of time (years, days, or any other measure) in the current literature simply reflects the longevity aspect of the meaning of life years in survival. The longevity, however, reflects only one component of the utility of quantity of life. The utility of quantity of life, if viewed in terms of meaning of life time in survival, can be viewed as the achievement of life plans. People develop, by adolescence, life plans. These life plans may be less detailed for the long-term than for the short-term duration. Our life plans go through continuous revisions. A premature death results not only in the loss of longevity or expected normal life, but also in the loss of opportunity to complete the life plans that give meaning and coherence to a person's life.[33] Thus, the quantity of life as measured by a unit of time in the current QALY measure may not reflect the true preferences of an individual.

Kamlet points out that the concept of life plan, and not the longevity of life expectancy, becomes an important issue when an individual has advance knowledge about the timing of future health outcomes.[15] In Figure 16.4, scenario one, an individual is informed that he will have an illness in five years that will require him to make a decision between surgery and no surgery at that time. He can do nothing until then. Five years from now, if he elects to have surgery, he will have a .5 chance of living an additional five years. However, he may also die on the operating table. If he decides not to have surgery, he will have six months to live. In scenario two in Figure 16.4, the individual is faced with the same decision, but he has to make the decision now. It is possible that this individual may prefer surgery in scenario one but may prefer no surgery in scenario two, although both scenarios have the same odds. As Kamlet points out, the individual may prefer the option of having six months of added life with certainty "if he feels his affairs are not in order and it is essential that he brings them into order during his remaining time."[15]

ISSUES IN THE MEASUREMENT OF Q

It is commonly recognized that the vNM utility theory is a normative theory and not a descriptive theory.[34] Even Weinstein, one of the pioneers who articulated the concept of QALY, stated in 1986 that: "[e]vidence from

FIGURE 16.4. Alternatives of Delayed Death vs. Immediate Death

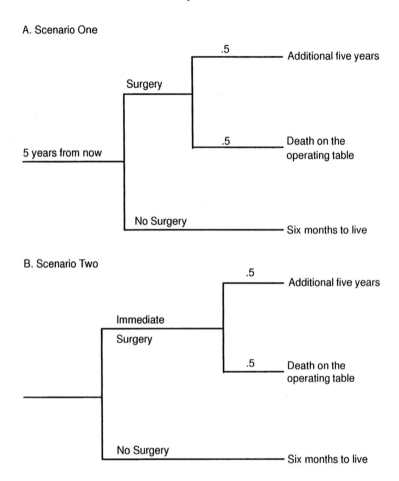

A. Scenario One

B. Scenario Two

clinical studies confirms the findings from psychological experiments, that patients' preferences do not seem to fit the simple model suggested by expected utility theory."[35]

Besides the commonly recognized problems of violation of the three normative axioms of the vNM theory, a bias is introduced in measuring the health status utility due to the use of the SG method with death as a reference health state. The present emphasis on the probability equivalence approach in the SG method for measuring health state utilities is biased toward risk-averse behavior; hence, higher utility scores for a given health state are obtained using the SG technique as compared to VAS or TTO.[36,37] In other words, the present approach results in the underestimation of the utility improvement resulting from the use of a pharmaceutical or any other technology. Fortunately, McCord and de Neufville have proposed an alternate approach–a lottery equivalence approach–that can be considered to reduce the bias using the SG as a tool as shown in Figure 16.5.[36] Basically, the McCord and de Neufville procedure proposes that each alternative be presented as a lottery with death (or the least preferred health state) being a part of both alternatives. According to McCord and de Neufville, utility value–using the approach presented in Figure 16.5–can be calculated as follows: $0.5\ U(HS_i) + 0.5\ U(H_0) = p\ U(H^*) + (1-p)\ U(H_0)$. Thus, $U(HS_i) = 2p$. This approach results in a less risk-averse function and has yet to be tested in the health care setting. The lesson to be learned from McCord and de Neufville's approach is that many approaches can be adopted to obtain utility scores using the SG technique. What is needed is comparison of the results obtained from the manipulation of different parameters involved in the application of the SG technique.

Another question that is still debated in the literature is whose preferences should be incorporated in the QALY calculations used for societal resource allocation decisions. Although it is commonly recognized that Q weights should reflect patient preferences, studies have used weights for different disease states from healthy subjects, health care experts (such as

FIGURE 16.5. The McCord-de Neufville Lottery Equivalence Procedure

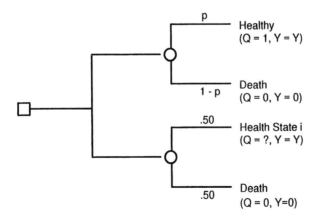

physicians), and community experts. Are these appropriate? It has been shown by various studies that patient preferences differ markedly from those of the other groups.[38,39]

Even if patient preferences are used to arrive at Q weights, the variability of utility scores at the individual level is still a problem. Sackett and Torrance indicate that individual differences among the general public for same health state on the 0-1 utility scale result in a standard deviation of scores of approximately 0.30.[40] This variability is found to be less (0.18) for subjects who were more homogeneous and more knowledgeable about the health state.[31] For example, the mean daily health state utility for home dialysis for the general public was 0.40, and the standard deviation was .42 (derived from SE of .031 and $n = 187$). These results indicate that if we add or subtract one standard deviation from the mean, individual utility scores could range from .02 to .82! While using the standard error of mean at the group level the error of .031 may be tolerable, the variability at the individual level may not be acceptable. Note that in terms of QALY measurement the results could vary 40 years of survival duration, from 31.6 to 0 QALYs (assuming no fate worse than death) for individuals for the same health state of home dialysis. By the way, the same criticism could be leveled against Q weights derived from the use of any quality of life instruments.

In addition to the potential intra-instrument variability of Q values using the SG technique, there is a problem of interinstrument correlations of Q values. A correlation analysis of six measures of Q (SIP, IWB, SG, TTO, VAS, and QWB) used among chronic renal failure patients showed that correlations between these measures ranged from .094 to .519.[41] It was also found that, at the individual level, results varied depending upon the index used. Thus, if one index shows no improvement, treatment may be rejected. But use of another index may suggest that the program be adopted!

This problem of low intercorrelations between instruments measuring Q is further magnified since the arrival of new instruments such as CRBRS and LSI. Although these instruments do not measure utility (i.e., strength of preference under risk), the use of these instruments is justified on the basis of the argument that the QOL weights based "across-program" methods such as QWB and IHQL are less sensitive to changes in elderly people's health states than the program-specific methods, such as CRBRS, which are commonly used in the field of evaluating long-term care.[42] Unfortunately, the weights derived from these "program-specific" methods are not comparable with the utility weights derived from the standard gamble method. Also, many of these new instruments do not reflect the trade-off decisions of the respondents between the quantity and quality of life and hence may not be appropriate weights for QALY calculations needed for resource allocation decisions. When weights used in arriving at QALY calculations are based upon different instruments, the results are not comparable. This is the reason why Weinstein lamented: "A QALY is a QALY is a QALY–or is it"?[43] In other words, are all Qs created equal?

Finally, there are two psychometric theory-based concerns related to the calculations of Q weights for the QALY measurement that require attention. These two issues are the approach used to establish validity of the multiattribute utility theory (MAUT) based weights and the measurement of error term in the vNM theory based utility scores.

Although it is recognized that health is a multidimensional construct, there are only a limited number of QALY studies published using the MAUT-based weights. All of these studies are from the McMaster group. The fundamental problem with the MAUT approach, however, is with the procedure used for establishing the convergent validity of selected attributes. "The present approach of establishing convergent validity for the MAUT procedure using holistic preferences basically tells us that the sum of the parts is correlated with the whole, i.e., overall utility is a function of utility weights derived for selected attributes."[44] Hence, Stillwell and Barron argue that: "If the goal of MAU procedure is to reproduce the holistic weights, then they are a waste of time . . . "[45] In other words, the MAUT weights need to be validated against some external criteria.

Another thorny problem with the vNM utility scores is the underlying assumption that there is no error term in the calculation, or the error, if any, may be due to model specification. However, as von Winterfeldt has noted: "[E]ven after you go through the process of model elimination and selection, you will still have to make up your mind about the possible trade-offs between assessment error and modeling error."[46] Veit and Ware are even more critical and point out that, like holistic designs, the MAU approach "does not provide any way to validate the weights, the utilities, or the model and thus any prescribed outcomes; nor is there any way beyond definition of knowing what the scale properties of the numbers are."[47]

One of the reasons for this frustration is that there are no other assessment procedures available that can be used to compare the MAUT-based weights or utility scores as described by Keeney and Raiffa.[48] After recognizing that there is a need to use more than one method to assess preferences in the context of health care, Mehrez and Gafni concluded: "[I]n spite of this criticism, to the best of our knowledge, no one has yet proposed better tools for revealing individuals' desires."[11] There is an alternative. McCord and Leotsarakos have proposed an alternative method to Keeney and Raiffa's approach for generating multiattribute utility functions.[48,49] Because they used their new technique for generating a bivariate utility function, they called it an "assessment cube," with the third dimension representing the range of probabilities. On the basis of the results obtained using the assessment cube, they concluded that "the utility functions do, indeed, depend on the values of the assessment parameters and that the 'pricing out' method can lead to invalid results."[49]

ISSUES IN THE MEASUREMENT OF QALY

Besides the issues involved in the measurement of the Y and Q components of QALY, there are some inherent problems in the measurement of QALYs for representing individual preferences. Figure 16.6 depicts the problem of preference reversal as described by Gafni and Mehrez.[11] Figure 6 shows that an individual assigns a utility value of .65 to health state A with a five-year survival and a utility value of .5 to a ten-year survival in health state B. Hence, the utility scores based on the vNM theory seem to indicate that this individual prefers health state A to health state B. However, the QALYs associated with health state A are 3.25 (.65 × 5) years, whereas he or she receives five QALYs (.5 × 10 years) from health state B, reflecting that he or she has a preference for health state B. One reason for this preference reversal is that QALY is a utility weighted index, and it is alleged to be a utility function. However, this is true only under very restrictive assumptions that are beyond those required by the vNM theory. It should be noted that this particular example used by Gafni and colleagues has been criticized by Johannesson, Pliskin, and Weinstein.[50] While Mehrez and Gafni recognize why there may be confusion in the interpretation of this example, their hypothetical examples were created to alert the reader to the possibilities of preference reversal due to differences in the assumptions underlying the measurement of utility scores based on the vNM theory and the QALY scores which require additional assumptions beyond those required for the vNM theory.[51]

A more serious problem with using the QALY as a measure to select a therapeutic intervention is that it is biased against interventions designed to improve quality of life due to acute conditions for short duration. For example, consider a cancer patient on chemotherapy who experiences severe episodes of emesis for 24 hours after each round of therapy. The patient receives therapy six times during a year. The patient assigns the utility value of 0.60 to his or her health state with cancer, but 0.00 (i.e., death) for the 24-hour emesis period after each treatment. Let us also assume that a drug is invented that completely avoids the episodes of emesis after each treatment. The value of the drug in terms of QALY is: .60 × 6/365 = .0098 QALY. This drug has provided an insignificant improvement in QALY, so it will have a low priority because the CUA ratio will be prohibitive for this drug. However, because we know that patients are willing to pay significant amounts to cure (or avoid) acute conditions of short duration, it can be concluded that the technique used to arrive at QALY is highly restrictive and may result in undervaluing the contribution of a health care technology and misallocation of resources.

There are two major reasons for the low QALY values associated with acute conditions of short-term duration. First, contemporary utility theory is designed to measure "utility in use" or utility based on experience, and it does not take into account "anticipated utility (or disutility)" of a health state. Second, the risk neutrality assumption restricts the conversion of ill

FIGURE 16.6. Preference Reversal Problem

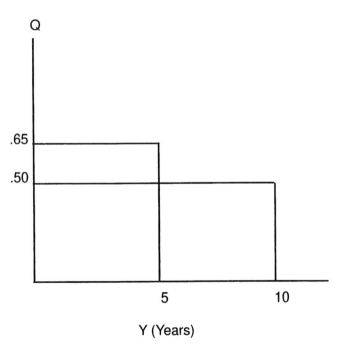

Y (Years)

health time into "full health" time in a linear fashion only, resulting in an additive formula for calculating the lifetime health profile.[52] The net effect of this inherent limitation of the QALY method is that it underestimates the potential value of health care technologies for acute conditions.

Even for a chronic condition, the linearity assumption results in over-valuation of the QALYs associated with the current health state and, hence, underestimation of the potential value of health care technologies. Let's look at an example. Assume that for an individual, survival time is 40 life years and that the utility for the current health state is 0.75. For this individual, the QALY is 30 years under the risk neutrality assumption, and it is only 15 years (derived from the indifference curve) under the risk-averse assumption (Figure 16.7).

The empirical justification for the risk neutrality assumption is based on the original published report by Pliskin, Shepard, and Weinstein.[32] They reported the results of two studies. The first study consisted of ten respondents (three physicians and the rest were economists and statisticians). They found that five respondents were risk neutral, three respondents demonstrated risk-seeking attitude, and two respondents demonstrated risk aversion in terms of their willingness to sacrifice longevity for relief from angina pain. While they realized that a linear function may be "unacceptably restrictive," they concluded that "when remaining longevity and health status are the overriding consequences, it is helpful to take advan-

FIGURE 16.7. Impact of Risk Neutrality and Risk Aversion on the QALY Calculations

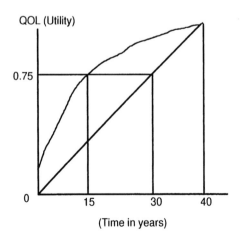

(Time in years)

tage of the flexibility offered by the family of constant proportional risk posture utility function for remaining life years."[32] They did not report the distribution of the attitude toward risk of the Coronary Artery Bypass Graft (CABG) patients in the study in their 1980 article. Loomes and McKenzie provide additional evidence indicating that the linearity assumption is not appropriate for health care decisions.[53]

Loomes and McKenzie also question the constant proportional trade-off assumption required for the QALY calculations.[53] They question this assumption based on their review of several studies. McNeil, Weichselbaum, and Pauker, in their study of laryngeal cancer, also found that their study subjects were willing to accept some decrease in long-term (25 years) survival with impaired speech to maintain normal speech, but very few subjects were willing to accept any decrease when survival with impaired speech was less than five years.[54] This pattern clearly violates the constant proportional trade-off assumption. In effect, the results of this study could be interpreted to violate the mutual independence assumption also.

ALTERNATIVE APPROACHES

Although there are many unresolved issues with the current approaches used in the measurement of QALY in its present form, there is still a great deal of interest in developing measures of output of health care programs that combine the impact on both quantity and quality of life of those affected by the programs. To address this need, a new generation of alternative approaches has emerged.

Healthy years equivalent (HYE) is one approach that has been recently proposed by Mehrez and Gafni as an alternative to QALY.[11] The originators of this approach claim that numbers represented by the current QALY measures do not represent the "real" preferences of the patients because when we use QALYs we must assume that the number we use to represent the quality of life for a particular health state is independent of the time spent in the state and that patients are risk neutral. The HYEs, on the other hand, "fully represent patients' (or other individuals') preferences, stemming from the way they are calculated from each individual's utility function. In other words, unlike the situation with QALYs, assumptions are not needed to equate the HYE with utility."[11] These claims have generated a heated debate in the literature from the defenders of both concepts. Regardless of the point-and-counterpoint debate about these two concepts, it is obvious that the measurement procedure for obtaining the HYE values is more complex and perhaps more costly because it requires asking two lottery questions compared with the one lottery question needed to obtain weights for calculating QALYs. Unfortunately, there are not many studies yet available comparing the results obtained from the use of the HYE approach and the QALY approach.

Miyamoto and Eraker have proposed another approach based upon the "generic utility theory," which weakens some of the "strong" assumptions of the vNM theory.[55] They indicate that a multiplicative utility function of $U(Y,Q) = F(Y) \cdot G(Q)$ is supportable. Unfortunately, both the theory and scaling of utility functions for the given outcome domain are more complicated in the generic utility framework than under the expected utility (EU) theory.

Another approach is to recognize that there is no *single* QALY formula. There are many bivariate functions for QALY, and depending upon which underlying assumption holds for a given study, the appropriate QALY function may be different. Technically speaking, there are three major assumptions for deriving a bivariate utility function: (A) utility independence (including mutual utility independence); (B) constant proportional trade-off; and (C) risk neutrality in life years. If only the first two assumptions hold and the assumption of risk neutrality does not hold, then power or logarithmic functions may be more appropriate. If only the assumption of mutual independence holds (which is viewed by Pliskin and colleagues as very likely) in health care situations, then the function will be as follows:

$$U(Q,Y) = a \cdot U(Q) + b \cdot U(Y) + (1 - a - b) \cdot U(Q) \cdot U(Y)$$

where a and b are constants. This is a quasi additive form. But, it should be noted that it is still different from the present approach used in the literature, which states that $QALY = U(Q) \cdot Y$. It is interesting to note that if the assumption of value independence holds, then $a + b = 1$, and the above equation provides us with an additive function. However, this is very unlikely for a bivariate utility function consisting of quantity and quality of life.

There is a third possibility that has not been recognized in the health care literature. The bivariate utility function could be defined as follows:

$$U(Q,Y) = [\alpha + \beta \cdot U(Q)] [\gamma + \delta \cdot U(Y)].$$

In fact, there are many other utility functions that can be considered assuming that: (1) neither attribute is utility independent of the other; (2) only Y is utility independent of Q; and (3) only Q is utility independent of Y.[48]

CONCLUSIONS

There are many other issues related to the QALY measure that are not considered in this chapter. Some of these issues are: measurement of QALYs for patients encountering multiple disease states and multiple therapies, accounting for the intra- and interindividual "spillover" effects in the measurement of QALYs, implications of the relationship between health and other domains of life for the measurement of QALYs, and above all, the question of link between preferences determined from judgmental responses and the final choice. Regardless of many of these unresolved issues, it is clear that the technology of measuring QALYs is still in its evolutionary stage. Hence, at this time, QALY, if used, should be viewed as only one more input that is available to assist decision makers in making resource allocation decisions.

One must also recognize that regardless how carefully "real" preferences are measured, they are not choices, nor do they always materialize in choices. Hence, decisions to allocate resources based on preference measures alone require faith in inferential leaps.

Even in terms of measurement of preferences for health outcomes, the current debate clearly indicates that QALYs may not represent "real" preferences and may be only another numerical abstraction of preferences. Fryback recently concluded: "This debate has underlined, in public, the fact that any measure of health care output combining quality of life and length of life is a fiction. And, as a consequence, the whole cost-effectiveness enterprise may be built on sand."[1] The fact still remains, however, that we must devise some "fiction" that is useful for resource allocation decisions because decisions will be made regardless of the debate about which measure of health care output is methodologically sound. The challenge, then, as Weinstein puts it, "is to understand more about what patients, and potential patients, value about health care. It is clearly naive to assume that patients wish to maximize quality-adjusted life expectancy. But what do they wish to maximize? The more we learn about this question, the more acceptable will be the prescriptive models that seek to guide allocations of medical resources."[35]

REFERENCES

1. Fryback DG. QALYs, HYEs, and the loss of innocence. Med Decis Making 1993;13:271-2.

2. Mishan EJ. Cost benefit analysis. London: George Allen and Unwin, 1975.

3. Mooney GH. The valuation of human life. London: Macmillan, 1977.

4. Drummond MF, Stoddart GL, Torrance GW. Methods for the economic evaluation of health care programmes. Oxford: Oxford University Press, 1987.

5. Torrance GW, Feeny D. Utilities and quality-adjusted life years. Int J Technol Assess Health Care 1989;5:559-75.

6. Weinstein MC, Stason WB. Foundations of cost-effectiveness analysis for health and medical practices. N Engl J Med 1977;296:716-21.

7. Patrick DL, Bush JW, Chen MM. Methods for measuring levels of well-being for a health status index. Health Serv Res 1973;8:228-45.

8. Bush JW, Chen M, Patrick DL. Cost-effectiveness using a health status index: analysis of the New York State PKU screening program. In: Berg R, ed. Health status index. Chicago: Hospital Research and Educational Trust, 1983:172-208.

9. Chen M, Bush JW, Patrick DL. Social indicators for health planning and policy analysis. Policy Sci 1975;6:71-89.

10. Kaplan RM, Bush JW. Health related quality of life measurement for evaluation research and policy analysis. Health Psychol 1982;1:61-80.

11. Mehrez A, Gafni A. Quality-adjusted life years, utility theory, and healthy-years equivalents. Med Decis Making 1989;9:142-9.

12. Mehrez A, Gafni A. The healthy-years equivalents: how to measure them using the standard gamble approach. Med Decis Making 1991;11:140-6.

13. Commonwealth of Australia. Draft guidelines for the pharmaceutical industry on preparation of submission to the Pharmaceutical Benefits Advisory Committee: including submissions involving economic analysis. Canberra, Australia: Department of Health, Housing, and Community Services, 1990.

14. Ontario Ministry of Health. Guidelines for preparation of economic analysis to be included in submission to Drug Program Branch for listing in the Ontario Drug Benefit Formulary. Draft 6. Toronto, Ontario: Drug Programs Branch, Ministry of Health, 1991.

15. U.S. Department of Health and Human Services. Public Health Service. Office of Disease Prevention and Health Promotion. Kamlet MS. A framework for cost-utility analysis of government health care programs. Washington, DC: U.S. Department of Health and Human Services, 1992.

16. von Neumann J, Morgenstern O. Theory of games and economic behavior. 2nd ed. Princeton, NJ: Princeton University Press, 1947.

17. von Winterfeldt D, Edwards W. Decision analysis and behavioral research. New York: Cambridge University Press, 1986.

18. Gafni A. The standard gamble method: what is being measured and how it is interpreted. Health Serv Res 1994;29:207-24.

19. Thompson MS. Willingness to pay and accept risks to cure chronic disease. Am J Public Health 1986;76:392-6.

20. Reardon G, Pathak DS. Assessment of a contingent valuation technique with utility estimation models. J Res Pharm Econ 1989;1(3):67-89.

21. Mitchell RC, Carson RT. Using surveys to value public goods: the contingent valuation method. Washington, DC: Resources for the Future, 1989.

22. Fisher GW. Utility models for multiple objective decisions: do they accurately represent human preferences? Decis Sci 1979;10:451-79.

23. Veit CT, Rose BJ, Ware JE Jr. Effects of physical and mental health on health-state preferences. Med Care 1982;20:386-401.

24. Froberg DG, Kane RL. Methodology for measuring health-state preferences–I: Measurement strategies. J Clin Epidemiol 1989;42:345-54.

25. Kaplan RM, Bush JW. Health related quality of life measurement for evaluation research and policy analysis. Health Psychol 1982;1:61-80.

26. Wilkins D, Masiah T, Jolley DJ. Changes in behavioral characteristics of elderly populations of local authority homes and long stay hospital wards, 1976-7. Br Med J 1978;2:1274-6.

27. Luker KA. Measuring life satisfaction in an elderly female population. J Adv Nurs 1979;4:503-11.

28. Rosser R, Allison R, Butler C et al. The Index of Health-Related Quality of Life (IHQL): a new tool for audit and cost-per-QALY analysis. In: Walker SR, Rosser RM, eds. Quality of life assessment: key issues in the 1990s. Boston: Kluwer Academic Publishers, 1993:179-84.

29. Rosser R, Sintonen H. The EuroQuol quality of life project. In: Walker SR, Rosser RM, eds. Quality of life assessment: key issues in the 1990s. Boston: Kluwer Academic Publishers, 1993:197-200.

30. Feeny D, Torrance GW, Goldsmith CH, et al. A multi-attribute approach to health status. McMaster University Centre for Health Economics and Policy Analysis Working Paper Series (Paper 94-5), February, 1994.

31. Torrance GW. Measurement of health state utilities for economic appraisal: a review. J Health Econ 1986;5:1-30.

32. Pliskin JS, Shepard DS, Weinstein MC. Utility functions for life years and health status. Operations Res 1980;28:206-24.

33. Brock D. Quality of life measures in health care and medical ethics. In: Nussbaum MC, Sen A, eds. The quality of life. Oxford: Clarendon Press, 1993:95-132.

34. Schoemaker PJH. The expected utility model: its variants, purposes, evidence and limitations. J Econ Lit 1982;20:529-63.

35. Weinstein MC. Risky choices in medical decision making: a survey. Geneva Papers Risk Insurance 1986;11:197-216.

36. McCord M, de Neufville R. Lottery equivalents: reduction of the certainty effect problem in utility assessment. Manage Sci 1986;32(1):56-60.

37. Torrance GW, Sackett DL, Thomas WH. Utility maximization model for evaluation of health care programs. Health Serv Res 1972;7:118-33.

38. Jachuck SJ, Brierley H, Willcox PM. The effect of hypotensive drugs on the quality of life. J R Coll Gen Pract 1982;32:103-5.

39. Boyd NF, Sutherland HJ, Heasman KZ, Tritchler DL, Cummings BJ. Whose utilities for decision analysis. Med Decis Making 1990;10:58-67.

40. Sackett DL, Torrance GW. The utility of different health states as perceived by the general public. J Chronic Dis 1978;31:697-704.

41. Hornberger JC, Redelmeier DA, Peterson J. Variability among methods to assess patients' well-being and consequent effect on a cost-effectiveness analysis. J Clin Epidemiol 1992;45:505-12.

42. Donaldson C, Atkinson A, Bond J. Should QALYs be programme-specific? J Health Econ 1988;7:239-57.

43. Weinstein MC. A QALY is a QALY is a QALY–or is it? J Health Econ 1988;7:289-90.

44. Pathak DS, MacKeigan LD. Assessment of quality of life and health status: selected observations. J Res Pharm Econ 1992;4(4):31-52.

45. Stillwell WG, Barron FH. Evaluating credit applications: a validation of multiattribute utility weight elicitation techniques. Organiz Behav Hum Perform 1983;32:87-103.

46. von Winterfeldt D. An overview, integration, and evaluation of utility theory for decision analysis. SSRI Research Report, 75-9. Los Angeles, CA: University of Southern California, 1975.

47. Veit CT, Ware JE Jr. Measuring health and health care outcomes: issues and recommendations. In: Kane RL, Kane RA, eds. Values and long term care. Lexington, MA: Lexington Books, 1982.

48. Keeney RL, Raiffa H. Decision with multiple objectives: preferences and value tradeoffs. New York: John Wiley & Sons, 1976.

49. McCord MR, Leotsarakos C. Investigating utility and value functions with an "assessment cube." In: Munier BR, ed. Risk, decision and rationality. Norwell, MA: D. Reidel Publishing Company, 1988:59-75.

50. Johannesson M, Pliskin JS, Weinstein M. Are healthy-years equivalent an improvement over quality-adjusted life years? Med Decis Making 1993;13:281-6.

51. Mehrez A, Gafni A. Healthy-years equivalents versus quality-adjusted life years: in pursuit of progress. Med Decis Making 1993;13:287-92.

52. Mehrez A, Gafni A. Preference based outcome measures for economic evaluation of drug interventions: quality adjusted life years (QALYs) versus healthy years equivalents (HYEs). Pharmacoeconomics 1992;1:338-45.

53. Loomes G, McKenzie L. The use of QALYs in health care decision making. Soc Sci Med 1989;28:299-308.

54. McNeil BJ, Weichselbaum R, Pauker SG. Fallacy of five year survival in living cancer. N Engl J Med 1978;229:1397-401.

55. Miyamoto JM, Eraker SA. A multiplicative model of the utility of survival duration and health quality. J Exp Psychol 1988;117(1):3-20.

PART IV:
PRICES AND PRICING

This section begins with an international comparison of public pricing policies by Huttin. It is followed by a description of some of the practical effects of policy, in this case Medicaid, in the chapter by Kotzan and Carroll. Economics and the practicing physician are the subject of chapters by Kolassa, by Miller et al., and by Kotzan, Perri, and Wolfgang. The section concludes with a chapter by Jackson, containing the description of theoretical models that might explain pricing strategies and perspectives on the U. S. environment.

Chapter 17

Price Control Policies in the Pharmaceutical Industry: A Selection of Case Studies

Christine Huttin

INTRODUCTION

Pharmaceutical price control regulation is a major topic of interest in the EEC (European Economic Community), the U.S., and Japan. Common economic pressures push each government at the national, federal, or EEC level to develop different price control strategies.

This chapter provides an analytical view of alternative drug policy models in use in different countries. Price legislation is under considerable debate since there is no evidence of absolute advantages of liberal frameworks versus more administrative forms of control. This chapter compares various forms of legislation used to control prescription drug prices and points out the interesting features of more highly regulated markets that could be useful to U.S. policymakers in devising price policy tools.

THE U.K.: A MANAGED COMPETITION

The concept of managed competition is developed by Einthoven, especially in health care services. The role of insurance companies in particular

This information was presented at an International Business Communications conference, "Price Control & Pricing Strategies: Pharmaceutical & Biotechnology Companies," held in Washington, DC, February 28-March 1, 1991.

Previously published in *Journal of Research in Pharmaceutical Economics*, Vol. 4(3), 1992.

leads the major purchasers of services to devise monitoring schemes since competitive behaviors such as sensitivity to prices or access to information are largely imperfect.

The case of the U.K. in the area of health care is interesting since the introduction of competition in the market for health services lead to a managed competition within the National Health Service. In particular, the National Health Service combines competition with a public insurance system for the coverage of pharmaceutical costs. In that respect, it may give U.S. policymakers some ideas about the way to manage competition starting from an administrative environment. This paper describes the major pattern of the price control strategy in the U.K., the major changes that are introduced with the implementation of the medical control system, and some conclusions on the impact of firms' strategies.

The National Health Service has existed since 1948 in the U.K., and the administration intervenes both on the supply side and on the demand side of health services. For pharmaceutical companies, three main drug policy tools exist: the Prescription Price Regulation Scheme (PPRS), the drug lists, and the drug tariff.

The PPRS was begun in 1957. It is a collective agreement regularly discussed with the profession. It is discriminatory since each manufacturer negotiates individually with the U.K. administration. Within the scheme, an upper limit is set on the manufacturers' profit, on a maximum level of promotion expenditures, and on a level of research and development (R&D) expenditures.

This price control mechanism has been quite successful, and the industry has, over time, kept a reasonable price level, a high level of R&D expenditures, and a strong international diffusion of products (Tables 17.1 and 17.2). The contribution of G. Thomas on the international competitiveness of pharmaceutical products shows a comparable rate of diffusion for the U.S. and the U.K. The U.K. system's cost of delivery–another performance criterion–is the lowest of the four drug systems under study.[1]

At a time when the U.S. is devising a new policy in the area of price control with the new Medicaid legislation, we can point out some of the major aspects of the PPRS success: the low number of the key actors in the industry, which allows a "fair" setting of the rules for the players; a long tradition of cooperation and discussion with the Department of Health; and the size of the market, which makes it manageable for an administration. It would probably be more difficult for U.S. policymakers, even for limited segments such as Medicaid, to organize such collective agreements, or at least such agreements should be decentralized at the level of the various state administrations. Moreover, it supposes a business culture

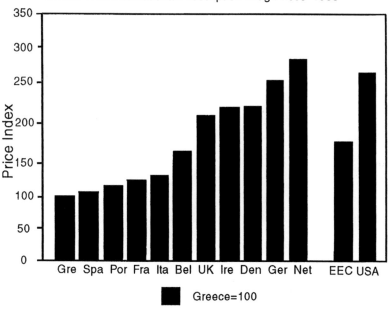

TABLE 17.1. International Prescription Drug Prices–1988*

■ Greece=100

*U.S. versus EEC drug prices of 25 identical drug products
Source: *Farmindustria*

where firms are used to discussion with the Department of Health on a regular basis to exchange strategic information.

Another interesting characteristic of the price regulation in the U.K. that can be relevant to the U.S. is the existence of the drug tariff and the regulation of generic competition. Generics were first introduced in hospitals and are now widespread in the outpatient prescription drug market (estimated at about 15% of the U.K. market). Generics were encouraged by the U.K. government as a tool to promote price competition with brand name products. Before 1975, there was only the PPRS legislation for the pharmaceutical manufacturers. However, the generic producers were not really taking part in the agreement because they were too small. The Department of Health could not agree with such players on a "fair" conduct. The administration has decided to take the generic drugs out of the PPRS and to devise a specific legislation for them. The aim of such legislation is to set a level of reimbursement for the generic products.

Drug tariff prices are determined with the major players in the generic industry. These players can be manufacturers, but they can also be the

TABLE 17.2. Diffusion Range of Product Discoveries

N	USA	THE U.K.	JAPAN	GERMANY	FRANCE
2	28%	25%	77%	49%	60%
3-5	28%	24%	14%	33%	26%
6-12	58%	44%	9%	18%	13%

N: number of countries
Source: G. Thomas, 1989

major wholesalers, such as Vestric and Unichem. The objective of such a regulation is to guarantee a level of remuneration for all retailers. In the U.K., if the coverage for drugs were determined at the level of the lowest generic price, some pharmacists' margins would be sharply cut because they do not have access to the same commercial conditions as the major chains in the U.K. This kind of legislation limits price competition; however, it does not impede a sharp decline of both prices and market sales for the incumbent firms.

Another specificity of the U.K. drug price regulation is a rebate system that allows the Department of Health, through a regular survey, to take a percentage of the discount amounts the retailers can get on the ingredient costs of the drugs. Again, such a regulation appears very similar to the new Medicaid legislation. Major differences, however, are that the survey is managed directly by the Department of Health and that the level of the rebates is on a national basis, not negotiated with each firm.

Finally, the last element of the U.K. price control policy that could be useful for policymakers in the U.S. concerns the latest legislation for medical control. Such reforms and the kinds of informative instruments that are devised could be useful for managed care organizations in the U.S., which also have access to all types of information, especially on prices and costs, and which have registered doctors and pharmacists.

The huge reform of the National Health Service undertaken in the U.K. includes major changes for the organization of primary care. The main principles of the reforms have been to increase the role of local authorities, to introduce business managers at the national level for devising the new health policy, and to give more autonomy to individuals–in particular, the physicians–to manage health care services. Concerning the drug policy, the reform will mainly change the relations between doctors and their local administrative unit, the Family Health Authority (FHA). First, the computerization of the information on each prescription will be delivered regularly to each doctor. The information delivered is illustrated in Table 17.3. Dr. Sample's practice, in this example, is clearly over the Family Practitioner Committee Average (FPCA) by more than 84%. Such an indicator will be used in the future by medical advisers recruited in each FPC to discuss with each general practitioner the reasons for overprescribing and also to try to influence the practitioner's behavior. The idea of the change, therefore, is not only to deliver the information to each doctor but also to deliver it to each Family Health Authority (FHA is the new name for FPC), which will analyze the information, set its own standards, and devise its own policy to influence doctors' prescribing. The public policy change implies, then, a decentralization of decision at the level of local authority.

What lessons can be useful for the U.S.? First, the way the information is structured and the type of information that is delivered to each doctor illustrate major similarities between the FHA and the formularies used in health maintenance organizations (HMOs). However, FHAs can provide an empirical assessment on the whole population of the U.K., contrary to HMOs, where often adverse selection problems can bias the representativity of the behavioral changes observed. The various issues that are already discussed by the industry can provide interesting reactions on the system. Such a use of information by the U.K. administration on drug prescription creates a new institutional environment, and for firms, it is a source of knowledge about the competition for general practitioners. Firms are then very concerned about the kind of information that will be delivered to doctors. The PACT information can be misleading if measurement problems impede a fair representation of effective prescribing behavior. When the government was just delivering information without budget ideas, firms were not so active in trying to intervene in the process of change.

With the budget idea, the PACT information becomes crucial. Firms seem ready to cooperate and share part of their knowledge on doctors' behavior. They are also very concerned by the management problem that the Department of Health will face in monitoring control of the prescription bill. In particular, can one or two pharmacist facilitators easily manage the number of transactions they will have with doctors? In case of lack of resources, firms question the kind of decisions that managers from FHAs will make. They already have various possibilities for exerting subtle pressures on doctors. For instance, they can refuse to pay for a doctor's attendance at a conference abroad, or they can reduce the budget for modernizing the practice premises.

Another response of firms to such a change is to consider the new marketing target they will face with medical advisers who are recruited in the FHAs.

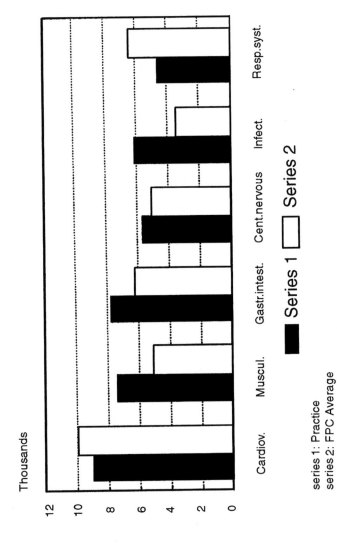

TABLE 17.3. Prescription Pricing: Prescribing Information Level 2

Thousands

Series 1 ■ Series 2 □

series 1: Practice
series 2: FPC Average

Firms are using their representative networks to build information on the population of medical advisers and model a new marketing policy. Another major change for the firms may be easier access to cheap versions of prescription drugs. This influential scheme for changing doctors' behavior, focused on cost issues, may accelerate a great deal the substitution of generics. The U.K. industry leaders are facing major changes now or in the coming years because of patent expiration (e.g., drugs such as Amoxil® for Beecham, Tagamet® for Glaxo).

The role of pharmacists and medical advisers is going to be essential in successful implementation of the scheme. Firms will be very active in their attempts to countervail the information provided by the FHAs. Alternative sources of analysis and delivery of information to doctors may emerge, for instance, through the Royal College of General Practitioners. Such a use of strategic information will probably lead to major reshuffling of bargaining positions among key actors, and from an international perspective, it will be a key experience for drug policymakers to follow.

THE GERMAN PRESCRIPTION DRUG SYSTEM

Germany has known a major reform from 1989 since the last Blum Plan. Before the *Festbetrager,* Germany was as well-known as the U.S. for its philosophy of the liberal market. Manufacturers, in particular, were free to set their own price, and the insurance funds were ready to pay the published wholesale price and to pay for the pharmacist's services.

The wholesale system in Germany is under the control of full-range wholesalers who agree to deliver most of the drugs available on the prescription drug market. There is a maximum decreasing margin system, which limits the price level at this stage and impedes potential effects of collusion on prices.

Contrary to the French retailing system, competition among pharmacists exists because there is no limitation of entry and, since 1958, any pharmacist is free to set up a pharmacy. However, if there is a free entry, the remuneration of pharmacies is highly dependent on the levels of margins fixed by the Ministry of Health.

German patients contribute to price control through a copayment system. The patient pays three deutsche marks per prescription when he or she buys the drug. This copayment system on prescription drugs has, however, changed with the introduction of the *Festbetrager* scheme. For such price regulated drugs, the patient is not contributing anymore, which means that he or she has a strong incentive to ask the doctor to substitute a drug that is covered by the *Festbetrager* for any drug outside the system. German physicians are very tightly controlled in their practice and remuneration. However, in prescribing policy, the German medical profession is less controlled. There is an ex post facto control on prescription volume, and positive or negative incentives exist to limit prescription volume. Insurance funds have also recruited pharmacists to influence doctors' prescribing behavior. However, such tools remain at a limited scale (not more than 60 pharmacists, for instance, employed by the insurance funds) and do not represent major components of the German price policy. This could, however, be in question in the future since negotiations are taking place with the medical profession to reinforce the rationalizing of prescriptions.

Finally, the federal organization of the health system in Germany has generated various insurance funds. However, they do not compete on the level of reimbursement, which is unique for prescription drugs.

The most interesting lesson from the German system lies in the huge change of policy with the implementation of an administrative price control. In 1989, a major reform took place with the implementation of the *Festbetrager* system. Several factors can explain it:

- There is a strong increase in German sales (both in volume and in value) (Table 17.4).
- German prices are the highest in the EEC.
- Large price differences exist among major drugs with the same ingredients.
- There are changes in the behavior of the medical profession because it realizes that its share of health care expenditures is declining in comparison with expenditures for pharmaceuticals.

The reform adopted by Germany aimed to develop some methodology for clustering drugs into three classes:

Class I   All drugs with identical ingredients.
Class II   All drugs with different ingredients that have pharmacologically therapeutically comparable active substances.
Class III   All drugs that have pharmacologically therapeutically comparable effects, especially drug combinations.

After the grouping of the drugs, the system adopted consists in developing a methodology to represent the pricing strategies of the firms. The way to do this is to represent through a regression model the various drugs in the same group, but present in different packaging and dosage forms. An example, oxazepam, is given in Table 17.5. This regression line does not

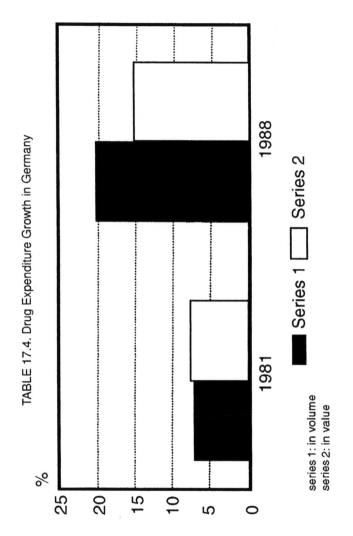

TABLE 17.4. Drug Expenditure Growth in Germany

series 1: in volume
series 2: in value

■ Series 1   □ Series 2

provide a figure for the prices, but it provides the combination linking various dosage forms and packages for drugs in the same group.

The final decision on the level of the reimbursement price is, however, made independently by a board composed by the insurance funds. The chosen reference price combines one of the lowest level with the need to cover the entire market at such prices. Generally, the reference price represents a substantial cut from the average prices before the implementation of the scheme.

What are the lessons that can be useful at this stage to U.S. policymakers? First, it is interesting to understand the firms' pricing responses and why what happens in such a liberal environment is different from what seems to happen with the new Medicaid legislation in the U.S.

The major response to the implementation of the control system is that the firms cut their prices. In most cases, for the drugs in Group I, firms have decided to align their prices at the level of the *Festbetrager,* which can represent a cut in prices ranging from 40% to 60% of initial prices. The major difference from the U.S. case is the bargaining power of the German insurance funds. Even if there are several insurance funds, the funds agree on a unique reference price system and fix a price for all markets for the various groups of drugs (Class I drugs represent 35% of the German drug market).

Two other responses–from the patient and from the medical profession–

TABLE 17.5. Explanation of the German Festbetrager System

THE CASE OF OXAZEPAM

Value	10MG	15MG	20MG	50MG
Package size	20 50 100	10 20 50	10 20 50	10 20 50
Praxiten Adumbran	15	6 11 26		14 25 47
Sigacalm	10 17			6 11 22
Uskan	4 8		4 7 14	
Oxazepam	3 6 13			9 18

Source: Wido, abstract of the German Festbetrager System

are also interesting. The physician has to inform the patient about the change of policy. If the drug is not covered by the *Festbetrager,* the patient will have to pay the three deutsche marks per item (as before the reform). If the drug is under the scheme, the patient will not pay anything. It is interesting to see that the general behavior of the medical profession has been to prescribe drugs covered by the *Festbetrager* to avoid problems with the patient. However, this is a transitional step because beginning in 1992, the patient will have to contribute a fixed amount of 15% per prescription.

The success of the scheme from the short-term insurance view can be explained by a number of factors. Politically, there was a coalition of interests among the strongest actors implementing the change: the insurance funds, the Ministry of Labor, and, to a lesser extent, the medical profession. These groups were interested in finding ways to contain drug prices and to avoid an increase in social contributions in comparison with the level of wages. The Board of Sickness Funds is a key actor in determining prices. The German administration does not take part in the decision process. However, the *Bundeskartelamt* plays a role in controlling the decision process on price fixing.

The long-term impact can, however, be relevant for all players, especially the U.S. administration. First, the global impact of prices seems to be tied to the average German price index. However, even if the rest of the market is to be submitted to such a price control, the new drugs will not be covered by the system and the German administration is faced with the same problem as U.S. policymakers concerning the price level of originator drugs.

A perverse effect of the legislation has been the creation of mistrust in the public and the medical profession in the face of firms cutting their prices on such a scale. In the long run, it will be more difficult to develop coalitions interested not only in the cost of drugs but also in the value for the country of keeping the German pharmaceutical industry based in Germany.

THE JAPANESE PRICE REGULATION SYSTEM: AN INFLATIONARY SYSTEM

The Japanese system is one of the most expensive systems, accounting for almost 30% of health insurance expenditures (versus about 10% in Western countries). As in Europe, pharmaceutical companies' actual sales depend on reimbursement under the National Health Insurance (NHI) scheme, which covers the entire Japanese population. The reimbursement prices are determined by the Ministry of Health and Welfare (MHW) according to guidelines established by the Central Social Insurance Medical

Council. A prescription drug cannot be marketed unless its price is listed under the NHI system.

The distinguishing feature of the Japanese system lies in the central role of physicians, who not only prescribe, but also sell drugs. Doctors can benefit from a margin that is the difference between the NHI price and their purchase price. This source of income for doctors is a major incentive for Japanese firms to cut their prices. Low prices will entice physicians to select a company's products and so increase the physicians' margins and income. Contrary to the system in European countries, the prescribing patterns of Japanese physicians are not controlled by government. According to the principle of professional freedom of physicians, neither the government nor other third parties interferes in the physician-patient relationship.

For the practitioner, the margin he or she can get on pharmaceutical prices provides a profitable and secure source of revenue. Such a price policy is an incentive for physicians to select products not only for their therapeutic efficiency, but also for their high profit. So, the pricing system provides a strong incentive to expand the Japanese pharmaceutical market for the financial benefit of the physician.

Because the way the physician is remunerated is a central element of the price control policy of the Japanese government, it is important to examine it carefully to understand the implications for drugs. The Japanese physician is basically reimbursed on a fee-for-service basis, and fees are determined by government in consultation with the medical association and other interest groups such as the consumer. However, it is a regulated point system. Two basic components are taken into account: the skill component and the material component. The skill point measures the technical difficulty of medical treatment, and the material point measures the cost of materials, such as drugs. One of the major problems with the system for drugs is that evaluation of the cost and the value of new development is difficult. This is done by a committee of representatives from government, the medical profession, and consumers, but the committee cannot keep up with the pace of the changes. In many cases, it does not assign points quickly enough, or it assigns points that are much lower than what they should be. This system is an inflationary one, since under the point system, physicians have no control over prices, but they have discretion over the use of drugs. The combination of these two characteristics of the system has resulted in excessive use of drugs.

Usually physicians do not compete on prices, but they often compete for patients by advertising or by quality competition. Moreover, a third factor that explains the excessive cost of drugs is that the physician can use his discretionary power over drug prescribing for recovering the high cost of equipment. This practice of generating revenues from prescribing drugs occurs especially when the skill point is set at such a low level that physicians have to recover revenues by cross subsidizing the skill point with the material point.

Other actors in the drug system in Japan are not key actors for price control mechanisms. Wholesalers can compete on margins and rebates. The reimbursement price of the NHI does not prevent them from competing with each other. The outpatient prescription market is dispensed by pharmacies mainly managed by medical groups, since it is the physicians who deliver the drugs. There are a limited number of independent pharmacies in Japan (doctors and hospitals dispensing 90% of all ethical drugs sold). They mainly sell over-the-counter (OTC) products.

Japanese patients contribute via the public third-party system. However, as in France, there are complementary and voluntary insurance schemes that cover the share not covered by the NHI. Fees paid directly by the patient usually vary from 30% to 50%.

Facing such an inflationary system, what are the measures undertaken by the Japanese government? The Japanese government controls prices by drastically cutting the NHI reimbursed prices. For instance, between 1980 and 1986, prices have been cut by 44%. Such measures hurt both manufacturers and physicians' margins. Official cuts in drug prices have mainly hit the antibiotics, which are heavily prescribed and the drugs most highly discounted to doctors. Despite these cuts, however, and chiefly prior to the 1980s, generous reimbursement rates in Japan served as an indirect support mechanism for the domestic industry. Even if the price control policy of the Japanese government is to cut prices, the Ministry of Health and Welfare favors innovative products by giving them more favorable reimbursement prices.

The major concern for U.S. policymakers is to foresee the impact of Japanese policy on the strategic responses of Japanese companies. The fixing of a high reimbursement price and the incentive this high price represents for the producer and the physician have encouraged expansion of the pharmaceutical market in Japan and favored the domestic producers. For a long time, the Japanese firms have not been pushed to export, and contrary to many other sectors, the pharmaceutical industry is an area where they are not so visible in international markets.

Another component of the Japanese drug price policy has been differentiation of reimbursement levels according to therapeutic segments the government wished to promote or according to the innovative characteristics of the drug. This seems to have contributed to Japanese strength in the antibiotic segment, where new antibiotics are being developed using fermentation technology.[2]

From the early 1980s, however, successive cuts of ethical drug prices had two major effects on firms. First, the cuts pushed them out of the domestic market and accelerated their process of internationalization. Fujisawa established joint tie sales with Smith and Kline to market Fujisawa's antibiotics. Takeda and Abbott are jointly training a U.S. sales force. Moreover, Japanese firms do not simply sign license agreements, but form partnerships, thereby gaining useful marketing know-how and access to the market. They can also keep 50% of the profits in such operations. As Japanese firms, however, did not prove as innovative in the past as U.S. companies, one strategy in the U.S. market has been to enter the industry by the generic business (for instance, Fujisawa acquired a 30% interest in Lyphomed). Finally, an interesting effect of the Japanese drug policy has been to stimulate the growth of the OTC market: OTC sales increased 2.7 times from 1975 to 1985. The successive NHI price cuts have also given prescription drugs in Japan a relatively short life span. Over 26% of all ethical sales were accounted for by drugs introduced after 1980.

CONCLUSION

These three case studies can provide insight into the various tools used by governments in the area of drug prices. The cases of the U.K. and Germany–two of the major pharmaceutical producers in Europe–show that the EEC is moving toward stronger cost policy measures to respond to the pressure on the social contribution. In the Japanese case, which is distinguished mainly by the role of physicians, the system is a very inflationary one, and not much of a control system is in place except for direct cuts by the National Health Insurance. Tougher policies on cost reduction both in Europe and Japan are of concern to U.S. policymakers since they push Japanese firms or other actors to expand abroad to find new returns. This situation may also create some spillover effects on other geographical markets.

REFERENCES

1. Huttin C. The pharmaceutical distribution systems: an international survey. J Soc Admin Pharm 1989;6:184-96.

2. Yoshikawa A. The other drug war: U.S.-Japan trade in pharmaceuticals. Calif Manage Rev 1989;31(2):76-90.

Chapter 18

Why Medicaid Pays More: A Comparison of Private Payment and Medicaid Prescription Prices, Quantities, Product Mix, and Dosage Forms

Jeffrey A. Kotzan
Norman V. Carroll

INTRODUCTION

Third-party prescription plans are an increasingly important reality of the current pharmaceutical market. It is anticipated that in less than seven years nearly half of all prescriptions dispensed in the United States will be administered by third-party prescription plans.[1] The federal-state Medicaid prescription benefit program is the largest national third-party prescription plan. The number of eligible recipients was approximately 23 million unduplicated recipients in both 1987 and 1988. Those recipients annually consumed approximately $3 billion worth of pharmaceutical products.[2,3] Prescription drug benefits are the most popular form of medical treatment for Medicaid recipients. Approximately 80% to 90% of eligible Medicaid recipients utilize prescription benefits. This can be compared with the 65% of Medicaid recipients who visit physicians or the 15% who receive hospital benefits.[4]

Individual states responsible for administration of the Medicaid program are confronted with large aggregate sums of expenditures for significant proportions of their populations. For example, the 1988 Georgia Medicaid

This research was sponsored by the Georgia Department of Medical Assistance.
Previously published in *Journal of Research in Pharmaceutical Economics*, Vol. 3(2), 1991.

prescription program provided over seven million prescriptions at a cost of $118 million for slightly more than 400,000 recipients.[5] The state imposed a limit of six prescriptions and strongly encouraged one-month quantities as a means of prescription utilization control. Formulary management was not in place, with the exception of federal- and state-imposed maximum cost provisions. Pharmacists were reimbursed on the basis of average wholesale price (AWP) less 10%, with a $4.16 professional fee per Medicaid prescription. A prior approval process was in place for those Medicaid recipients requiring more than the limit of six prescriptions per month.

The State of Georgia was concerned with the rapidly increasing incremental costs of the Medicaid prescription benefit program. For example, the average prescription cost per Medicaid recipient utilizing prescription services increased 11% between 1986 and 1987 and 9% between 1987 and 1988.[6] An initial analysis of the Georgia program indicated that the overall average prescription price for the Medicaid patient exceeded the price for the private payment patients. For example, the average private payment prescription price for Zantac® was $37.81 in November 1988, and the average Medicaid price was $57.28.

The disparities in average prescription prices and the concern over the increasing costs per recipient spurred interest in pursing the project. It was understood that prescription consumption is related to cost of the drugs. For example, as the cost to the consumer of prescriptions increases with increased co-payments, the consumption of pharmaceuticals decreases.[7,8] Since Medicaid prescriptions in Georgia were without any copayment feature and cash prescriptions are a total cost to the consumer, per capita consumption of Medicaid recipients was expected to be greater than the consumption of private payment patients. However, per capita consumption of prescriptions was *not* the focus of the research. The overall purpose was to examine causes for differences between private payment and Medicaid average prescription costs within selected therapeutic categories.

A single study can be cited that examined the differences in Medicaid prescription prices and those prices determined by the competitive marketplace. Porter, Carroll, and Kotzan studied nine states without deductible features in the average wholesale price (AWP) base during March of 1985. The overall results indicated considerable variance among the states. The results from Georgia pharmacies described a 0.25% underpayment for Medicaid prescriptions compared to the usual and customary market price. Unfortunately, the study was limited to only 13,000 doses (tablets, capsules, ounces, etc.) for the Georgia comparison.[9] The price differentials described in the Porter study may have limited utility for the current pharmaceutical market. Only nine states currently reimburse Medicaid prescriptions on the basis of the full AWP. However, six of the nine states are considering a change to reduce the full AWP reimbursement base, and one state is under litigation.[10]

It is evident that differences in average prescription prices can be attributed to a limited number of causes. For example, pharmacies may charge more for Medicaid prescriptions than the usual charges for private payment patients. A second cause may be differences in the quantities of doses received. Finally, Medicaid patients may consume the more expensive products and dosage forms within selected therapeutic categories.

The first objective of the research study was to compare prices paid for Medicaid prescriptions with prices paid for identical private payment prescriptions. The second objective was to determine the factors responsible for prescription price discrepancies between private payment and Medicaid patients. For purposes of the study, the first factors were defined as differences in quantities received for the same products. The second and third factors were defined as product mix and dosage form differences within therapeutic categories.

METHODOLOGY

A data set representing 320 Georgia pharmacies for November 1988 was purchased from Pharmaceutical Data Services, Inc. (PDS). The data included information regarding price, trade name, strength, dosage form, and quantities for each of 1,653,593 prescriptions dispensed in November 1988. All preparations and analysis of the data were accomplished with the Statistical Analysis System.[11] A 40% univariate random sample was taken to reduce the mainframe computer resources and to minimize the expenses of subsequent analyses (Figure 18.1). Also, the 40% sample produced a quantity of prescriptions approximately equal to the quantity of Medicaid prescriptions available for the month. The univariate sample procedure produced 599,299 prescriptions for all of the prescriptions on the PDS tape.

All prescriptions in the PDS data set were categorized as cash, Medicaid, or other third-party prescriptions. The cash, or private payment prescriptions, were analyzed to determine the most utilized therapeutic categories. Antispasmodics, antiarthritics, calcium channel blockers, and nitrate vasodilators were selected on the basis of total volume of prescriptions and total cost of each of the categories.

The next phase of the process committed to analysis all Georgia Medicaid prescriptions dispensed during November 1988. The cash prescriptions from the PDS sample were merged with the Medicaid prescriptions on the

FIGURE 18.1. Methodology for Comparison of Private Payment and Medicaid Prescriptions

METHODOLOGY

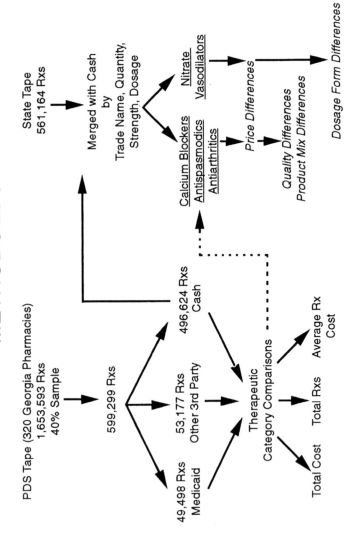

basis of identical trade name, quantity, strength, and dosage form. Package size was excluded from the analysis. Only those prescription combinations of quantity, strength, and dosage form that appeared for both the Medicaid and private payment prescriptions were included in the analysis of price differences.

The projected private payment price for each product combination of quantity, dosage form, and strength was calculated for the matched Medicaid prescription. For example, 830 Tagamet® 300 mg tablet prescriptions in quantities of 100 were dispensed to Medicaid recipients for the month. The 830 prescriptions were matched with 551 private payment Tagamet® prescriptions in quantities of 100 for the 300 mg tablets. The average price of the 830 Medicaid prescriptions was $48.86, compared to $49.22 for the private payment prescriptions. Thus, if the 830 Medicaid prescriptions had been dispensed at the private payment rate of $49.22 rather than the actual rate of $48.86 per prescription, the net reduction in total price for the Tagamet® prescriptions in quantities of 100 would have amounted to $0.36 per prescription for a total difference of $298.80 (830 × $0.36). In an analogous fashion, all combinations of products and quantities for identical strengths and dosage forms were matched, verified, and programmed to determine the individual projected difference between the private payment and Medicaid prices. Finally, the data were summed by trade name and category and subjected to analysis of variance.

The quantity comparisons were calculated by categorizing the products within three of the four therapeutic categories into quantities of dozens.* The nitrate vasodilators represented a special case and were withheld from the quantity analysis for subsequent evaluation for differences in dosage form consumption between the private payment and Medicaid patients. The three remaining categories (antiarthritic, antispasmodics, and calcium channel blockers) were subjected to a comparison between private payment and Medicaid patients by quantities of dozens. The resulting data were subjected to an analysis of categorical data. Projections of cost differences between the two categories were calculated on the basis of differences in consumed quantities between the two patient populations.

The last stage of the analysis was similar to the comparison of quantity differences. In this stage, the three therapeutic categories were grouped by trade name. Again, comparisons were calculated for the differences be-

---

*Upon preliminary examination of the quantity data, it was decided to pursue a categorical approach to better describe the irregular distributions. Initial trials with various quantity categories indicated that dozens produced the most homogeneous descriptions across the products and therapeutic categories.

tween the two patient populations on the basis of differences in consumption of trade names. Further, the results were submitted to a categorical analysis, and projections of cost differences were computed on the basis of differences in utilization of trade-name products.

The nitrate vasodilators represented a special case. Because the mix of dosage forms represented significant differences in overall prices, the products were categorized by the dosage form factor. The results were analyzed in a manner similar to the quantity and product mix procedures.

RESULTS

The results for the price differences for matched products are represented in the analysis of variance (Table 18.1, Figure 18.2). The trade-name factor was nested within the therapeutic class for the analysis of variance. All factors of patient type, therapeutic class, and trade name were significantly different. These results indicate that, in addition to the expected differences in product prices and therapeutic class prices, the differences between prices received in Medicaid reimbursements and private payment receipts were significantly different. A visual scan of the printed data revealed that, in almost all cases, the prices received by the pharmacies for Medicaid prescriptions were lower than private payment prices for comparable products, quantities, strengths, and dosage forms. The results presented in Figure 18.2 show the overall difference in prices received for matched prescriptions for the four therapeutic categories. The price difference was greatest for the antispasmodics at $1.93 per prescription and lowest for the calcium channel blockers at $0.99 per prescription.

The results for the quantity analysis are presented in Table 18.2 and Figure 18.3. The nitrate vasodilators were not dispensed in significant quantity differences (dozens). However, differences in the quantities dispensed among the three remaining therapeutic categories were significantly different in terms of private payment and Medicare aid patients. Thus, the quantities of doses of antiarthritic, antispasmodic, and calcium channel blocker prescriptions dispensed to private payment patients were not similar to those dispensed to Medicaid patients. The largest chi-square presented in Table 18.2 is 421.28, which represented the antispasmodic category. Figure 18.3 reveals that private payment patients received greater proportions of products for one, two, three, four, and nine dozen quantities. Medicaid patients, however, received greater proportions of prescription for five, six, seven, eight, ten, and greater than ten dozen quantities. In a similar manner, calcium channel blockers and antiarthritic products were dispensed in greater quantities for Medicaid patients.

TABLE 18.1. Analysis of Variance Table for Differences in Prescription Price Received for Identical Products from Private Payment versus Medicaid Patients

Source	DF	Type III SS	F Value	Pr > F
Payment*	1	227.64	40.42	0.0001
Therapeutic class†	3	5079.75	4.95	0.0056
Trade name (therapeutic class)	36	12307.58	60.71	0.0001

*Payment is represented by private "cash" payment and Medicaid payments.
†Therapeutic classes are represented by antispasmodic, antiarthritic, nitrate vasodilator, and calcium channel blocker.

FIGURE 18.2. Comparison of Identical Prescriptions at Private Payment (Cash) and Medicaid Reimbursement Rates

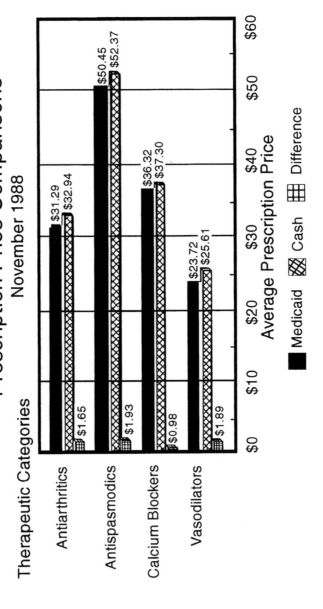

Prescription Price Comparisons
November 1988

Prescriptions are matched on the basis of trade name, dosage form, quantities, and strength.

TABLE 18.2. Categorical Analysis of Contrasts Between Private Payment and Medicaid Patients

Category	DF	Chi-Square	Pr > 0
Quantity Differences			
Antiarthritics	1	37.73	0.0001
Antispasmodics	1	421.28	0.0001
Calcium channel blockers	1	45.17	0.0001
Nitrate vasodilators	1	0.12	0.7288
Product Mix Differences			
Antiarthritic	1	420.92	0.0001
Antispasmodics	1	2.95	0.0860
Calcium channel blockers	1	0.25	0.6140
Dosage Form Differences			
Nitrate vasodilators	1	6.51	0.0107

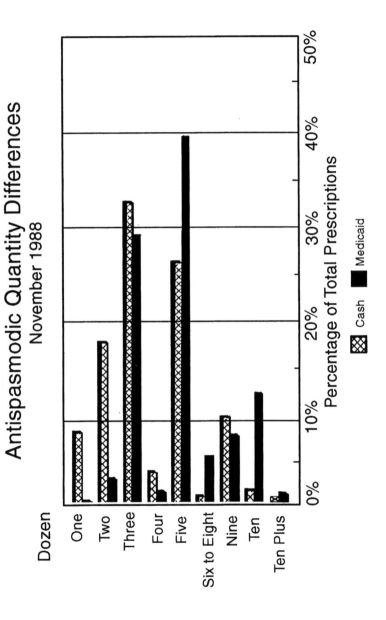

FIGURE 18.3. Quantity Comparisons for Medicaid and Private Payment Antispasmodic Prescriptions

Antispasmodic Quantity Differences
November 1988

The results for the differences in products between the private payment and Medicaid patients are presented in Table 18.2 and Figure 18.4. Only the antiarthritic category displayed a statistically significant difference between the private payment and Medicaid patients. Feldene® was the leading product for the Medicaid population, and the generic ibuprofen was the market leader for the private payment market. Also, the ibuprofen equivalent, Motrin®, was more than twice as popular for private payment patients as for Medicaid patients. The results indicate that the less expensive generic antiarthritic products are more likely to be prescribed for private payment patients than for Medicaid patients.

The last row of Table 18.2 presents the results of the categorical analysis for dosage form differences for the nitrate vasodilators. Again, the results were significantly different, indicating that private payment and Medicaid patients do not consume nitrate vasodilators in the same proportion of dosage forms. Figure 18.5 presents the results, which indicate that the patches were dispensed to Medicaid patients for almost 60% of the total vasodilator prescriptions. The private payment patients received much greater quantities of nitrate vasodilator prescriptions in the sublingual, tablet, and capsule dosage forms than the Medicaid recipients.

The differences in total prices for the four categories are presented in Table 18.3. The differences represent the projected costs for the Medicaid program if the Medicaid patients had received quantities, product mixes, or dosage forms identical to those received by the private payment patients. The difference in utilization of dosage forms for the nitrate vasodilators represented the greatest percentage difference between the cost of the Medicaid rate and the private payment rate. The largest dollar differences were attributed to antispasmodic therapy. In the antispasmodic category, $167,981 more was expended for Medicaid patients than by the private payment patients. The difference represented a 17.50% increase in total cost for the category.

DISCUSSION AND CONCLUSIONS

A third-party prescription system that encourages monthly supplies without copayment or deductible provisions creates a prescription drug market unlike that of the private sector. Other studies have demonstrated that such systems will induce increased per capita consumption of legend pharmaceuticals. This study demonstrated that the quantity of the dosage forms received for the Medicaid prescriptions greatly exceeded the quantity received for private payment prescriptions. The size of the quantity differences was not anticipated. It may be that a monthly prescription limit

FIGURE 18.4. Market Share for Medicaid and Private Payment Antiarthritic Prescriptions

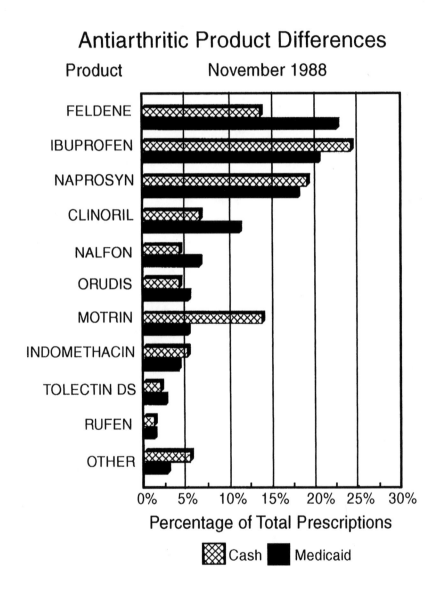

FIGURE 18.5. Dosage Form Comparisons for Medicaid and Private Payment
Nitrate Vasodilator Prescriptions

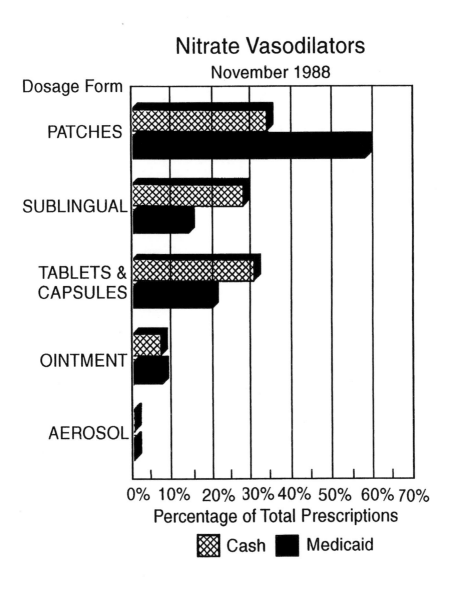

TABLE 18.3. Projected Total Medicaid Costs for Significant Differences at Private Payment Rates

Category	Medicaid Costs	Projected Costs	Difference	Percent
Quantity Differences				
Antispasmodics	$959,769	$791,788	$167,981	17.50
Antiarthritics	738,329	615,271	123,058	16.67
Channel blockers	336,725	304,340	32,385	9.62
Total	2,034,823	1,711,399	323,424	15.89
Product Mix Differences				
Antiarthritics	738,329	624,515	113,814	15.42
Dosage Form Differences				
Nitrate vasodilators	231,415	163,866	67,549	29.19

induces physicians to prescribe greater quantities of prescriptions to ensure that recipients do not use any of the limit for refill prescriptions. Thus, the prescription limit may be self-defeating as a mechanism for cost containment. In summary, the purpose of the study was to determine why Medicaid recipients had higher average prescription costs than private payment patients. The results indicated that Medicaid patients had higher drug costs because they consumed greater quantities of more expensive products. The quantity, dosage form, and mix differences more than offset the lower prices paid for prescriptions by the Medicaid administration.

The increased utilization of the more expensive products and dosage forms was a significant element contributing to the higher costs. Not surprisingly, Feldene, as a once-a-day dosage regimen, was the most popular antiarthritic agent for the Medicaid patient. Available generic antiarthritic products–less expensive but more inconvenient in terms of daily doses–were not prescribed in proportions equal to those for the private payment patients. In a strikingly similar case, the nitrate vasodilator patches were more frequently prescribed for Medicaid patients. Private payment patients tended to rely upon the less expensive oral forms of vasodilators. In both cases, the more expensive and more convenient products were prescribed for the Medicaid recipients. The behavior and resulting increased costs to the Medicaid prescription program may result from the absence of any cost incentives. Neither the prescribing physician nor the Medicaid patient has any direct compensation or gratification for prescribing or using less expensive therapeutic agents. Thus, the prescription benefit program is employed to the fullest potential in terms of convenience as measured by quantities, dosage forms, and products.

This study, although employing a greater number of patients and prescriptions, is not without limitations. The single state available for analysis may not be representative of other states. The lack of formulary and copayment structure further limits the comparisons.* Little patient information regarding the private payment category was available from the PDS tapes. Demographic differences very likely exist between the Medicaid and private payment patients. The Medicaid population consists of recipients from the Aid to Families with Dependent Children and the Supplemental Security Income programs, which include the blind, dis-

---

*In January 1990, the Georgia Department of Medical Assistance imposed restrictions upon the prescription program. Prior approval was required for patented nonsteroidal antiarthritic agents. Additionally, the H_2 antagonists (anti-spasmodics) were limited to a 90-day supply for the year, and sucralfate was limited to a 60-day supply per year.

abled, and aged. Thus, the Medicaid and, most likely, the private payment populations are not homogeneous in terms of patient characteristics.

In conclusion, the results further illuminate the differences attributable to free versus cash prescription programs. The impact of price sensitivity has been demonstrated. These results suggest that private payment exerts a degree of price sensitivity into the prescription purchase decision. Private payment patients appeared less willing or unable to purchase the most expensive products and largest quantities. They may express their unwillingness to procure the more expensive products directly to the pharmacist who, in turn, contacts the physician for alternative therapy. They may also state their need for less expensive therapy directly to the prescribing physician, who accommodates the request by prescribing generically available products at a minimum quantity. Whatever the process, the results indicate that Medicaid prescription programs without cost-containment mechanisms including formulary and copayment provisions are inherently more expensive than similar therapy for private payment patients. They are more expensive even though, as was the case in Georgia, the pharmacies were reimbursed at a lower than the private payment charges.

REFERENCES

1. APhA Policy Committee on Public Affairs, American Pharmaceutical Association, Washington, 1989.

2. Anon. Social Security Bulletin: annual statistical supplement, 1988. np: Social Security Administration, 1989.

3. Anon. Social Security Bulletin: annual statistical supplement, 1989. np: Social Security Administration, 1990.

4. Howell EM, Baugh DK, Pine PL. Patterns of Medicaid utilization and expenditures in selected states: 1980-84. Health Care Fin Rev 1988;10(2):1-16.

5. Johnson A. Annual report of the Department of medical Assistance. Atlanta, GA: Georgia Department of Medical Assistance, 1988.

6. Leibowitz A, Manning WG, Newhouse JP. The demand for prescription drugs as a function of cost-sharing. Soc Sci Med 1985;21:1063-9.

7. O'Brien B. The effect of patient charges on the utilization of prescription medicines. J Health Econ 1989;8:109-32.

8. Wolfgang AP, Perri M. III. Consumer price sensitivity toward prescriptions. J Res Pharm Econ 1989;1(4):51-60.

9. Porter BH Jr., Carroll NV, Kotzan JA. A comparative study of current Medicaid prescription reimbursement (MAC/EAC) with prescription reimbursement based on a competitive market. J Pharm Market Manage 1988;3(2):37-46.

10. Anon. NACDS issues profile. Alexandria, VA: National Association of Chain Drug Stores, 3 April 1990.

11. SAS Institute, Inc. SAS user's guide. Cary, NC: SAS Institute, Inc., 1988.

Chapter 19

Physicians' Perceptions of Prescription Drug Prices: Their Accuracy and Effect on the Prescribing Decision

E. M. Kolassa

INTRODUCTION

Health care costs are currently the focus of considerable attention by all facets of society. Physicians, as the primary decision makers and resource allocators within the health care system, must bear a large share of the responsibility for controlling health care costs while providing the best possible care for their patients. Balancing these two responsibilities can only be accomplished when prescribers are made aware of the costs associated with the treatments they select for their patients.

While diagnosis and selection of the most appropriate therapy are the main focus of physician training, little, if any, attention in this training is paid to the cost of health care and the role of cost in affecting treatment choices. Efforts to contain health care costs, however, cannot be successful until the decision makers within the system–physicians–are cognizant of costs and consider them in their decisions. Several studies performed in the past found physicians, in general, to be unaware of and unaffected by the price of the medications they prescribe. Zelnio and Gagnon, in a review of studies spanning over 25 years, found physicians to be consistently unaware of the prices of the medications they prescribed.[1] The current focus of attention on rising health care costs should, it would seem,

Previously published in *Journal of Research in Pharmaceutical Economics*, Vol. 6(1), 1995.

be expected to increase prescribers' concern for and knowledge of the costs incurred due to the treatments they prescribe. To assess the accuracy of physicians' knowledge of the cost of prescribed drug products, a survey of primary care providers was undertaken. Primary care physicians were chosen because of the higher likelihood that costs would play a role in their decisions and that they would be aware of the costs of selected therapies.[2]

The objectives of this study were threefold: to assess primary care physicians' current levels of price awareness in comparison with previous findings, to measure these physicians' attitudes about the cost of pharmaceuticals, and to identify the common sources of medication price information used by physicians.

METHODOLOGY

Between February 1 and 12, 1993, primary care physicians were contacted by telephone and asked to participate in this study. Their names and telephone numbers were drawn from a nationwide list of physicians who had responded previously to telephone surveys conducted by the contracted interviewing agency.[3] Five hundred physicians were contacted in total, with 100 agreeing to respond without receiving honoraria. The remaining 400 would agree to respond only in exchange for monetary compensation. Since none was offered or available for this study, those physicians requiring honoraria did not participate.

The physicians who did participate were asked to estimate their monthly use and the retail prices of 16 commonly prescribed pharmaceuticals and to state their level of confidence in their estimate. They were then queried as to sources and accuracy of price information and asked to respond to a series of statements dealing with health care costs and their own prescribing decisions. Their price estimates were compared with average retail prices paid by patients and third-party payers. These averages were acquired from IMS Americas' *Basic Data Report,* which is a virtual census of retail pharmaceutical activity.

Frequency distributions and cross tabulations of the data were generated and analyzed. When appropriate, statistical tests, including chi-square analysis and analysis of variance, were performed to determine differences among respondent types.

STUDY LIMITATIONS

Since the sample was drawn from physicians who had previously responded to telephone surveys, the sample cannot be considered random and, therefore, may not be representative of the entire population of primary care physicians. Additionally, only 20% of this sample agreed to participate, providing, in total, two potential sources of nonresponse bias. Still, the consistency of these findings with those of previous studies, which will be discussed, would appear to limit nonresponse bias as a source of error.

RESULTS AND DISCUSSION

A total of 100 primary care physicians participated in this study. The distribution of physicians by practice type, subspecialty (e.g., IM, GP, FP), age, gender, years in practice, and patient load is shown in Table 19.1. A qualitative comparison of these data with national-level information on family practitioners suggests this sample was approximately representative of primary care physicians as a whole.[4] The respondents were also asked to estimate the proportion of their patient loads that belong to HMOs, health maintenance organizations (either IPA or staff model organizations).

Table 19.2 presents the drugs included in the study, the average physician estimates of the number of prescriptions written monthly for each agent, physicians' average estimate of daily drug cost (retail cost to patient), the actual national average daily costs for these agents, and the average level of physicians' confidence of the accuracy of their estimates of cost.[5] Respondents were asked to estimate the costs of only the drugs

TABLE 19.1. Physician Characteristics

		n			n
Specialty:	FP	26	Practice Type:	Solo	45
	GP	38		Group	33
	IM	31		Hospital Staff	21
	Other	5		HMO Staff	2
	Total	100			

		n			Average
Gender:	Female	13		Age:	48.3
	Male	87	Monthly Patient Load:		366

Percentage of Patients Belonging to HMOs:	
None	16%
25% or less	44%
26% to 50%	38%
51% to 100%	2%

they prescribed. No significant differences in accuracy, confidence, or attitudinal questions were found among physicians according to age, gender, specialty, practice setting, patient load, or intensity of HMO patient load. Only in the area of drug price information sources were differences found among respondent types, with staff physicians more likely to receive price-related information from pharmacists and less likely to receive patient feedback than private practice physicians.

All but one of the agents selected for this study are leaders in their respective classes and are likely to be frequently prescribed by primary care physicians. The one agent not fitting this description is Lotensin® (benazepril, CIBA-GEIGY), which was selected due to its unique positioning in the marketplace as a low-cost alternative to its competition. It was felt that the promotional attention given this agent might provide prescribers with a product for which accurate pricing information was available. As can be seen from Table 19.2, physician estimates of the price of this agent, as with all others, were not accurate.

The final column of Table 19.2 presents the level of confidence the physicians had in their price estimates. Using a scale of 1 to 7, with 1 indicating they were not sure of the accuracy of their estimate and 7 indicating they were sure, the answers tended to cluster just above the point of neutrality. No differences were found to exist among physician specialties or practice types, and there was no statistical relationship between the level of confidence in a physician's estimate and the accuracy of the estimate.

To allow for a reasonable margin of error in the estimates, a +/− 20% range about the average actual price was used to evaluate the physician estimates. This same level of error has been used several times in previous studies and would accommodate variations in retail pricing structures for the branded products, although prices for generic products vary much more widely.[6,7] Table 19.3 presents the distribution of these estimates.

Previous studies found roughly one-third of physicians stated they had "no idea" of the prices of the drugs they prescribed.[5,6] A study performed by the American Medical Association in 1977 found 62% of the association's membership was similarly ignorant of drug costs.[8] Physicians responding to this current study were not provided the opportunity to simply avoid estimating drug costs. Those failing to estimate the costs agreed to the statement that they did not care about the costs of the agents they prescribed. In total, 16% (16) of the physicians participating stated they did not care about these costs. The remaining 84 offered estimates for those agents they prescribed.

As would be expected, the relative error in the physicians' price estimates was significantly higher for medications priced at the lower end of

TABLE 19.2. Physician Estimate of Drug Prices, Actual Prices, and Confidence in Estimates

Product and Daily Dose	Number of Prescribing Physicians*	Average Monthly Prescriptions Written**	Average Estimate of Daily Cost (Std. Deviation)	Actual Patient Cost	Average Confidence ***
Generic HCTZ 25 mg QD	78	21.0	$0.36 (0.32)	$0.09	4.7
LANOXIN 0.25 mg QD	78	22.1	$0.58 (0.36)	$0.12	4.5
LASIX 40 mg BID	84	25.0	$0.86 (0.68)	$0.22	4.5
PREMARIN 0.625 mg QD	72	24.0	$0.82 (0.48)	$0.35	4.0
Generic Ibuprofen 600 mg TID	80	20.5	$0.83 (0.56)	$0.56	4.2
LOTENSIN 10 mg QD	40	8.7	$1.35 (0.55)	$0.84	3.8
VASOTEC 10mg QD	79	18.3	$1.38 (0.48)	$0.86	4.3
MICRONASE 5 mg BID	76	19.1	$1.24 (0.66)	$0.98	4.1
APAP w/ Cod #3 Q4h	65	25.0	$0.91 (1.05)	$1.06	4.3
ZANTAC 150 mg QD	94	22.1	$1.21 (1.28)	$1.45	4.6
MEVACOR 20 mg QD	78	13.6	$1.98 (0.90)	$1.74	4.2
PROCARDIA XL 60 mg QD	80	16.2	$1.78 (0.59)	$1.85	4.4
FELDENE 20 mg QD	65	11.5	$1.63 (0.60)	$2.25	4.4
VOLTAREN 50 mg TID	69	13.1	$1.94 (0.72)	$2.51	4.3
CECLOR Susp 250 mg/ml TID	53	12.6	$3.47 (2.37)	$5.06	4.4
AUGMENTIN 250 mg TID	75	19.5	$3.01 (2.70)	$5.30	4.6

* Physicians were asked to estimate only the prices of those agents they had prescribed in the past month.
** Average number of prescriptions written monthly for the agent by those physicians who currently prescribed the product.
*** Confidence measured on a scale where 1 = "Not sure at all" and 7 = "Sure."

TABLE 19.3. Distribution of Physician Estimates of Drug Costs

Product and Daily Dose	Percentage Underestimating Cost	% of Estimates Within 20% of Average Actual Cost	Percentage Overestimating Cost	Percentage Stating "Don't Care"*
Generic HCTZ 25 mg QD	2.5%	10.3%	71.8%	15.4%
LANOXIN 0.25 mg QD	1.3%	2.7%	79.5%	16.5%
LASIX 40 mg BID	3.6%	3.6%	73.8%	19.0%
PREMARIN 0.625 mg QD	1.4%	7.0%	70.8%	20.8%
Generic Ibuprofen 600 mg TID	21.3%	22.5%	41.3%	15.0%
LOTENSIN 10 mg QD	2.2%	17.4%	65.2%	15.2%
VASOTEC 10mg QD	2.5%	25.3%	54.4%	17.8%
MICRONASE 5 mg BID	15.8%	32.9%	32.9%	18.4%
APAP w/ Cod #3 Q4h	60.0%	13.9%	12.3%	13.9%
ZANTAC 150 mg QD	9.5%	27.7%	45.7%	17.0%
MEVACOR 20 mg QD	17.9%	35.9%	30.7%	20.5%
PROCARDIA XL 60 mg QD	26.3%	37.5%	17.5%	18.8%
FELDENE 20 mg QD	55.4%	27.7%	6.1%	10.8%
VOLTAREN 50 mg TID	62.3%	21.7%	5.8%	11.6%
CECLOR Susp 250 mg/ml TID	60.4%	11.3%	11.3%	17.0%
AUGMENTIN 250 mg TID	72.0%	10.7%	8.0%	9.3%

*Physicians were required to estimate the price of the medications they prescribed or state they "don't care" about the cost of pharmaceuticals.

the range studies, since a small absolute difference in an estimate for a low-priced agent would render a larger relative difference than for a more costly agent. Table 19.4 provides a breakdown of estimates that were within $0.50 of the actual average daily price. This table does not include those physicians stating they did not care about the cost of medications. As can be seen, the pattern of overestimating the cost of less costly agents and underestimating the cost of those priced higher is also apparent here.

As with previous studies, physicians, in general, tended to overestimate the costs of medications; in this case, 48.2% of the estimates given were more than 20% higher than the mean actual cost.[5,6] These overestimations were not consistent across all agents studied, however, since physicians consistently overestimated only the costs of those medications that are used for chronic disorders that are relatively asymptomatic, such as hypertension and hypercholesterolemia. The price estimates of medications for acute disorders, such as infections and pain, as well as those for more symptomatic diseases, such as arthritis, tended to be low. Since this study, as well as those previously cited, found patient feedback to be the physicians' primary source of drug price information, it might be hypothesized that patients are more prone to complain of the cost of medications for which they feel little benefit from therapy, while medications offering relief from acute symptoms are less likely to generate these complaints. Tables 19.3 and 19.4 provide the percentage of responses that fell below, within, and above the range of prices for the specific agents while Table 19.5 provides the physicians' reported acquisition of drug price information from various sources and the perceived accuracy of the information provided by each source. Table 19.6 contrasts the responses of private practice physicians with those who are staff employees of hospitals or HMOs.

Physicians claim to receive price information from pharmaceutical company sales representatives and patients on a fairly regular basis and believe patients to be accurate in their assessments of prices. Differences between practice types did emerge in this area of questioning, as shown in Table 19.6, with physicians who are staff employees of hospitals and HMOs being significantly less likely to receive price information from sales representatives ($p = .04$) or patients ($p < .01$) than physicians in private practice. The solo practitioners differed from staff physicians in the extent of their belief in the accuracy of price information provided by pharmacists, with staff employees appearing to trust pharmacists' price information more than the solo practitioners ($p = .016$). These differences may be due to the lack of individual patient follow-up and repeat visits within a staff employee's

TABLE 19.4. Accuracy of Physician Estimates of Drug Costs for Physicians Offering Estimates

Product and Daily Dose	n	Percentage Underestimating Cost by More than $0.50	% of Estimates Within +/- $0.50 of Average Actual Cost	Percentage Overestimating Cost by more than $0.50
Generic HCTZ 25 mg QD	66	0%	86.4%	13.6%
LANOXIN 0.25 mg QD	65	0%	63.1%	36.9%
LASIX 40 mg BID	68	0%	48.5%	51.5%
PREMARIN 0.625 mg QD	67	0%	64.9%	35.1%
Generic Ibuprofen 600 mg TID	68	79.4%	11.8%	8.8%
LOTENSIN 10 mg QD	39	0%	41.0%	59.0%
VASOTEC 10mg QD	65	0%	55.4%	44.6%
MICRONASE 5 mg BID	62	6.5%	67.7%	25.8%
APAP w/ Cod #3 Q4h	56	41.1%	46.4%	12.5%
ZANTAC 150 mg QD	78	3.8%	46.2%	50.0%
MEVACOR 20 mg QD	63	9.5%	63.5%	27.0%
PROCARDIA XL 60 mg QD	65	32.3%	49.2%	18.5%
FELDENE 20 mg QD	58	62.1%	31.0%	6.9%
VOLTAREN 50 mg TID	62	69.3%	24.2%	6.5%
CECLOR Susp 250 mg/ml TID	65	96.9%	0%	3.1%
AUGMENTIN 250 mg TID	68	82.4%	5.9%	11.7%

TABLE 19.5. Sources and Perceived Accuracy of Drug Price Information

n = 100	"How often do you get drug price information from:"					"How accurate or trustworthy is this information?"			
Source	Always	Often	Seldom	Never		Very	Somewhat	Not	No Opinion
Drug Company Sales Person	12.1	47.5	30.3	10.1		26.0	63.5	8.3	2.1
Patient	8.1	48.5	41.4	10.1		59.6	26.6	11.7	2.1
Pharmacist	4.0	16.2	51.5	28.3		58.1	23.7	2.2	16.1
Published Source	1.0	17.2	55.6	26.3		32.6	43.2	8.4	15.8
Colleagues	1.0	21.2	57.6	20.2		9.6	56.4	20.2	13.8

practice and the staff employee's greater exposure to pharmacists on a regular basis.

Even with these differences in the manner in which the physicians may receive price information and their assessments of the accuracy of this information, there were no differences in the accuracy of the price estimates offered by physicians in the various practice settings.

As mentioned previously, the error in price estimates appeared to follow a pattern, with physicians overestimating the costs of some medication types and underestimating others. Additionally, there was a distinct pattern of overestimation of the costs of less expensive agents, such as Lanoxin®, Lasix®, and generic products, while there was underestimation of the costs of antibiotics and NSAIDs (nonsteroidal anti-inflamatory drugs, such as Feldene® and Voltaren®). While the overestimation of drug costs has been deemed acceptable by previous researchers, since this overestimation may limit the use of these products to only those cases where they are truly necessary, the underestimation of the costs of some agents may then lead to their overuse or to failure to consider similar products with lower costs.[6] This pattern of overestimation of the costs of some agents and the underestimation of others leads to an examination of the distribution of the estimates.

While only four of the 15 agents included in the study were priced between $1.00 and $2.00 per day, 59.3% of all price estimates fell within that range. Might one, then, generalize that the responding physicians assume that the "typical" drug costs between $1.00 and $2.00 per day? This assumption would allow the physician's stated concerns about health care costs to be reconciled with his or her ignorance of the actual costs.

TABLE 19.6. Comparison of Drug Price Information Source for Private Practice and Staff Physicians, Average Ratings

$n = 100$	"How often do you get drug price information from:" (1 = "Always" 4 = "Never")			"How accurate or trustworthy is this information?" (1 = "Very" 3 = "Not")		
Source	Private Practice	Staff	p value (chi-sqr.)	Private Practice	Staff	p value (chi-sqr.)
Drug Company Sales Person	2.31	2.64	.04	1.86	1.67	.40
Patient	2.40	3.00	< .01	1.49	1.61	.45
Pharmacist	3.12	2.77	.09	1.39	1.15	.19
Published Source	3.09	3.00	.40	1.72	1.68	.30
Colleagues	2.97	2.96	.70	2.11	2.16	.09

BELIEFS AND OPINIONS

Included in the survey instrument was a group of statements dealing with health care cost issues. Physicians were asked to assess their degree of agreement with these statements using a 1 to 7 scale, with "1" indicating very strong disagreement and "7" indicating very strong agreement. The findings from this section are presented in Table 19.7.

Physicians registered strong agreement with most questions concerning health care costs and the role of cost in prescribing. There was, in fact, general agreement with every statement dealing with the use of cost information and the concern for the cost impact of decisions. At the same time, physicians indicated a weak disagreement with statements concerning their own knowledge of drug prices, partly acknowledging their own lack of knowledge. The only difference between practice types in this set of statements was, again, between solo practice and staff physicians, who differed in the amount of patient complaints they hear concerning price ($p < .01$). Such a finding would be expected, since staff physicians would be less likely to treat the same patient on an ongoing basis and, hence, be less likely to receive feedback.

The responses to several of these statements appear to be contradictory, and many responses are refuted–effectively–by the inaccuracy of the price estimates provided by the physicians.

The high level of agreement with the statements "Patients should get the best treatment possible, regardless of cost" and "I prescribe lower cost

TABLE 19.7. Physician Beliefs and Opinions

	Solo (n = 45)	Group (n = 30)	Practice Type (Mean Response) Staff (n = 25)	Total (n = 100)
The cost of health care is a major concern for my patients	6.0	6.6	6.0	6.1
The prices of new medications are in line with their value	3.8	3.3	2.7	3.4
I am very concerned about the cost of treatments I prescribe	6.0	6.4	5.8	6.1
The cost of health care is too high	5.5	5.5	6.3	5.7
I wish I knew more about the costs of the drugs I prescribe	5.2	4.3	4.9	4.9
Drug company profits are appropriate for the risks they take	4.1	3.9	3.5	3.9
My patients often complain about the cost of medicines	6.0*	5.5	4.5*	5.5
I change prescriptions when patients complain about costs	4.9	5.1	4.4	4.8
I am satisfied with my knowledge of drug costs	3.8	3.9	3.2	3.7
The government should take steps to control drug costs	3.4	3.1	4.4	3.5
Pharmacists are a good source of price information	4.8	5.3	5.6	5.1
I prescribe lower cost drugs for patients with low incomes	5.3	5.3	4.4	5.1
Patients should get the best treatment, regardless of cost	5.8	5.2	5.1	5.5
I often seek out drug price information	4.4	4.5	4.4	4.4
Pharmacists often contact me to recommend lower priced drugs	2.2	2.1	2.0	2.1
I often warn patients that a drug I prescribe will be expensive	5.5	6.2	4.8	5.6
Cost controls should NOT be a concern for physicians	2.9	3.1	2.0	2.7
Drug company sales reps are good sources of price information	4.1	3.8	3.5	3.8
The cost of pharmaceutical research excuses high drug prices	3.5	3.6	3.4	3.5
The cost of a drug has a great influence on my prescribing	4.8	4.9	4.8	4.8

Measured on a scale where 1 = Strongly Disagree and 7 = Strongly Agree
* $p < .01$ using analysis of variance, Scheffé test

315

drugs for patients with lower incomes" may either be contradictory or reveal an area of medical practice where beliefs and behavior are contradictory. The agreement with the statement of prescribing lower cost drugs for patients with lower incomes, however, cannot reflect actual behavior, given the lack of drug price knowledge demonstrated by the respondents.

Still, the physicians in this study agreed strongly that costs do, at least in part, guide their prescribing. These costs, it must be assumed, are the physician's perceptions of costs as opposed to the actual purchase prices.

Several previous studies have also found that physicians claim to consider the cost of medications to be a key consideration in their selection.[9-11] Whether this stated consideration is actually based on the prescriber's perception of drug costs, as discussed above, or is simply a case of normative bias compelling the respondent to answer these questions in the affirmative is unknown. But the lack of accuracy of the estimates of cost, taken in light of these statements of cost concerns, implies that prescription decisions are being made without full consideration of all implications of those decisions and that the stated concerns over costs are, indeed, manifestations of normative bias.

This position is supported by the results of a study of physicians conducted in 1975 in the State of Washington, where less than 2% of responding physicians identified drug costs as an area where they believed more information was needed.[12] While that study was conducted some 18 years ago, there appears to be no evidence that the findings are no longer valid. Another, more recent study solicited physicians' views on the importance of cost considerations, then went on to assess the value of this information to prescribers.[13] While there was general agreement that cost is, indeed, an important consideration in prescribing decisions, the researchers concluded that physicians would not be willing to pay to acquire this information. One would assume that if costs were truly a determinant of selection, information on these costs would be deemed necessary by prescribers.

Unless and until physicians become aware of the costs of treatments they prescribe and use the information on these costs as they already claim to, control of health care spending is not likely to occur.

CONCLUSION

The physicians participating in this study claimed to consider the cost of medications when prescribing, but failed to estimate those costs accurately. These cost estimates, which may or may not affect prescribing behavior, indicated patterns of grouping most drugs into a narrow price range. It cannot be assumed that these findings can be generalized across the universe of prescribing physicians due to the small sample, but should these findings reflect the larger population, the inaccuracy of the cost estimates must lead to questions of the adequacy of any cost-containment measures that do not include the attainment of accurate price knowledge by physicians and physician commitment to consider this factor in making decisions.

REFERENCES

1. Zelnio RN, Gagnon JP. The effects of price information on physician prescribing patterns–literature review. Drug Intell Clin Pharm 1979;13:156-69.

2. Greenfield S, Nelson EC, Zubkoff M, Manning W, Rogers W, Kravitz RL, Keller A, Tarvlov AR, Ware JE, Jr. Variations in resource utilization among medical specialties and systems of care. JAMA 1992;267:1624-30.

3. Market Insight, Inc., of State College PA.

4. Facts about family practice. American Academy of Family Physicians, 1991.

5. Data provided by IMS, International. 3rd quarter 1992 basic data report. Prices of products that experienced price changes between the gathering of these data and the fielding of the survey were adjusted to reflect the new, more current, prices.

6. Fink J, Kerrigan D. Physicians' knowledge of drug prices. Contemp Pharm 1978;18(1):18-21.

7. Kaine R, O'Connell E. Physicians' appreciation of drug charges to the patient. Clin Pediatr 1972;11:665-6.

8. How MDs and pharmacists view mutual problems. AMA News 1978;20(5).

9. Chinburapa V, Larson LN. Predicting prescribing intention and assessing drug attribute importance using conjoint analysis. J Pharm Market Manage 1988;3(2):3-18.

10. Harris P, Savage H. Physicians' prescribing practices and decision making methods. Ill Pharm 1989;(Apr):9-12.

11. Epstein AM, Read JL, Winickoff R. Physician beliefs, attitudes, and prescribing behavior for anti-inflammatory drugs. Am J Med 1984;77:313-8.

12. Smith G, Sorby D, Sharp L. Physician attitudes toward drug information resources. Am J Hosp Pharm 1975;32:19-25.

13. Kotzan JA, Perri M, Wolfgang AP. An exploratory study of physician perceptions of drug price information and a prescription price newsletter. J Pharm Market Manage 1990;4(3):3-13.

Chapter 20

Does Drug Insurance Influence Physician Prescribing?

David W. Miller
Sylvie Poirier
Judy S. McKay
Ming-haw Liu
Donnell L. Harris
Stuart S. Speedie

INTRODUCTION

When the now defunct Medicare Catastrophic Coverage Act was being deliberated on Capitol Hill, a recurrent issue was the effect of prescription drug coverage on the quantity of prescriptions used by the potential beneficiary population. It was estimated that such coverage would increase demand for prescription drugs anywhere from 3% to 60%.[1] Although the act was repealed, the concept of a system of national health insurance remains. Such a system would likely include a provision for the coverage of prescription medicines.[2,3] It therefore seems important to evaluate the impact of a prescription drug benefit plan on the use of medications.

Coverage of prescription drugs by public or private third-party programs has the effect of lowering the price of the drug products to the consumer.[4] Under economic consumer behavior theory, such a decrease in price should increase the demand for drugs if all other factors are held equal. It is instructive to note, however, that this theory assumes that the consumer is the decision maker. With prescription drugs, the consumer makes the decision to purchase, but the decision to order the medication is the prescriber's. Unfortunately, economic theory provides little guidance

Previously published in *Journal of Research in Pharmaceutical Economics*, Vol. 5(2), 1993.

on the effect of price on demand in situations where consumption decision making is shared.

Investigations of the effect of price on prescription drug demand have focused largely on changes in drug use associated with the implementation of a drug insurance program. These studies have been conducted either as natural experiments by measuring prescription use before and after the implementation of such a program for a known population or by using a case-control design whereby the use of drugs by persons with drug coverage is compared to the use by persons without coverage.

In 1968, Greenlick and Darsky investigated the impact of a third-party drug program on prescription use in Windsor, Ontario.[5] This case-control study compared prescription use of persons covered by a drug benefit plan and those paying prescription prices entirely out-of-pocket. Patients with drug coverage received more prescription drugs per person per year than the comparison group. In addition, prescription expenditures per person per year were higher for drugs covered by the program. The authors did not control for adverse selection among their comparison groups; therefore, it is plausible that patients with prescription drug coverage were more ill than those without such coverage.

Weeks studied the use of prescriptions before and after the implementation of a United Auto Workers (UAW) drug insurance program.[6] He found that after the introduction of the program, physicians prescribed more medications per patient visit and prescribed for a higher proportion of patients. The study results, however, indicate that patients may have been aware of the future implementation of the program and may have delayed their prescription purchases until after the program was introduced. In addition, statistical analyses of the reported differences in prescription use were not provided.

Smith and Garner evaluated prescription drug use three months before and after the implementation of a Medicaid program in Mississippi.[7] Both prescriptions per patient and drug expenditures per patient increased after the introduction of the plan.

Johnson and Azevedo, however, determined that the introduction of a prepaid drug program for a medically indigent population in Oregon did not change the use of drugs over a three-year period when use was measured by prescriptions per person.[8] The percentage of program beneficiaries using prescription drugs, however, did increase slightly.

Lech, Friedman, and Ury examined the characteristics of a population of heavy and light prescription drug users enrolled in a health maintenance organization (HMO) in California.[9] A smaller percentage of the heavy drug users had prescription coverage than the light prescription users. The authors state that they could find no relationship between heavy drug use and prepayment for prescription drugs.

The RAND Health Insurance Experiment studied the effect of cost sharing on the demand for prescription drugs in a randomized controlled experimental design.[10] The researchers randomly assigned varying coinsurance amounts for prescriptions to the study population and measured the effect on drug expenditures per person and prescriptions per person. The results demonstrated that both drug expenditures and prescriptions per person increased as the coinsurance liability for the patient decreased.

Similarly, Eng used data from the National Medical Care Utilization and Expenditure Survey to determine that–except for those persons receiving free drugs–as the percentage of coinsurance decreased, both prescriptions per person and expenditures per person increased.[11] The author states that the persons receiving free drugs may not have had adequate access to the health care system because of limited financial resources.

With the exception of the RAND study, these investigations suffer from inherent weaknesses. Those studies based on a before-and-after design do not account for any effects due to extraneous sources. Research using case-control designs suffers from the possible lack of similarity between the two groups. This is especially troublesome in those studies where health status may predispose persons to be covered by drug benefit plans. Hence, differences in prescription drug use between those with and those without insurance may reflect differences in health status between the two groups.

In addition to reports on the impact of drug price on patient prescription use, the influence of medication price on physician prescribing has been investigated. Among the various factors studied, drug price was not found to affect the practitioner's decision to order a specific medication.[12-17] The effect of drug price on the number of drugs prescribed, however, was not addressed in any of these reports.

The consumer behavior model predicts that concurrent with an increase in demand for a product after its price declines is a decrease in demand for economic substitutes of the product. There is empiric evidence suggesting that over-the-counter (OTC) drugs are such substitutes for prescription medications.[18,19] With some exceptions, drug benefit plans typically do not cover nonprescription drugs. As a result, the cost of a prescription drug to the insured may be lower than the cost of a nonprescription substitute. Hence, it seems reasonable that if prescription and OTC drugs are substituted for each other, then patients with drug coverage would use more prescription than nonprescription medications because the out-of-pocket cost would be lower.

The literature on the effect of drug coverage on the use of noncovered OTC drugs, however, reveals conflicting conclusions. Bush and Rabin reported that persons who have prescription drug coverage are less likely to be users of nonprescription medications.[19] This finding supported the authors' hypothesis that consumers use nonprescription drugs as substitutes for prescription drugs. In a report from the RAND Health Insurance Experiment, however, Leibowitz demonstrated that persons with more generous prescription drug coverage purchased more of both prescription and (noncovered) nonprescription medications.[20] In addition, persons in poorer health purchased more of each class of drugs. Leibowitz remarks that these results suggest that OTCs are an adjunct, rather than a substitute, for prescribed drugs.

Similar to the studies analyzing the effect of drug insurance on prescription demand, these nonprescription versus prescription investigations have measured the impact of drug coverage on patient medication use and have largely ignored any effects on physician prescribing. In addition, the RAND study indicated the need to control for health status to detect a difference in OTC or prescription drug use after the implementation of a drug insurance program.[20] Hence, although there is little consensus among the reports, the effect of drug insurance on the demand for prescription and nonprescription medications as measured by patient use has been examined in the literature. Little has been documented, however, regarding the role of drug insurance on physician prescribing. This study examined the effect of a public drug benefit program on the number of drug orders–both prescription and OTC–prescribed per patient visit. Economic theory predicts that those with drug coverage will receive more prescription drug orders and fewer nonprescription drug orders than those without such coverage.

METHODS

Data for this project were provided by the 1985 National Ambulatory Medical Care Survey (NAMCS), a national probability sample survey conducted by the Division of Health Care Statistics of the National Center for Health Statistics.[21-23] The physician sample for the NAMCS was selected with the cooperation of the American Medical Association and the American Osteopathic Association. Participating physicians were requested to submit information on office visits occurring during a specified nine-day period between March 1985 and February 1986. A copy of the patient record, the data collection instrument used in the survey, can be obtained from the authors.[21]

Information was collected on patient, physician, and visit characteristics, such as reason for visit, diagnosis, and medication and nonmedication therapy. Physicians were asked to report nonprescription and prescription medications, to distinguish between new and continued medications, and to indicate whether the drug was intended for the principal diagnosis associated with the visit or was used for some other reason.[21] Hence, unlike previous studies, this survey measured drug demand by physician orders. Medications reported on the data collection form will hereafter be referred to as drug mentions or drug orders. A total of 71,594 patient records were collected, and at least one drug mention was made for 61% of these visits.

Sample Selection

To test the study hypotheses, the sample selected from the NAMCS data set had to meet two objectives: (1) included patients had to be suffering from the same condition and (2) included patients either paid out-of-pocket for the drugs or were covered by a drug insurance program. The first criterion afforded homogeneity among the selected patients with regard to the therapy ordered. The second criterion allowed comparison between the two payment groups to test the hypothesis that those with drug insurance would receive more prescription and fewer nonprescription drugs than those without such coverage.

The similar medical conditions of the patients were cough or diseases of the respiratory system. These often-related conditions were selected because they are amenable to both prescription and OTC drug therapies. In addition, cough ranked as the eighth and cold as the fourteenth most prevalent reason for visit among the total NAMCS data set; thus, common conditions that afforded a sample size large enough for statistical analysis were chosen.

Patients suffering from cough or cold were identified by the relevant reason-for-visit code on the patient record. Although the patient initiated the physician office visit with symptomatology related to these illnesses, the principal diagnosis by the physician may or may not have been the same as the patient's principal reason for the visit. Therefore, only patients with principal diagnoses of cough (identified by an ICD-9-CM code of 786.2) or diseases of the respiratory system, including cold, (identified by ICD-9-CM codes of 460.00 through 519.00) were included in the patient sample.

Drugs included in the analysis were restricted to those that were ordered for the primary diagnosis of the patient. Coding of the drugs as either prescription or OTC status was conducted by pharmacists involved on the project. Seventy of the drug mentions (5%) were classified as unknown. This class resulted from the prescribing of an unknown or illegibly specified drug on the patient record.[23]

Patients without drug coverage were defined as those indicating "self-pay" on the patient record as their only payment method for the physician visit. Because it is unlikely that these patients would have drug insurance without physician visit coverage, it was assumed that self-pay patients paid for their medications entirely out-of-pocket. Patients with drug insurance were defined as those with Medicaid as their only payment source for the office visit. In 1985, Medicaid beneficiaries were covered by a prescription drug program in all states but Alaska and Wyoming.[24] Because the proportion of Medicaid enrollees in these states to the total U.S. Medicaid population is only 0.2%, all Medicaid beneficiaries in this analysis were considered covered by a drug insurance program.[25] In some states, Medicaid pays for selected OTC drugs, such as aspirin, acetaminophen, and insulin. Few Medicaid programs, however, cover the types of OTC drugs used to treat cough or cold.[24] Thus, the Medicaid beneficiaries in this study were assumed to be confronted with paying out-of-pocket for any nonprescription drugs ordered.

Because the medical conditions under consideration were universal to all age groups, sexes, and racial identities, most of these data were left intact. Native Americans, Asians, and Alaskan Natives, however, were excluded from the sample because these groups were underrepresented in the NAMCS database.

Analytic Methods

The Statistical Package for the Social Sciences (SPSS-X) was used for all data analysis.[26] Because the literature suggested that age, sex, and race affect the use of prescription and nonprescription drugs, the numbers of prescription and nonprescription drugs ordered per patient were regressed on each of these variables, along with method of payment, using standardized multiple regression analysis.[11,27,28] The effect of patient payment method was determined by entering age, sex, and race first into the regression model, followed by method of payment. This forced entry of the independent variables allowed the effect of payment status to be established after accounting for the influences of the other three patient covariables. An analysis of residuals was conducted to test for violations of the assumptions of multiple regression analysis. The likelihood of receiving a nonprescription drug order among self-pay and Medicaid patients was determined using multiple logistic regression. As with the standardized multiple regression analysis, the patient covariables of age, sex, and race were entered into this model first, followed by method of payment.

RESULTS

Sample Characteristics

Within the sample selected, self-pay patients represented 80% (n = 666) and Medicaid patients constituted 20% (n = 162) of the total sample. The distributions of ICD-9-CM codes between the two groups were similar. Sociodemographic characteristics of the sample are described in Table 20.1. Males represented 46% among self-payers and females 54%. Forty percent of the Medicaid patients were males and 60% females. Medicaid and self-pay patients presented differences in age and race. The average age for the self-payers was nearly 14 years greater than the average age for Medicaid patients (26.2 vs. 12.6 years, t = 7.06, df = 826, p < 0.001). Whites constituted 94% of the self-pay sample but only 68% of the Medicaid group (chi-square = 19.17, df = 1, p < 0.001).

TABLE 20.1. Sociodemographic Characteristics of Study Sample

Age	Self-Pay (n = 666)	Medicaid (n = 162)	Total (n = 828)	
0-5	196 (29.4%)	71 (43.8%)	267 (32.2%)	
6-10	52 (7.8%)	29 (17.9%)	81 (9.8%)	
11-20	71 (10.7%)	28 (17.3%)	99 (12.0%)	
21-44	185 (27.8%)	24 (14.8%)	209 (25.2%)	
45-64	117 (17.6%)	10 (6.2%)	127 (15.4%)	
> 65	45 (6.7%)	0 (0%)	45 (5.4%)	
average	26.2	12.6	23.5	*p < .001
Sex				
Male	303 (46%)	64 (40%)	367 (44%)	
Female	363 (54%)	98 (60%)	461 (56%)	**n.s.
Race				
White	626 (94%)	110 (67%)	736 (89%)	
Black	40 (6%)	52 (32%)	92 (11%)	***p < .001

```
*    t = 7.06, df = 826
**   chi-square = 1.89, df = 1
***  chi-square = 89.82, df = 1
```

Data Analysis

A total of 1,362 drug mentions were recorded for the 828 patients, resulting in a mean of 1.64 drug mentions per patient visit. Table 20.2 shows the frequency distribution of the number of drug mentions per patient visit by method of payment. Among the drug mentions, 40.2% were antibiotics, 14.5% antihistamines, 22.6% cough medications, and 22.7% other medications.

Standardized multiple regression was conducted to determine the effect of method of payment on the number of prescription and nonprescription drugs ordered per patient visit after accounting for differences in age, sex, and race. Table 20.3 shows the results of regressing the number of prescription drugs against age, sex, race, and method of payment. The model was statistically significant ($p < .001$). Age and method of payment were the most important predictors of the number of prescription drug orders. Age was positively associated with the number of prescription orders; older patients tended to receive more prescription drug orders than younger patients. The direction of the association between the number of prescription drug orders and the method of payment indicated that Medicaid coverage was predictive of fewer prescription drug orders than self-pay status in the sample. The variance explained by the four independent variables was only 6.9%.

Table 20.4 shows the results of regressing the number of nonprescription drug orders against age, sex, race, and method of payment. The model

TABLE 20.2. Number of Drug Mentions Per Patient by Method of Payment

Drug Mentions per Patient	Frequency		
	Self-Pay n (%)	Medicaid n (%)	Total n (%)
0	43 (6.5%)	8 (4.9%)	51 (6.2%)
1	274 (41.1%)	77 (47.5%)	351 (42.4%)
2	242 (36.3%)	65 (40.2%)	307 (37.1%)
3	82 (12.31%)	7 (4.3%)	89 (10.7%)
4	17 (2.6%)	3 (1.9%)	20 (2.4%)
5	8 (1.2%)	2 (1.2%)	10 (1.2%)
Total	666 (100%)	162 (100%)	828 (100%)

TABLE 20.3. Standardized Multiple Regression Analysis of Prescription Drug Orders

Variable	B	Beta	p-value
Payment	−.212006	.080352	.0085
Age	.008740	.225201	.0000
Sex	−.057980	−.032964	.3312
Race	.127211	.045755	.2007
Constant	1.212706	- - - - - -	.0000

$F = 15.30419$ (df = 4, 823)
$p < .001$

$R^2 = .06923$
Standard error = .84551

Coding of categorical variables:
    Self-pay = 0
    Medicaid = 1

    Female = 0
    Male = 1

    White = 0
    Nonwhite = 1

was significant ($p < .001$). Among the independent variables, method of payment and race were statistically significant in predicting the number of OTC drugs ordered per patient visit. Examination of the regression weights indicated that black patients tended to receive more OTC orders per visit than white patients. Medicaid coverage was also predictive of more nonprescription drug orders than self-pay status. This model accounted for only 5.1% of the variance in the number of nonprescription drug orders.

Because of the large difference in the number of Medicaid and self-pay patients in the sample, an analysis of residuals was conducted to determine the effect that this disparity may have had on the results. Plots of residuals versus predicted values of the dependent variable did not demonstrate any discernable heteroscedasticity for either model. In addition, a Goldfeld-Quant test determined that the variances in the dependent variable associated with Medicaid and self-pay patients were not statistically different. [29]

TABLE 20.4. Standardized Multiple Regression Analysis of Nonprescription Drug Orders

Variable	B	Beta	p-value
Payment	.158548	.136540	.0002
Age	−.001392	−.068036	.0536
Sex	−.023961	−.025841	.4506
Race	.152798	.104246	.0040
Constant	.189923	. . . .	.0000

F = 11.00798 (df = 4,823)
$p < .001$

R^2 = .05078
Standard error = .45015

Coding of categorical variables:

    Self-pay = 0
    Medicaid = 1

    Female = 0
    Male = 1

    White = 0
    Nonwhite = 1

Multiple logistic regression demonstrated that method of payment was a significant predictor of an OTC drug order (Table 20.5) after accounting for the other patient covariables. Specifically, patients covered by Medicaid were 1.90 times more likely to have an OTC drug ordered than self-pay patients in the study sample. Among the three additional patient covariables, only age contributed to the prediction of an OTC drug order. For every one-year increase in age, the likelihood of receiving a nonprescription order declined 0.9889 times.[30]

DISCUSSION

This investigation was undertaken to determine the effect of patient payment status on the number of prescription and nonprescription drugs

TABLE 20.5. Logistic Regression Analysis of Nonprescription Drug Orders

Variable	Coefficient	Standard Error	Coefficient/ Standard Error	p-value	Odds Ratio
Age	−.0117	.0048	−2.321	.0215	.9889
Sex	−.0867	.1931	−.4492	.6559	.9169
Race	.4088	.2747	1.488	.1400	1.505
*Payment	.6443	.2269	2.839	.0049	1.905
Constant	−1.718	.1410	−12.19	.0000	.1794

Log-likelihood = −361.757
Chi-square goodness of fit = 263.418, p = .268 (df = 250)
*Improvement in chi-square = 7.754, p = .005 (df = 1)

Coding of categorical variables:

No nonprescription drug ordered = 0
Nonprescription drug ordered = 1

Self-pay = 0
Medicaid = 1

ordered by physicians for ambulatory patients with similar conditions. Standardized multiple regression analysis demonstrated that payment method significantly affected the number of prescription and nonprescription drugs ordered per patient. With each type of drug ordered, however, the directions of the associations between method of payment and the number of orders were contrary to the hypothesis that Medicaid coverage would increase the number of prescription orders and reduce the number of nonprescription drug orders for ambulatory patients with cough and cold. Our results showed that Medicaid patients received fewer prescription and more nonprescription drug orders per visit for cough and cold than self-pay patients.

Multiple logistic regression analysis demonstrated that method of payment exerted an influence on the likelihood of a patient receiving a nonprescription drug order. But again, the direction of this effect was contrary to the hypothesis. Patients with Medicaid coverage were almost twice as likely to receive an over-the-counter drug order per patient visit as self-pay patients.

Because previous research had shown age, sex, and race to be associated with the number of prescription and nonprescription drugs used by patients and because age and race were not distributed equally between the self-pay and Medicaid groups, these covariables were evaluated in each model as additional explanations of the number of drug orders per visit. The results indicated that age was positively associated with prescription drug mentions and that being black was predictive of receiving more nonprescription orders. The remaining covariables did not significantly account for additional variance in the dependent variable of each model.

The unexpected findings of the analysis may have several alternative explanations. As illustrated in Table 20.6, ten state Medicaid programs had prescribing or dispensing caps in 1985 that restricted the number of drug orders per patient per month.[24] These restrictions would tend to reduce the number of prescriptions ordered per Medicaid patient in the study sample. Thus, the finding that Medicaid coverage predicted fewer prescription orders and more nonprescription orders may be an indicator of the effectiveness of these limitations. The extent to which physicians restrict the number of drugs prescribed per patient per month to comply with these caps, however, is not known. Because pharmacists are presumably not reimbursed for drugs dispensed beyond the restrictions, it seems likely that compliance with such limitations occurs predominantly at the pharmacy level. If so, these caps would have little effect on the number of drug mentions in the NAMCS data set for Medicaid patients.

TABLE 20.6. States with Prescribing/Dispensing Caps in 1985

State	Restriction
AR	Four prescriptions per patient per month
FL	Coverage restricted to $22 per patient per month
GA	Six prescriptions per patient per month
MS	Four prescriptions per patient per month
MO	Five prescriptions per patient per month
NV	Three prescriptions per patient per month (does not include prescriptions for family planning or prenatal care)
NC	Six prescriptions per patient per month
OK	Three prescriptions per patient per month
SC	Three prescriptions per patient per month
TN	Seven prescriptions and/or refills per patient per month

Source: National Pharmaceutical Council. *Pharmaceutical Benefits Under State Medical Assistance Programs.* Reston, VA: National Pharmaceutical Council, September, 1985.

Another possibility is that physicians, although aware of their patients' socioeconomic standing, were unaware of their patients' payment status during the visit. It is conceivable, then, that physicians would order fewer prescription medications for patients they perceived as belonging to a group less able to pay for medications. And it follows that these same patients would receive a higher proportion of less expensive medications such as OTC drugs.

Alternatively, it is reasonable that self-pay patients expect more out of physician visits than Medicaid patients and hence, implicitly or explicitly insist on orders for prescription–as opposed to nonprescription–drugs. Such patient demand has been found to be an important factor in inappropriate drug prescribing by physicians.[15] Because the cost of a physician visit for Medicaid patients is minimal, patients may expect less from their physician visits.

Physicians in the analysis may not have recorded all OTC drug mentions.[23] The effect of any missed OTC mentions on the findings presented here is not known. In addition, this study was limited fundamentally by an inability to determine if patients in the self-payment group were beneficiaries of drug insurance plans. Nevertheless, it can be assumed that the Medicaid patients in the study sample experienced fewer out-of-pocket direct costs for their prescription orders than patients in the self-payment group. Furthermore, it should be recognized that this analysis was limited to a sample group with conditions related to the respiratory system. The use of a 1985 database may present some limitations because of the change during that year of some cough and cold medications from prescription to OTC status. There is little reason to suggest, however, that these switches would affect the generalizability of these findings by affecting the payment groups differently.

The low variance explained by the four independent variables of each model suggests that additional factors are influencing the number of prescription and nonprescription drugs ordered per patient visit. Severity of illness may be such a factor. To eliminate the effects of comorbidities, only patients with single conditions (i.e., cough or cold) were included in this analysis. Nevertheless, it is recognized that presentation of a cough or a cold can vary in severity. The effect of this variance on the results obtained here is not known.

In summary, these findings provide evidence that third-party drug coverage does not induce physician prescribing for prescription drugs. Indeed, the results indicate that, despite the prescription drug coverage that Medicaid provides, there is a fundamental difference between the types of pharmaceuticals prescribed for indigent patients and those prescribed for self-pay patients. Any effect of this difference on the health outcomes of the respective groups awaits further research.

REFERENCES

1. Wilensky GR, Neumann PJ, Blumberg LJ. The Medicare Catastrophic Drug Benefit: an analysis of the cost estimates. Washington, DC: Project HOPE, September 1987.

2. Anon. Catastrophic care act repealed by both chambers despite 11th hour rescue attempt in Senate. FDC Rep: The Pink Sheet 1989;51(48):10-11.

3. Anon. Prescription drug coverage is a minimum national health benefit. FDC Rep: The Pink Sheet 1990;52(31):T&G 1.

4. Feldstein PJ. Health care economics. New York: Wiley & Sons, 1988.

5. Greenlick MR, Darsky BJ. A comparison of general drug utilization in a metropolitan community with utilization under a drug prepayment plan. Am J Pub Health 1968;58:2121-36.

6. Weeks HA. Changes in prescription drug utilization after the introduction of a prepaid drug insurance program. Am Pharm 1973;NS13:205-9.

7. Smith MC, Garner DD. Effects of a Medicaid program on prescription drug availability and acquisition. Med Care 1974;12:571-81.

8. Johnson RE, Azevedo DJ. Examining the annual drug utilization of a cohort of low income health plan members. Med Care 1979;7:578-91.

9. Lech SV, Friedman GD, Ury HK. Characteristics of heavy users of outpatient prescription drugs. Clin Toxicol 1975;8:599-610.

10. Leibowitz A, Manning WG, Newhouse JP. The demand for prescription drugs as a function of cost-sharing. Soc Sci Med 1985;21:1063-9.

11. Eng HJ. Economic analysis of the demand for prescription medicine in the United States. Ann Arbor, MI: University Microfilm International, 1985.

12. Hemminki E. Review of the literature on the factors affecting drug prescribing. Soc Sci Med 1975;9:111-5.

13. Miller RR. Prescribing habits of physicians. Part I-IV. Drug Intell Clin Pharm 1973;7:492+.

14. Miller RR. Prescribing habits of physicians. Part VII-VIII. Drug Intell Clin Pharm 1973;8:81-90.

15. Schwartz RK, Soumerai SB, Avorn J. Physician motivation for nonscientific drug prescribing. Soc Sci Med 1989;28:577-82.

16. Zelnio RN, Gagnon JP. The effects of price information on physician prescribing patterns. Drug Intell Clin Pharm 1979;73:156-9.

17. Becker MH, Stolley PD, Lasagna L, McEvilla JD, Sloane LM. Differential education concerning therapeutics and resultant physician prescribing patterns. J Med Educ 1972;47:118-27.

18. Dunnell K, Cartwright A. Medicine takers, prescribers, and hoarders. London: Routledge and Kegan Paul, 1972.

19. Bush PJ, Rabin DL. Who's using nonprescribed medicines? Med Care 1976;14:1014-23.

20. Leibowitz A. Substitution between prescribed and over-the-counter medications. Med Care 1989;27:85-94.

21. U.S. Department of Health and Human Services. Public Health Service. National Center for Health Statistics. McLemore T, DeLozier J. 1985 summary: National Ambulatory Medical Care Survey. Advancedata No. 128. Hyattsville, MD: NCHS, 23 January 1987.

22. U.S. Department of Health and Human Services. Public Health Service. National Center for Health Statistics. Koch H, Knapp DE. Highlights of drug utilization in office practice, National Ambulatory Care Survey, 1985. Advancedata No. 134. Hyattsville, MD: NCHS, 19 May 1987.

23. U.S. Department of Health and Human Services. Public Health Service. National Center for Health Statistics. Koch H. The collection and processing of drug information, National Ambulatory Medical Care Survey, 1980. Vital and Health Statistics. Series 2, No. 90. Washington, DC: NCHS, March 1982.

24. National Pharmaceutical Council. Pharmaceutical benefits under state medical assistance programs. Reston, VA: National Pharmaceutical Council, Inc., 1985.

25. Garwood AN, ed. Almanac of the 50 states: basic data profiles with comparative tables. Newburyport, MA: Information Publications, 1986.

26. SPSS Inc. SPSS-X user's guide. 3rd ed. Chicago: SPSS Inc., 1988.

27. Kotzan L, Carroll NV, Kotzan JA. Influence of age, sex, and race on prescription drug use among Georgia Medicaid recipients. Am J Hosp Pharm 1989;46:287-90.

28. Benrimoj SI, Chua SS. Predictors of nonprescription medication use. J Pharm Market Manage 1990;5(1):3-27.

29. Kelejiam HH, Oates WE. Introduction to econometrics. New York: Harper and Row, 1989.

30. Hosmer DW, Lemeshow S. Applied logistic regression. New York: John Wiley & Sons, 1989.

Chapter 21

An Exploratory Study of Physician Perceptions of Drug Price Information and a Prescription Price Newsletter

Jeffrey A. Kotzan
Matthew Perri
Alan P. Wolfgang

INTRODUCTION

Examination of various strategies designed to contain health care costs, including those for ethical pharmaceutical products, is an area of much interest to providers, fiscal intermediaries and other third-party payers, and consumers alike. Interest in the evaluation of those strategies will undoubtedly grow in the future with rapidly escalatuing costs for medical services. Expenditures for personal health care topped $435 billion in 1987 and are expected to increase to almost $1.4 trillion in the year 2000.[1]

As ethical pharmaceuticals play a larger role inpatient care, personal expenditures for pharmaceuticals and devices are projected to increase from $33 billion in 1987 to $103 billion in 2000.[1] Estimating pharmaceutical expenditures accurately may be difficult because of the influence of new product introductions, biotechnology research and development, and innovations in pharmaceutical marketing, such as direct-to-consumer prescription drug advertising. These and other factors are likely to have unpredictable effects on drug use.[2] It is predictable, however, that new drug therapies will command premium prices and that the cost of drug therapies will continue to increase.

Previously published in *Journal of Pharmaceutical Marketing & Management*, Vol 4(3), 1990.

One strategy for containing future expenditures for pharmaceuticals is to persuade physicians to prescribe the most cost-effective product for a given condition by providing physicians with accurate drug cost information. An information strategy such as this has appeal but may not be successful because it is generally accepted that physicians are poorly informed about the cost of the pharmaceuticals they prescribe. In general, physicians have demonstrated poor overall accuracy for predicting prices for prescriptions.[3] They tend to greatly overestimate the prices of the less expensive legend drugs and to greatly underestimate the more expensive products. This study also provided evidence that physicians who claim they are confident about prescription costs are generally no better estimators of prices than those physicians who are less confident. Furthermore, medical residents who indicated that they relied on price information from pharmacists were more accurate estimators of prescription prices than practicing physicians who relied on information from manufacturers' representatives.[3] This finding implies that the source of price information may also be a factor affecting the accuracy of physician price predictions.

If an information strategy for reducing prescription expenditures is to be effective, physicians should perceive significant need for price information and be willing to alter their prescription writing habits in response to drug cost information. Physicians appear to be growing more receptive to the idea of incorporating price information into the decision process. In a study reported in 1954, physicians expressed little interest in considering price in the prescription decision process.[4] More recent evidence suggests, however, that physicians will accept and use price information in managed health care environments. In one study, providing drug price information to physicians in managed care settings in a bulletin or newsletter format was shown to reduce overall costs by as much as 30%.[5]

The primary objective of this investigation was to develop an understanding of how an information strategy would be accepted by physicians. To accomplish this objective, we set out to answer several basic questions. First, do physicians believe there is a need for accurate drug cost information, and are they willing to use this information in prescribing decisions if it is provided? Next, what sources do physicians currently use for drug cost information, and how satisfied are they with these sources? Finally, are physicians willing to pay for drug cost information?

METHODOLOGY

A preliminary questionnaire was developed from an initial pool of items developed by the investigators. This was informally tested on a small group of physicians, resulting in some minor changes in phraseology. The final version of the instrument contained three sections (available from the authors). The first section was a cover letter identifying the sponsor and explaining the voluntary nature and purpose of the study. The second section displayed a graph and tabular data of actual average prescription prices for the most frequently prescribed quantities of the top seven nonsteroidal, antiinflammatory agents. The drug products included in the graph were selected based on dollar volume. The prices and quantities presented to the physicians were derived from a Medicaid data base containing over 700,000 prescription charges for a one-month period. The final section of the questionnaire contained attitudinal items and several questions designed to assess physicians' sources of and satisfaction with drug price information and to assess physician demographics. The instrument was individually signed by one investigator and was designed so that after completion it could be easily folded to expose a business return reply address.

Two copies of a current mailing list composed of a random sample of 1,344 Georgia physicians were purchased commercially, facilitating an initial mailing and a follow-up mailing ten days later. Surveys that were completed and returned were reduced into machine readable form, verified, uploaded to a central computer system, and analyzed with the Statistical Analysis System.[6]

RESULTS

The overall response rate was 22.6%, and 304 usable questionnaires were collected. Two-thirds of the responding physicians reported that they practiced in a group practice setting. About one-half (56.3%) had been in practice less than 15 years, and 43.8% were in practice for 15 years or more. The responding physicians were almost evenly divided between primary care (53.1%) and specialty (46.9%) practice.

Perceived Need for Drug Price Information

Physicians' responses to individual survey items indicated that there was significant need for drug cost information in medical practice. This is evidenced by the fact that 82% of the physicians indicated that they needed more drug cost information than they currently receive. Most of the responding physicians agreed that patients are concerned about drug costs (85%) and expect physicians to know about drug cost information

(57%). Further, 59% of the respondents agreed that cost was a factor in patient compliance.

Use of Drug Price Information

Of the physicians surveyed, 82% agreed that if they did know more about drug cost, they could save their patients money on prescription drugs, and 68% agreed that they would use drug cost information if it were more accessible. A total of 82% of the physicians agreed that health care administrators are concerned about drug prices. Of the physicians who responded, 87% indicated that they frequently use drug cost information in making prescribing decisions; however, 62% indicated that they believed cost should not be a consideration in the selection of a drug therapy.

Drug Price Bulletin

A large majority of the respondents (90%) agreed that the newsletter concept was a good idea for providing physicians with drug cost information. Only 46%, however, indicated that they would be willing to pay for information in this format. Physicians' willingness to pay for the service on an annual basis was categorized as $0, $0-30, $31-$50, $51-$70, and more than $70. Only a few respondents indicated that they were willing to pay more than $30 per year for the service; therefore, the item was dichotomized into those who expressed a willingness to pay something (46%) versus those who expressed no interest in paying for the service (54%).

Sources of Information and Satisfaction

Figure 21.1 and Figure 21.2 show that physicians reported that they seek price information most frequently from patients, followed by pharmacists, pharmaceutical representatives, and finally, fellow medical practitioners. The survey results also indicated that physicians were most satisfied with the information received from patients and pharmacists and less satisfied with the information received from fellow practitioners and pharmaceutical representatives.

Physician Characteristics and Willingness to Pay

The results of the categorical analysis are presented in Table 21.1. This analysis produces a table similar to analysis of variance procedures with

FIGURE 21.1. Sources of Prescription Price Information and Their Frequency of Use

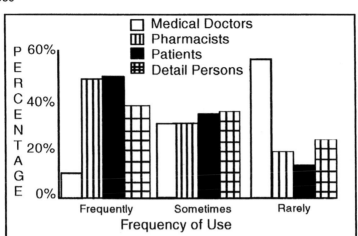

reported chi-square values in place of the customary F-ratios. The results indicated a significant relationship between the willingness to pay for the price information and the two variables of years in practice and patient expectations. The interaction between the years in practice variable and the patient expectation variable proved insignificant. No relationship was noted between willingness to pay for the prescription price information and physician specialty.

The individual effects of years in practice and patient expectations are reported in Figures 21.3 and 21.4. Those physicians who believed patients expect them to be knowledgeable about prescription prices were more willing to pay for the service. Also, those younger physicians who had been in practice for less than 15 years were more willing to pay.

DISCUSSION

Perceived Need for Drug Price Information

The results of this survey supported previous findings which indicated that physicians are poorly informed regarding prescription price information. Few medical practitioners stated that accurate drug price informa-

FIGURE 21.2. Satisfaction with Sources for Prescription Price Information

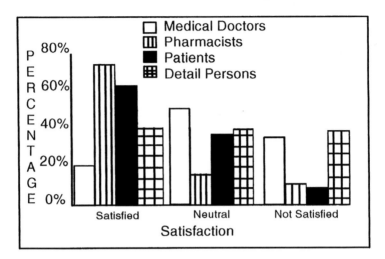

tion was readily available to them in their practices. Physicians reported that they tend to rely upon and are satisfied with drug price information gathered from patients. However, drug price information received from patients should be interpreted cautiously. The information received from patient sources may be anecdotal, imprecise, or simply incorrect. Furthermore, drug price information provided by patients cannot easily be organized in a manner allowing the practitioner to compare similar products within a single therapeutic category.

The results of the survey also provided evidence to support a relationship between patients expecting their physician to be aware of drug price information and physicians' willingness to pay for drug price information. Younger physicians also were significantly more willing to pay for a drug price information bulletin. This could be due to heightened sensitivity to patient expectations since younger physicians would be at a stage in their careers when they would be building practices, or perhaps this is simply a product of society's recent movement toward cost containment in health care.

Feasibility of a Drug Price Bulletin

Based on the results of this study, an informational cost-containment strategy for pharmaceuticals that relies upon voluntary subscriptions by phy-

TABLE 21.1. Categorical Model Analysis of Willingness to Pay for Years in Practice and Patient Expectations of Price Knowledge

Source	DF	Categorical Analysis Chi-Square	Probability
Intercept	1	154.84	0.0001
Years in Practice[1]	1	5.17	0.0230
Patient Expectations[2]	2	12.23	0.0022
Interaction of Years in Practice and Patient Expectations	2	2.92	0.2323
Residual	0	0.00	1.0000

[1]Less than 15 years in practice is coded "A," and 15 years or more is coded "B."
[2]Patients expect the physician to have prescription price information is coded "A" for agree, "D" for disagree, and "N" for neutral.

sicians for drug price information should be approached cautiously. Physicians indicate that they need accurate drug price information and that they will incorporate this information into their decision-making process and prescription-writing habits, thus providing an incentive to pursue this concept. However, many physicians were simply not willing to pay for this type of information service. If it is assumed that willingness to pay for a service such as this is an indicator of perceived worth, these results indicate a general reluctance to support a drug price information service. However, as noted above, physicians who are more sensitive to patient expectations–younger physicians, for example–are willing to pay for a drug price bulletin.

Considering recent trends in health care consumerism and innovative patient behaviors, such as "doctor shopping" where patients actively seek out a practitioner who will accommodate their needs and desires in a physician, the perceived worth of a drug price information bulletin should increase. The question remains whether providing this information to physicians will have any impact on their prescription-writing habits. A drug price information bulletin may be very effective in containing costs in managed care settings where savings can result in economic incentives for the physician. But what about fee-for-service physicians in private practice? The incentive for these professionals may be minimized because patient complaints may be deferred (e.g., to pharmacists) and probably will not be directly attributed to the prescriber.

It seems that a drug price information service will most effectively influence physician prescribing habits in situations where there are incen-

FIGURE 21.3. Perceived Patient Expectation for Prescription Price Information Knowledge

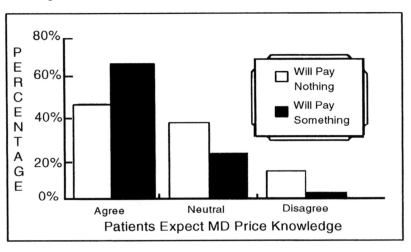

FIGURE 21.4. Willingness to Pay for Prescription Price Information and Years in Practice

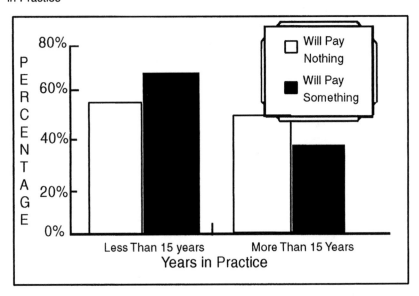

tives for cost containment. For example, risk-sharing contracts between physicians and managed health care provider groups might provide such an incentive. Arrangements such as these could limit prescription expense by passing a portion of the savings back to the physician, making price information necessary for attaining financial objectives.

Physicians perceive the need for drug price information and realize that many patients may want them to be knowledgeable about prescription prices. But is a general knowledge acceptable, or do patients want physicians to be able to make specific price comparisons? Managed-care and other cost-containment strategies are on the rise, providing an incentive for physicians to learn about drug prices. Fee-for-service physicians may currently have less incentive to be well informed about drug prices, but as the cost-conscious consumer begins to demand prescription price sensitivity from the physician, this, too, may change.

LIMITATIONS

This study was limited by the self-reported nature of the data and the limited exposure physicians have to drug price information. The response rate was only approximately 23%, indicating that nonresponse bias could be a significant factor in this investigation. The results obtained could be biased because physicians who are more concerned about drug prices might be more likely to respond to a survey such as this one. Although the low response rate and potential for bias are of great concern, this response rate should be sufficient to provide insight into this issue.

REFERENCES

1. Division of National Cost Estimates, Office of the Actuary, Health Care Financing Administration. National health expenditures, 1986-2000. Health Care Fin Rev 1987;8(Summer):1-36.

2. Lipton HL, Lee RL, Freeland MS. Drugs and the elderly. Stanford, CA: Stanford University Press, 1988.

3. Oppenheim GL, Steven HE, Asworth C. The family physician's knowledge of the cost of prescribed drugs. J Fam Pract 1981;12:1027-30.

4. Caplow T, Raymond JJ. Factors influencing the selection of pharmaceutical products. J Marketing 1954;19:18-9.

5. Fendler JF, Gumbhir AK, Sall K. The impact of drug bulletins on physician prescribing habits in a health maintenance organization. Drug Intell Clin Pharm 1984;18:627-31.

6. SAS Institute, Inc. SAS user's guide: statistics version 5 edition. Cary, NC: SAS Institute, Inc., 1985.

Chapter 22

Toward an Understanding of Pharmaceutical Pricing Strategies Through the Use of Simple Game Theoretic Models

C. Daniel Mullins

INTRODUCTION

Pharmaceutical manufacturers argue the need to charge high prices for their innovative products to cover the costs of research and development. Reekie explains that companies with an innovative product often continue to charge a high price even after competitors enter the market.[1] Significant brand loyalty results in large-scale retention of market share by pioneers despite widespread gaps between the prices of pioneers and generic brands. Similar results about pioneer firm pricing strategies and brand loyalty have been demonstrated by Masson and Steiner and by Hurwitz and Caves.[2,3]

Pioneer drugs have a traditional practice of pricing high and taking modest price increases even after generic entry occurs. Antibiotic drugs provide the only well-documented exception. The high substitutability is the most obvious reason why manufacturers must compete on price in the antibiotic market.

Grabowski and Vernon discuss the effects of the Drug Price Competition and Patent Term Restoration Act of 1984 on the U.S. pharmaceutical market.[4,5] They find that the act has some effect on pricing but that pioneer firms generally do not lower their prices even though generic entry occurs more rapidly after patent expiration than it did in the pre-1984 period. Hudson considers pricing dynamics in the pharmaceutical industry.[6]

Previously published in *Journal of Research in Pharmaceutical Economics*, Vol. 6(3), 1995.

This chapter examines how firms in a monopolistically competitive pharmaceutical market can sustain high price strategies. The next section presents a simple model in which firms make a binary choice regarding pricing strategy. The model predicts that, under specified conditions, firms are best off when all firms price high. This result is not a Nash equilibrium, however, and a Nash outcome includes a positive fraction of firms using both strategies.

The following section proposes applications for this model across certain types of drug markets. Using hypothetical examples, I demonstrate how a two-player game might produce the predicted results. A final section provides some concluding remarks and logical extensions, including empirical applications.

PHARMACEUTICALS PRICING MODEL

Consider a market for pharmaceutical products in which N identical firms compete for sales.[*] Each of the N firms selects a pricing strategy which can be adjusted in subsequent periods. For simplicity, let there be two pricing options for each firm, low (L) or high (H), so that the following describes the entire set of strategy options for an individual firm, y_i:

$$y_i \text{ selects } s_i \; \varepsilon \; \{L, H\}$$

$$where \begin{cases} L \text{ represents a strategy of pricing low} \\ H \text{ represents a strategy of pricing high} \end{cases}$$

Let n represent the number of firms that choose a low pricing strategy, L. Assume that the payoff associated with a firm's pricing strategy is a function of the total number of firms that choose the low pricing strategy, L, and describe the two payoff functions as:

$l(n)$ is the return to a firm using $s_i = L$ given that n firms use strategy L

$h(n)$ is the return to a firm using $s_i = H$ given that n firms use strategy L

---

[*]Firms are required to choose *ex ante* if they will participate in the market, knowing what the expected payoffs will be, but not knowing the degree of brand loyalty.

The payoff to an individual firm i given that n firms use strategy L is described by the following expected return, $r_i(n)$:

$$r_i(n) = r_i(s_i, s_{-i}) = \begin{cases} l(n) & if \ s_i = L \\ h(n) & if \ s_i = H \end{cases}$$

To graph the payoff functions, consider the extreme points. By definition, $h(0)$ is the payoff to a firm that chooses the high pricing strategy, H, when no firms choose L (i.e., when $n = 0$). Under this assumption, *all* firms receive the same payoff $h(0)$. It seems reasonable that under these assumptions an individual firm would expect a greater return if the firm were the only one to adopt a low pricing strategy. Thus, if $l(0)$ represents the payoff that the firm would receive if it were the only firm choosing strategy L, then $l(0) > h(0)$. Of course, $l(0)$ is not possible because as soon as one firm chooses L, then $n = 1$ so that the actual payoff is $l(1)$ rather than $l(0)$.

At the other extreme, we can examine a payoff for a representative firm when all firms choose strategy L. Let this payoff be represented by $l(N)$. Since the price-sensitive component of demand for pharmaceutical products relates to the availability of generically equivalent drugs and has little to do with generically different drugs, one would expect that $l(N) < h(0)$.[7] This simply means that if all firms price according to the same strategy, then the expected return is higher when they all price high than when they all price low. When all companies choose a low pricing strategy, the imposed price competition results in a low return for the typical firm. Thus, if N is not small, $l(N)$ may be very low, possibly close to zero.

As stated in the introduction of this chapter, Grabowski and Vernon and others have demonstrated that there is significant brand loyalty for many pharmaceutical products. It therefore seems reasonable that, in the presence of brand loyalty, if all other firms are using strategy L, an individual firm would be better off using strategy H.* While the firm would lose some of its customers to the lower priced firms, the increase in revenue from the patients who continue to purchase from the firm would more than balance this loss. We obtain the additional restriction that $l(N) < h(N)$. Note that $h(N)$ is not possible; as soon as one firm chooses strategy H, the actual payoff is $h(N - 1)$ rather than $h(N)$.

---

*It is important to note that this is a theoretical argument. We would not expect to observe a market where all firms were pricing low in the presence of significant brand loyalty. The fact that this has not been observed empirically supports the underlying assumption of this model.

Even with high brand loyalty, any degree of price sensitivity implies that not all customers who buy from a high-priced firm when its price is equal to that of all other firms would continue to buy from the firm when other companies sell at a lower price. The inequality $h(0) > h(N)$ provides the final condition necessary to describe the relationship among the four extreme points.

In summary, we have the following relationship:

$$l(0) > h(0) > h(N) > l(N)$$

One additional condition must be imposed to construct a graph of representative payoff functions. Assume that the payoff functions are linear in n.* This yields payoff functions as shown in Figure 22.1.

FIGURE 22.1

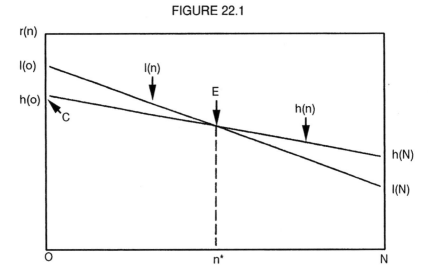

N   = total number of firms

n   = number of firms with a low price

h(n) = return to a firm with a high price

l(n) = return to a firm with a low price

E   = Nash equilibrium outcome

C   = agreed upon strategy under collusion

---

*This assumption can be relaxed without changing the basic results.

At this point, consider what would happen in a monopolistically competitive market for pharmaceutical products when collusion is not permitted. If all firms adopted a pricing strategy of H, then all firms would yield a return of $h(0)$. Each firm would recognize that it could do better by choosing strategy L since $l(0) > h(0)$. In fact, for any $n < n^*$ firms using strategy L will obtain a higher return than firms using strategy H. Firms using strategy H will respond to this by switching strategies until at least n^* firms choose L. If $n > n^*$, the exact opposite is true. Firms using strategy L will recognize that firms using strategy H are yielding a higher return and will therefore change their strategy, thereby reducing the value of n. As a result, n^* defines the Nash equilibrium number of low-priced firms in this model. The outcome with n^* firms using strategy L and $(N - n^*)$ firms using strategy H represents the unique (noncooperative) Nash equilibrium outcome.

Unique Nash Equilibrium Outcome in a Monopolistically Competitive Market:

$$s_i \, \varepsilon \, \{L, \, H\} \, s.t. \, \sum_{i=1}^{N} f(s_i) \, = \, n^*$$

$$where \, f(s_i) \, = \, \begin{cases} 0 \, if \, s_i \, = \, H \\ 1 \, if \, s_i \, = \, L \end{cases}$$

$$and \, l(n^*) \, = \, h(n^*)$$

Is there some other outcome that might result? If collusion were permitted and binding agreements could be made, any value of $n < n^*$ would yield *all* firms a higher return. If profits were not redistributed and all firms had equal bargaining power, we would expect the firms to agree upon a strategy in which all firms choose strategy H and obtain $h(0)$. Because any other set of strategies results in a lower payoff to any firm choosing strategy H, there would be some coalition that would object unless this collusive strategy were used.

Outcome Under Collusion with Binding Contracts, Equal Bargaining Power, and No Redistribution:

$$s_1 = s_2 = \cdots = s_N = H$$

and

$$r_i(0) = h(0) \ \forall \ i \ \varepsilon \ [1, \ldots, N]$$

Using strategy L is always harmful to other players but is beneficial to an individual player when $n < n^*$. The collusive outcome is therefore unstable. An intrinsic conflict arises because the collusive outcome represents a Pareto improvement for all players compared to the Nash equilibrium outcome described above, but each firm has an incentive to leave the coalition. This trade-off between what is good for the coalition as a whole and what is good for the individual firm at the margin presents a dilemma with roots in the Chamberlin tradition.*

APPLICATIONS AND OUTCOMES

We can examine several cases in which the described model has applications for the pharmaceutical industry. Three cases are presented in this section to illustrate the type of markets where we would expect the described outcomes. These examples are not meant to be an exhaustive list, and the specific numbers do not reflect empirical analysis. Rather, these three scenarios are meant to raise possibilities for future empirical work in this area.

The following examples will consider a strategic game being played by two players. To obtain the results presented in the previous section, redistribution must be possible.** For each of the three cases, certain conditions must be met. First, the combined payoffs of the two firms must meet the following condition—*Payoffs ranked from highest to lowest:*

---

*In his duopoly and oligopoly chapter of *The Theory of Monopolistic Competition,* Chamberlin asserts that the effect of uncertainty regarding rivals' actions is enough for an individual to go against what intelligence and farsightedness would dictate.[8] As Chamberlin states, "Any one seller may be perfectly aware of his own indirect influence upon the price, but uncertain as to how many of his competitors are aware of theirs. He will then be in doubt as to the effectiveness of his own foresight in maintaining the price, and therefore in doubt as to whether he should lower or maintain it."

**When a large number of players is involved, this simplifying assumption can be avoided. This chapter presents a two-player game for ease of illustration.

1. Both firms select strategy H.
2. One firm selects H, the other L.
3. The reverse of 2.
4. Both firms select strategy L.

In addition, for each case there must be a demand and profit associated with each outcome that is in line with general economic theory.* Finally, firms behave according to profit-maximizing behavior. Constant marginal costs are assumed in each of the examples so that profits are simply the product of demand and markup, where markup is the difference between price and marginal cost. In summary, the payoff for firm i is defined as follows:

$$\pi_i = (P_i - MC_i) \cdot D_i$$

$$where \begin{cases} \pi_i &= profits \\ P_i &= price \\ MC_i &= marginal\ cost \end{cases} for\ firm\ i$$

The prices that firms charge affect not only the demand observed by the respective firms, but also the total quantity demanded. The extent to which total demand declines as firms use a strategy of pricing high depends on the specific market being examined. Markets for which there are alternative therapies outside the defined market will be more price sensitive and therefore will see a greater drop-off in demand as firms switch from a strategy of pricing low to a strategy of pricing high.

Brand loyalty is the general term used to describe the ability of a firm to preserve a portion of the market when its price is higher than the price charged by its competition. Brand loyalty is exogenously determined and may be affected by the random order in which firms enter the market and the fact that individual consumers are not identical in their preferences.** This chapter provides examples of representative markets that reflect the brand loyalty described by each of the following cases.

---

*Demand should not be upward sloping, and competitor's prices should be negatively correlated with a firm's observed demand.

**The fact that individuals may be allergic to certain drugs would give competitors' products an inherent advantage. An allergic individual may therefore have "brand loyalty" to a product that does not produce side effects.

Case 1

Consider a market in which firms have the same marginal cost of production. Assume that both firms have the same extent of brand loyalty and that the market is fairly price sensitive. ACE inhibitors might provide such an example. There is a high substitutability within the ACE inhibitor market. Furthermore, there are beta blockers and calcium channel blockers that can be used to treat hypertension. The following conditions describe this market:

$$MC_1 = MC_2 = 12¢$$

$$(y_1, y_2) = (L, L) \Rightarrow \begin{cases} P_1 = 15¢ & P_2 = 15¢ \\ D_1 = 500M & D_2 = 500M \\ \pi_1 = \$15M & \pi_2 = \$15M \end{cases}$$

$$(y_1, y_2) = (L, H) \Rightarrow \begin{cases} P_1 = 15¢ & P_2 = 20¢ \\ D_1 = 700M & D_2 = 200M \\ \pi_1 = \$21M & \pi_2 = \$16M \end{cases}$$

$$(y_1, y_2) = (H, L) \Rightarrow \begin{cases} P_1 = 20¢ & P_2 = 15¢ \\ D_1 = 200M & D_2 = 700M \\ \pi_1 = \$16M & \pi_2 = \$21M \end{cases}$$

$$(y_1, y_2) = (H, H) \Rightarrow \begin{cases} P_1 = 20¢ & P_2 = 20¢ \\ D_1 = 250M & D_2 = 250M \\ \pi_1 = \$20M & \pi_2 = \$20M \end{cases}$$

The payoff matrix to the firms is summarized in Figure 22.2. Note that outcomes (L,H) and (H,L) are the only two stable Nash equilibria, while (H,H) provides the greatest combined profit for the market. A collusive agreement of (H,H) would provide a lower total demand. In the absence of collusion, the anticipated outcome is one of the two Nash equilibria. A priori, it is uncertain which of the two outcomes would occur. If, however, one firm credibly establishes its strategic position as setting a low price, the other firm is better off setting a high price. Such an outcome is stable, demonstrating that this market is characterized by first-mover advantage.

FIGURE 22.2

		PLAYER 2	
		L	H
PLAYER 1	L	15M 15M	21M 16M
	H	16M 21M	20M 20M

Case 2

Continue to assume that firms have the same marginal cost of production and that the market is fairly price sensitive. Assume, however, that firms enjoy different degrees of brand loyalty so that Firm 1 obtains a larger portion of the market when prices are the same. Calcium channel blockers might provide such an example. There is a substitutability within the calcium channel blocker market, but early entrance by Firm 1 may allow it greater brand loyalty. The following conditions describe this market:

$$MC_1 = MC_2 = 12¢$$

$$(y_1, y_2) = (L, L) \Rightarrow \begin{cases} P_1 = 15¢ & P_2 = 15¢ \\ D_1 = 600M & D_2 = 400M \\ \pi_1 = \$18M & \pi_2 = \$12M \end{cases}$$

$$(y_1, y_2) = (L, H) \Rightarrow \begin{cases} P_1 = 15¢ & P_2 = 20¢ \\ D_1 = 750M & D_2 = 150M \\ \pi_1 = \$21.5M & \pi_2 = \$12M \end{cases}$$

The payoff matrix to the firms is summarized in Figure 22.3. In contrast to Case 1, there is a unique Nash equilibrium of (H,L) with Firm 1 pricing high and Firm 2 pricing low. This result is logical because the brand

$$(y_1, y_2) = (H, L) \Rightarrow \begin{cases} P_1 = 20¢ & P_2 = 15¢ \\ D_1 = 300M & D_2 = 500M \\ \pi_1 = \$24M & \pi_2 = \$15M \end{cases}$$

$$(y_1, y_2) = (H, H) \Rightarrow \begin{cases} P_1 = 20¢ & P_2 = 20¢ \\ D_1 = 400M & D_2 = 100M \\ \pi_1 = \$32M & \pi_2 = \$8M \end{cases}$$

loyalty advantage allows Firm 1 to price higher. Note, however, that Firm 1 would still prefer outcome (H,H), which is the outcome associated with the highest total profits. If collusion were possible, the outcome (H,H) with a side payment between $7M and $8M from Firm 1 to Firm 2 would yield greater profits compared with the Nash equilibrium outcome (H,L) for both firms. As in Case 1, the collusive outcome results in lower total demand.

FIGURE 22.3

		PLAYER 2	
		L	H
PLAYER 1	L	18M / 12M	21.5M / 12M
	H	24M / 15M	32M / 8M

Case 3

Allow for individual firms to have different marginal costs of production. Assume that there is little brand loyalty and that the market is highly price sensitive. Further assume that the firm with a higher marginal cost offers some product advantage that is valued by consumers. An example of such a market is one in which one firm offers a time-release capsule so that the drug is taken once a day. The technology required to produce a time-release capsule would raise the marginal cost of production. The fact that the other product requires the patient to take the drug three or four times a day gives the time-release capsule some surplus value. The following conditions describe this market:

$$MC_1 = 10¢ \quad MC_2 = 12¢$$

$$(y_1, y_2) = (L, L) \Rightarrow \begin{cases} P_1 = 15¢ & P_2 = 15¢ \\ D_1 = 150M & D_2 = 850M \\ \pi_1 = \$7.5M & \pi_2 = \$25.5M \end{cases}$$

$$(y_1, y_2) = (L, H) \Rightarrow \begin{cases} P_1 = 15¢ & P_2 = 20¢ \\ D_1 = 400M & D_2 = 400M \\ \pi_1 = \$20M & \pi_2 = \$32M \end{cases}$$

$$(y_1, y_2) = (H, L) \Rightarrow \begin{cases} P_1 = 20¢ & P_2 = 15¢ \\ D_1 = 50M & D_2 = 900M \\ \pi_1 = \$5M & \pi_2 = \$27M \end{cases}$$

$$(y_1, y_2) = (H, H) \Rightarrow \begin{cases} P_1 = 20¢ & P_2 = 20¢ \\ D_1 = 100M & D_2 = 600M \\ \pi_1 = \$10M & \pi_2 = \$48M \end{cases}$$

The payoff matrix to the firms is summarized in Figure 22.4. The unique Nash equilibrium in this case is (L,H), with Firm 1 pricing low and Firm 2 pricing high. This result is logical because the product advantage of Firm 2 allows Firm 2 to charge a higher price to offset the associated surplus value. Note, however, that Firm 2 would still prefer the collusive outcome (H,H), and by making a side payment between $10M and $16M, both firms would see a net increase in profits. Again, the collusive outcome (H,H) would reduce total demand.

These results demonstrate the dilemma that firms face in setting prices when it is unclear whether competitors will behave cooperatively to achieve a collusive outcome. In each of the cases provided, at least one firm has an incentive to deviate from the collusive agreement. From a societal perspective, it may be detrimental to achieve a collusive outcome

FIGURE 22.4

PLAYER 2

		L	H

PLAYER 1	L	7.5M
		    25.5M
			20M
			    32M

	H	5M
		    27M
			10M
			    48M

when total demand is reduced. The fact that the collusive agreement is associated with a lower total demand in these three cases is a result of the hypothesized demand conditions, but this aspect of the results may well reflect real market conditions.

These three cases provide examples that demonstrate the difficulty of selecting a pricing strategy in the pharmaceutical industry and highlight the need for empirical testing of the theoretical model described earlier in this chapter. Empirical analysis is difficult because there are only a few examples in which companies have changed their pricing strategy significantly during the product life cycle. Furthermore, empirical studies that would meet the assumptions of the model would further limit the scope of application.

CONCLUSION

This chapter has discussed a theoretical model describing pricing strategies in a binary choice pricing game. It demonstrates that the predicted outcome is not one in which firms maximize total profits for the industry because such an outcome is not stable. The model explains that a stable outcome is likely to be one in which a fraction of drug manufacturers use a strategy of pricing high while the remainder use a strategy of pricing low. Further research could identify means by which one could predict the optimal fractions using each strategy and could incorporate a dynamic component allowing for market entry and exit.

The possibility for future empirical research to test the applicability of this model in certain drug markets is raised. Specifically, a case study of Motrin® and Rufen® might provide some useful insights even though the substitutability of these drugs is extremely high. Other examples should be identified and tested as well.

REFERENCES

1. Reekie WD. Price and quality competition in the United States drug industry. J Industrial Econ 1978;26:223-37.

2. Masson A, Steiner RL. Generic substitution and prescription drug prices: economic effects of state drug product selection laws. Staff report of the Bureau of Economics. Washington, DC: Federal Trade Commission, 1985.

3. Hurwitz M, Caves R. Persuasion or information? Promotion and the shares of brand name and generic pharmaceuticals. J Law Econ 1988;31:299-319.

4. Grabowski H, Vernon J. Brand loyalty, entry and price competition in pharmaceuticals after the 1984 Drug Act. J Law Econ 1992;35:331-50.

5. PL 98-417, September 24, 1984. United States statutes at large, pp. 1585-1605.

6. Hudson J. Pricing dynamics in the pharmaceutical industry. Appl Econ 1992;24:103-12.

7. Schwartzman D. Innovation in the pharmaceutical industry. Baltimore, MD: Johns Hopkins University Press, 1976.

8. Chamberlin E. The theory of monopolistic competition. 7th ed. Cambridge, MA: Harvard University Press, 1960.

Chapter 23

Pricing and Perspectives

Joseph D. Jackson

INTRODUCTION

The pharmaceutical industry is experiencing unprecedented pressure to moderate prices and to innovate. By using the budgetary process rather than the legislative process, Senator David Pryor (D-Ark.) engineered the passage of the Medicaid Pharmaceutical Prudent Purchasing Act (MPPPA) as a provision of the Omnibus Budget Reconciliation Act (OBRA) of 1990. Senator Pryor has succeeded in his attempts to make pharmaceutical prices a front-page issue. Many Americans believe that drug prices are bitter pills to swallow.

Four topics touching on value in the pharmaceutical and health care industry are developed in this chapter. The first addresses the responsibilities of the Health Care Financing Administration (HCFA), the states, and the pharmaceutical manufacturers under MPPPA; in other words, the Medicaid rebate law. The pharmaceutical industry and the elements that contribute to pricing practices are explored in the second section of the chapter. The third portion considers the global health care environment and the elements of cost in this environment. The closing section focuses on outcomes research, value in health care goods and services, and value pricing for pharmaceuticals. The importance of the free enterprise system to health care in the United States is endorsed.

This chapter was presented at an International Business Communications conference, "Price Control & Pricing Strategies: Pharmaceutical & Biotechnology Companies," held in Washington, DC, February 28-March 1, 1991.

The author acknowledges the assistance of Bob Freeman, G. D. Searle; Herbert Gladen, Valley Medical Center, Fresno, CA; Art Haymes, NPC; Rich Levy, NPC; Pat McKercher, Upjohn; Paul Meyer, Pfizer; Doug Morrow, HRPI; David Nash, Thomas Jefferson University Hospital; and Kent Thompson, Ernst & Young.

Previously published in *Journal of Research in Pharmaceutical Economics*, Vol. 4(1), 1992.

The central question asked by customers or consumers of health care in the United States today is: What value should be placed on drug therapy? This question is asked by physicians, payers, and patients alike. It is the responsibility of the pharmaceutical industry to provide answers to this important question. Perhaps if we had had the answer to the question on value, we might have avoided yet another major government program and its attendant bureaucracy.

THE MEDICAID REBATE PROGRAM

The MPPPA is designed to return $3.4 billion in state and federal pharmaceutical expenditures over the next five years by requiring manufacturers to rebate a percentage of the drug cost as a condition of coverage. To appreciate the size and scope of the program needed to accomplish this objective, a review of the major responsibilities of HCFA, the state Medicaid agencies, and the manufacturers is useful.

Under the Medicaid rebate law, HCFA has the responsibility of collecting the rebate agreements from manufacturers in the absence of previously negotiated state-specific rebate agreements that were in effect prior to November 1990. It also has the responsibility of preparing a data file of covered drugs that includes average manufacturer price, best price, and rebate amount. This drug-specific information must be supplied by national drug code (NDC). HCFA then provides these data to the states. HCFA has the authority under the law to survey manufacturers to ensure that the data are accurate; significant penalties exist under the law for manufacturers who supply false information concerning their prices to HCFA. Finally, HCFA has the responsibility for conducting and monitoring a series of mandated studies on aspects of pricing and drug utilization review.

States have a number of responsibilities under the new Medicaid law. They must prepare statewide summary data of drug use by NDC. They are required to organize invoices by manufacturer according to the use by NDC. Next, they submit the data and the invoices to the manufacturer while providing the same data to HCFA. Upon receipt of the invoice, the manufacturer has 30 days to pay the invoice, and it is the state's responsibility to track the receipt of the rebate dollars from the manufacturers. The final responsibility of the state is to return the federal financial participating (FFP) portion of the rebate to HCFA. The FFP portion is based upon the federal matching share within a specific state; for example, California's share would be 50%, whereas Mississippi's share could be as high as 80% federal, with 20% matching funds from the state.

The manufacturer also has a series of responsibilities under the new Medicaid law. First, it must sign the rebate agreement and submit it to HCFA. Quarterly, it must provide information to HCFA concerning its average manufacturer prices (AMP) and best prices. The manufacturer may elect to validate the state utilization information. Outside auditors at the local level will probably be needed to accomplish this task. When there are disputes over the appropriate rebate amount, it is the manufacturer's responsibility to adjudicate the dispute. This legislation puts the pharmaceutical industry on notice that in the future it will be required to give value for money to discourage regulatory solutions to rising health care and pharmaceutical costs.

In a larger context, the medical approach to the delivery of health care in the United States has been changing during the last 100 years. The medical credo of the preantibiotic era was *primum non nocere*, or "first do no harm." During the 1960s, the medical credo changed to "be complete." In jest, it was said of this era that a healthy patient was one who had been inadequately studied. Technological advances during the 1960s led to the current medical credo, "give value for money."[1] This credo reflects the need to balance the interests of the patient with those of society. It is important to distinguish in this context, however, the notion of cost containment as opposed to price containment. It would appear that the current initiative on the part of the federal government through the Medicaid rebate program is directed primarily at price containment and not at the overall issue of cost containment.

THE PHARMACEUTICAL INDUSTRY

Before exploring the structure of and the processes within the pharmaceutical industry and their relationship to price, two global missions of the industry should be recalled. The first is to facilitate the treatment of patients with prescription medicines that are effective, safe, and efficient. The second is to generate sufficient profits to survive and to innovate in an increasingly competitive environment. To underscore the competitive nature of the pharmaceutical business, note that the entire pharmaceutical industry would rank eighth on the list of Fortune 500 companies using 1986 data.[2] Ahead of the pharmaceutical industry on this list would be such names as General Motors, Exxon, Mobil, Ford Motor, IBM, Texaco, and Chevron. The pharmaceutical industry is also a very diverse industry, with no single company having more than an 8% market share.

During the 1980s, pressures on pharmaceutical prices increased steadily as a result of decreasing pharmaceutical product lives, increasing research expenditures, expanding out-of-pocket research costs, and the increasing cost of capital. In February 1989, *The Economist* published an article concerning the new world of drugs.[3] (Figure 23.1). In this article, increasing research and development (R&D) expenditures, eroding patent lives, and increased competition were the factors generating an uncertain future for the pharmaceutical industry.

The science-finance cycle within the pharmaceutical industry shown in Figure 23.2 highlights the developmental process for a pharmaceutical.[4] The area of maximum intervention by the authorities corresponds roughly to the area of maximum financial risk in the drug development process. In Europe, pricing and reimbursement are determined before the launch of the product. This is not currently the situation in the United States. The long development process means that the typical drug is in development for a large portion of its patent life.

In the United States, the time to approval–including the development time–has increased steadily over the last two or three decades. There are many reasons for this phenomenon; however, it is clear that with the increase in development time and time to approval, financial risk has also been increased. The stages of drug development and the approximate years within each stage are:

- Preclinical Testing   3 years
- Phase 1–Safety   1.5 years
- Phase 2–Efficacy-Safety   2 years
- Phase 3–Efficacy-Expanded   3 years
- FDA Approval Process   2.5 years
- Total   12 years

It presently takes about 12 years to bring a new pharmaceutical to market. It is, on average, a full three years before a new molecular entity is first tested in a human.

Research and development is a critical success factor within the pharmaceutical industry. Figure 23.3 lists world research and development expenditures by the pharmaceutical industry from 1980-1987, with the $7.9 billion figure representing 1987 U.S. dollar adjustments and, therefore, real growth in those seven years.

Western Europe, Japan, and the United States remain the principal areas of the world where pharmaceutical research is conducted. It is generally agreed that to promote pharmaceutical research, two characteristics are needed: a scientific infrastructure and a relatively user-friendly or pharmaceutical-friendly environment. At present, five countries in the world are thought to have these two characteristics and are therefore considered

FIGURE 23.1. The New World of Drugs

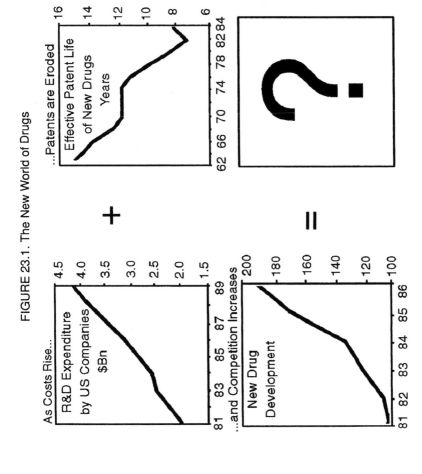

...Patents are Eroded

Effective Patent Life
of New Drugs
Years

As Costs Rise...

R&D Expenditure
by US Companies
$Bn

...and Competition Increases

New Drug
Development

Source: US FDA; WHO; *Pharmaceutical Journal; The Economist*, February 1989

FIGURE 23.2. The "Science-Finance" Cycle in the Pharmaceutical Industry

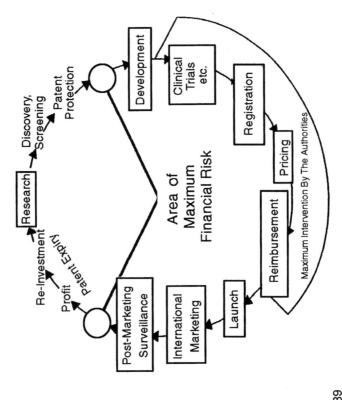

Source: Redwood, 1989

adequate to promote pharmaceutical development. They are the United States, the United Kingdom, West Germany, Switzerland, and Japan. Of course, there are exceptions to this phenomenon, such as Astra Pharmaceuticals in Sweden.

The pharmaceutical research results from 1975 to 1986 are listed in Figure 23.4.[4] Notice that of the 610 new chemical entities (NCEs) approved during this period, only 60 would be categorized as "world-marketed" new chemical entities. Among the world-marketed compounds, the United States has a disproportionate share. This U.S. advantage clearly has a beneficial effect on the U.S. trade balance. These figures support the statement that these five countries have environments conducive to pharmaceutical development. The ratio of all NCEs to world-marketed NCEs highlights the inherent risk in pharmaceutical development. Truly innovative compounds are not commonplace.

With respect to commercial attrition, single products should not be considered in isolation. The chain of attrition in the drug development process from synthesis through marketing is inherently risky (Table 23.1).[4] Commercially successful products in the pharmaceutical industry bear a disproportionate financial liability in the drug development process. Only one in 23 new molecular entities that make it to market is considered highly successful, with sales in 1988 dollars of more than $100 million per year.

Compounding uncertainty and expense in the drug development process over the last decade has been the shift away from therapies for acute diseases toward chronic care therapies. Research and development costs have risen dramatically during this period as a result of two major considerations: (1) chronic care diseases present a greater challenge to prove long-term efficacy; and (2) issues of safety are much greater with the long-term treatment of chronic care diseases. Presently, the cost per case in the typical Phase III protocol for the treatment of chronic care disease ranges from $5,000 to $10,000.

The most recent figures on the cost of development borne by marketed new chemical entities are fixed at $231 million dollars.[5] DiMasi found that out-of-pocket costs, cost of capital, and cost of drug failures have driven up the R&D costs associated with a successful new chemical entity to the $231 million figure, on average.

During the last decade, new developmental efforts by the pharmaceutical industry have focused on cardiovasculars such as calcium antagonists, ACE inhibitors, and renin inhibitors, and anti-infectives such as quinolones and immunoglobulins.[4,6] Intensified research and development efforts in the pharmaceutical industry have focused on antiulcer products,

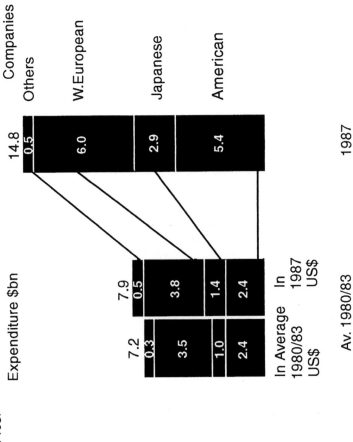

FIGURE 23.3. World Research and Development Expenditure by the Pharmaceutical Industry, 1980/83 and 1987

Source: American: Pharmaceutical Manufacturers Association. Other Data: Redwood, H. *The Pharmaceutical Industry.* Suffolk, England: Oldwicks Press, 1989.

FIGURE 23.4. Pharmaceutical Research Results: % of New Chemical Entities by Country of Origin, 1975-1986

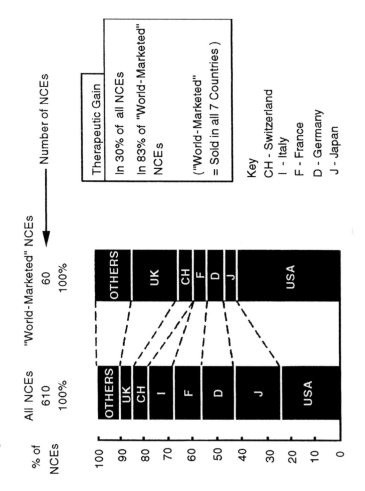

Source: BARRAL "Dix Ans De Résultats De La Recherche Pharmaceutique Dans Le Monde," 1985, and Update, 1987

TABLE 23.1. Chain of Attrition in Pharmaceutical Research and Development

Stage	Years Covered	Rate of Survival In Stage	Cumulatively
Synthesis, Screening[1]	1977-81	1 in 400	1 in 400
Clinical to Market[2]	1964-85	1 in 6.5	1 in 2,600
Commercial Attrition[3]	1961-83		
Moderately Successful*		1 in 8	1 in 21,000
Highly Successful**		1 in 23	1iln 60,000

* Sales Valued At > $20M
** Sales Valued At >$100M

Sources (1) Thesing, 1984; (2) Prentis, Lys, and Walker, 1988; (3) Redwood, 1988

fibrinolytics, antithrombolytics, antiarrhythmics, antianginals, dermatologicals for psoriasis, antivirals, beta-lactams, vaccines, anticancer agents such as hormonal products and immunostimulants, and neurologicals such as antimigraine products and brain function improvers. From the list of new and intensified research efforts, note the increasingly important role of biotechnology in the drug development process. The focus on biotechnology in pharmaceutical development is a relatively recent phenomenon, one that did not exist two decades ago. A manufacturer requires substantial expenditures in capital and labor to be competitive in this area. Frank Young, former Commissioner of the Food and Drug Administration, has stated that biotechnology represents the potential for "the third revolution in pharmaceutical sciences."[6]

At the same time, marketplace realities have forced diminished R&D effort in a number of product categories: vasodilators, penicillins, cephalosporins, macrolides, aminoglycosides, beta-lactamase inhibitors, systemic antifungals, antiparkinsonism products, antidepressants, and bronchodilators, to name a few.[4] Perhaps developmental trends represent better than any policy statement the tremendous challenge of new product development. Clearly, pharmaceutical R&D expenditures as a percentage of sales have risen steadily throughout the 1980s (Figure 23.5). The therapeutic developments for chronic care diseases and the efforts in biotechnology have led the way toward the need for more R&D expenditures.

FIGURE 23.5. Pharmaceutical Research and Development as % of Sales

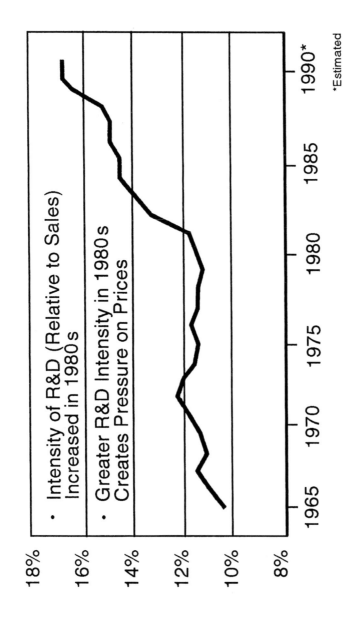

Source: PMA

THE U.S. HEALTH CARE ENVIRONMENT

In January 1989, the cover of *Newsweek* was titled, "Can You Afford to Get Sick?" The cover story highlighted the battle over health benefits and the contributors to cost in the health care industry. Health care expenditures and the factors that may contribute to these expenditures are important for understanding the need for pharmaceuticals and their development. Whether one considers health care expenditures in dollars or as a percentage of the gross national product (GNP), the rapid rise in expenditures during the 1980s is obvious (Figure 23.6).

Health care costs in 1987 consumed 11.1% of the GNP, approximately $540 billion. Dr. Victor Fuchs has written an insightful treatise on the health care sector's share of the GNP.[7] In this article, he explores the four decades of increase in health care expenditures at a rate of about 2.5% per annum. At this rate, health care expenditures in the year 2000 are anticipated to consume 14.3% of the GNP and by the year 2010, 17.6% of the GNP. In Europe, the last decade has seen increasing health care costs at a rate of 1.8% per annum.[7] Clearly, the United States, with its extensive reliance on private enterprise funding, will not continue to support increasing health care expenditures at a rate of 2.5% per annum.

Unlike European countries, the U.S. health care system is pluralistic as opposed to a largely centralized government function. Concerning the segments of U.S. health care spending, drugs and pharmacy services constituted 7% of health care expenditures while physician and hospital care together accounted for 59% of health care expenditures in 1986 dollars. These ratios have remained relatively constant for the past five years[8] (Figure 23.7). Rising health care costs provide the foundation for change in the U.S. health care system.

Demographics are also becoming more important as a progress factor in the cost of health care in the United States (Figure 23.8). Population cohorts over the age of 55 are expected to increase in number and in proportion until the year 2040.[9,10] These numbers are important because the elderly consume a disproportionate share of health care goods and services. This is especially true with pharmaceuticals, where the 12% of the population over the age of 65 consumes 30% of the prescription pharmaceuticals in this country.[11] The Medicare program is the primary funding source for the health care of Americans over the age of 65. The program covers 40% of the elderly's health care expenditures. However, these expenditures are not distributed uniformly among all of the elderly. Thirty percent of these dollars are accounted for by 6% of the elderly in their last year of life.[7]

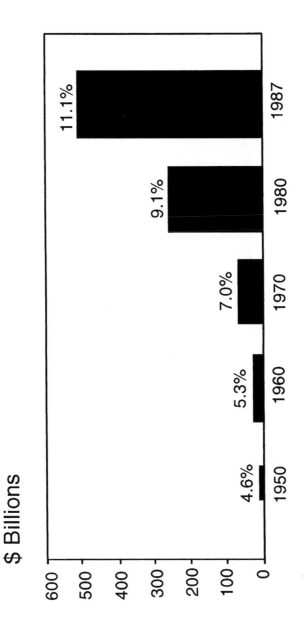

FIGURE 23.6. Healthcare $ and GNA %

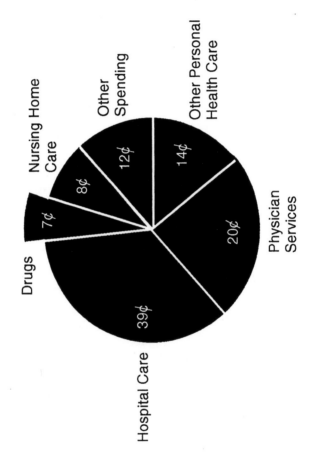

FIGURE 23.7. The Nation's Health Dollar by Expenditure Type, 1986

Hospital Care 39¢

Drugs 7¢

Nursing Home Care 8¢

Other Spending 12¢

Other Personal Health Care 14¢

Physician Services 20¢

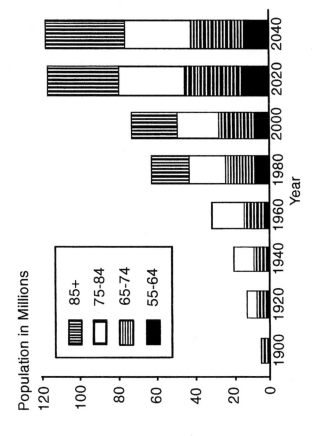

FIGURE 23.8. Population 55 Years and Over by Age: 1900-2040

Source: Current Population Reports, September, 1983 and May, 1984

The pluralism in the U.S. health care system is a significant factor in coverage for medical care. There has been a national trend away from major medical or first-dollar coverage in health care from 1982-1990[12] Figure 23.9).The shift away from major medical plans toward comprehensive plans with cost-cutting incentives such as deductibles, coinsurance, and other limits has been a rapidly growing phenomenon during the 1980s. As an increasing number of corporations become self-insured for medical benefits, this trend is likely to continue.

Labor costs are probably the single most important factor driving health care costs in this country. Dr. Fuchs has examined increases in both the quantity and the price of labor for the last four decades. Health care labor does appear to be resistant to recessionary forces in the United States economy[13] (Figure 23.10). During 1990, a recessionary year in the United

FIGURE 23.9. National Trend Away from 100% Medical Coverage

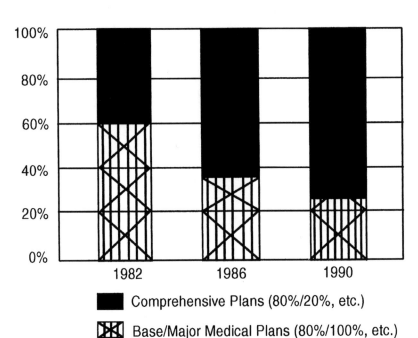

■ Comprehensive Plans (80%/20%, etc.)

▨ Base/Major Medical Plans (80%/100%, etc.)

Source: AT&T Flex Benefits, 1991

FIGURE 23.10. Defying Recession

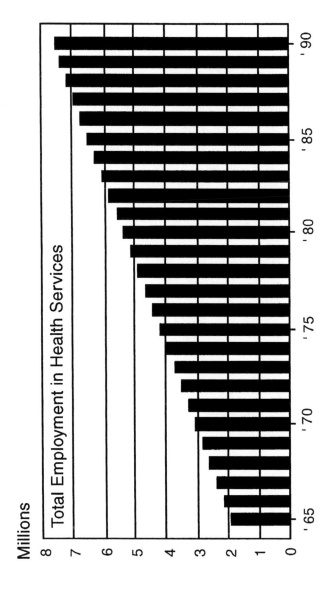

Source: Bureau of Labor Statistics, *The New York Times*, January 13, 1991

States, health care services accounted for 600,000 new jobs at a 7.7% rate of increase[13] (Table 23.2).

Of interest is the fact that hospital employment rose at a slower rate than the outpatient sector, especially in the home health care market. The need for increasing efficiency in health care could explain the shift to the outpatient and home health care sectors, where the growth rate was 19.2%. In the hospitals, according to statistics comparing the last six months of 1989 to the last six months of 1990, the number of admissions, average lengths of stay, and staffed beds were down, while outpatient visits had increased.[14] The search for efficiency in medical care may result in the downsiding of the in-hospital sector during the next decade.

The supply of physicians in the United States is another important factor in health care labor. In 1960, there were 144 physicians for every 100,000 Americans. In 1990, there were 230 physicians for every 100,000 Americans.[15] Dr. Philip R. Lee of the Institute for Health Policy Studies at the University of California at San Francisco has reconsidered a premise he originally supported as Assistant Secretary of Health, Education, and Welfare in the 1960s that expanding the supply of physicians could assist in controlling health care costs. Dr. Lee now admits that this was a mistaken notion.[16] In general, however, physicians work very hard to produce quality health care in the United States. They are actively searching for the most efficient means of delivering the health care product. Outcomes and effectiveness research may allow physicians to lead the way toward the delivery of more efficient health care in the future.

In the United States, 58% of the cost of health care is paid by private (nongovernment) sources; these figures are much lower for our European counterparts.[17] Private funding underscores the pluralistic nature of the

TABLE 23.2. The Employment Boom in Health Care: Number of New Workers Added in 1990

	Jobs Added	Percentage Increase
Total Health Services	600,600	7.7%
Hospitals	219,100	6.2
Doctors' Offices and Clinics	127,800	9.6
Nursing Homes	102,600	7.3
Home Health Care	50,800	19.2
Dentists' Offices and Clinics	19,500	3.8
Laboratories	16,900	10.0

Source: Bureau of Labor Statistics, *The New York Times*, January 13, 1991

U.S. health care system. As cost-containment efforts become more widespread, different patterns and approaches emerge among the payer profiles of our private institutions. Commercial carriers such as John Hancock, Aetna, and Prudential are working to support standards of health care that promote efficiency. "The Blues" are moving toward more stringent and centralized decision-making processes. Medicare remains the most rigid of all payers in the health care sector. Medicaid, as demonstrated by the rebate legislation, is undergoing revision. Also important are the state initiatives, such as the Oregon proposal to ration medical services.[18]

Further examples of pluralism are extant in the managed care sector. Managed care is expected to top 60% of the private-pay network during the 1990s. Managed care relies heavily on bureaucratic appeals processes to control delivery of health care goods and services. The following are examples of how managed health care seeks to control health care costs by limits on the delivery of goods and services:

Texas Instruments	– Requires physicians to seek approval before performing outpatient diagnostic procedures.
3M	– Requires doctors to seek approval before performing inpatient surgery.
General Electric	– Meets with doctors in communities with above normal treatment to discourage such excesses.
General Motors	– Pays bonuses to hospitals with low rates of hospital-related infections, mistakes, and inappropriate services.
Hershey	– Plans to use data on treatment patterns to determine which hospitals have the lowest costs and rates of complications and deaths.[19]

Counterbalancing efforts to cut costs are efforts to maintain benefits. Health care benefit packages have evolved into a potent strike issue in recent years. Health care benefits have become a key factor in preparing for a successful collective bargaining outcome in the nation's top corporations. With health care costs increasingly taking center stage as labor contracts expire around the country, several major unions have banded together with influential members of the business community to address rising health care costs. In 1990, 55 unions, corporations, and medical groups formed the National Leadership Coalition for Health Care Reform to develop proposals to overhaul the nation's health care system.[20]

Health care is now a factor in strike actions, causing increases in both the percentage of striking workers and the percentage of total strikes during the period 1988 through 1990[21] (Figure 23.11). Notice that health care was a factor for 78% of striking workers and in 60% of total strikes. These figures illustrate the larger unions' involvement in bargaining for better health care benefits.

SOLUTIONS:
OUTCOMES AND VALUE

One of the principal problems in addressing health care costs has been the challenge for doctors, patients, and payers to separate image from reality in judging which goods and services contribute to better, more efficient health care. This dilemma was featured as a cover story in *Time* (July 31, 1989).

The final segment of this chapter returns to the question of value in health care goods and services. One of the starting points in shaping a solution to the problem of health care costs may be patient data. Efforts are under way to use health care goods and services data in conjunction with outcomes data to pinpoint treatment gains.[22] Among the initial problems encountered with the use of patient data is control for the variables of disease severity and disease etiology.

Table 23.3 shows the different stages for one disease entity–bacterial pneumonia. Using Dr. Joseph Gonnella's disease-staging model, disease severity can be classified in Stages 1.1 to 3.8, ranging from pneumonia in one lobe to pneumonia with septic shock.[23,24] In Table 23.4, death rates are listed for bacterial pneumonia differing in etiology and severity. One can note a total death rate of 5.6% in Stage 1 pneumonia compared to a 33% death rate in Stage 3 pneumonia. Disease etiology also plays an important role in the understanding of death rates in pneumonia. Similar patterns exist for length of stay using the disease-staging system and disease etiology. Length of stay is the best proxy measure that exists for in-hospital health care costs (Table 23.5). Stage 1 pneumonia has an average length of stay of 7.5 days, whereas Stage 3 pneumonia has an average length of stay of 13.6 days. The national DRG length of stay for pneumonia (DRG 89) is approximately eight days. The evidence related to disease staging for severity highlights the complexity of using patient data and the need for application of appropriate controls.

How costs and care are distributed across patients in different disease entities is another fruitful area of research[25] (Figure 23.12). Lorenz curve analysis of DRG 127 (heart failure) plots the percentage of costs against the percentage of patients needed to generate the costs. This analysis is based upon the work of Dr. David Nash and is representative of most

FIGURE 23.11. Health Care Benefits as Factor in Strikes

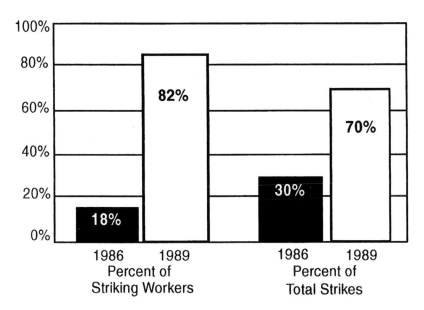

Source: Service Employees International Union, 1990

DRGs. Dr. Nash found that approximately 20% of the patients in DRG 127 accounted for roughly one-half of the costs. This is an important finding because it has implications for care patterns within a hospital. If restrictive formulary practices apply standard pharmaceutical care to all patients, regardless of their disease or their disease severity, then efficiency may suffer for a costly subset of patients. Sicker patients may require more aggressive, not less aggressive, pharmacological interventions. Practice guidelines and hospital-wide formulary practices must account for patient variability in disease severity to promote efficiency in aggregate treatment costs.

The outcomes movement that has recently emerged in medicine is characterized by terms such as practice guidelines, outcomes research, and medical effectiveness research. The historical background of this movement is based in rising health care costs, variation in practice patterns, and reports of inappropriate care.[26] The work of Dr. Jack Wennberg and others has brought attention to the need for some uniformity in medical practice.

The outcomes movement in the United States has gained considerable support in the medical care community. Table 23.6 lists the major players

TABLE 23.3. Clinical Criteria for Disease Staging

Disease: Bacterial Pneumonia

Stage		Stage	
1.1	Pneumonia in One Lobe	3.1	Pneumonia and Septicemia
1.2	Pneumonia with Small Areas in Multiple Lobes or Bronchopneumonia	3.2	Septic Arthritis
1.3	Atelectasis	3.3	Acute Osteomyelitis
2.1	Pneumonia with Bacteremia	3.4	Peritonitis or Subphrenic Abscess
2.2	Empyema	3.5	Pericarditis or Pericardial Effusion
2.3	Lung Abscess or Bronchopleural Fistula or Bronchopleural Cutaneous Fistula	3.6	Endocarditis or Meningitis
2.4	Diffuse Involvement of Multiple Lobes	3.7	Acute Respiratory Failure
		3.8	Septic Shock

TABLE 23.4. Death Rates for Bacterial Pneumonia Hospitalizations: National Hospital Discharge Survey (1987)

Disease Etiology	% In-Hospital Deaths Stage			
	1	2	3	Total
Pseudomonal Pneumonia	14.5	0.0	42.3	21.2
K. Pneumoniae Pneumonia	7.1	100.0	25.4	11.0
H. Influenzae Pneumonia	3.1	0.0	7.1	3.5
Staphylococcal Pneumonia	17.2	53.4	37.8	24.0
Streptococcal Pneumonia	2.8	5.3	12.2	4.0
Pneumonia, Organism Unspecified	5.0	2.8	35.2	7.8
Other Bactrial Pneumonia	9.0	38.3	44.2	14.1
Total	5.6	9.5	33.1	8.7

TABLE 23.5. Average Length of Stay for Bacterial Pneumonia Hospitalizations: National Hospital Discharge Survey (1987)

Disease Etiology	Average Length of Stay Stage			
	1	2	3	Total
Pseudomonal Pneumonia	12.9	13.8	23.3	14.8
K. Pneumoniae Pneumonia	8.8		22.9	10.7
H. Influenzae Pneumonia	7.7	7.2	16.4	8.7
Staphylococcal Pneumonia	10.2	6.0	17.0	11.9
Streptococcal Pneumonia	7.3	7.4	14.5	8.1
Pneumonia, Organism Unspecified	7.3	9.5	11.4	7.6
Other Bacterial Pneumonia	7.8	13.1	14.2	8.4
Total	7.5	9.4	13.6	8.1

Note: Hospital deaths have been removed from average lengths of stay calculations.

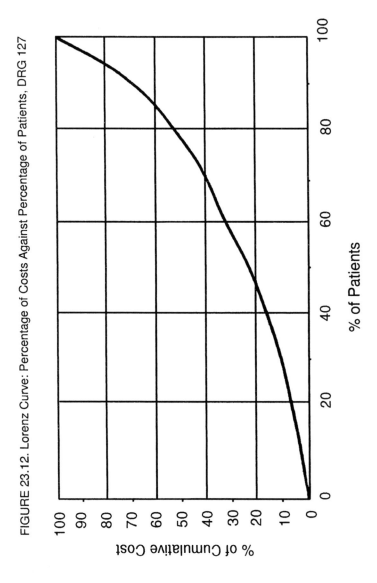

FIGURE 23.12. Lorenz Curve: Percentage of Costs Against Percentage of Patients, DRG 127

TABLE 23.6. Players (Outcomes Research)

• PHS (AHCPR)	• Hospitals
• Congress (GAO, OTA...)	• Insurers
• AMA	• Private Enterprises

• Medical Specialty Societies	– Interstudy
	  – Codman Research
	  – Value Health Services

• Academic Centers	
• Rand Corporation	• States (NJ, NY, ME, MA, OR)
• Institute of Medicine	

Source: Woolf, *Arch Int Med*, September 1990

in the outcomes research movement today. The leader of this movement today is probably the Agency for Health Care Policy and Research (AHCPR). This federal agency was formed in the last two years. Congress is also actively involved through the General Accounting Office (GAO), the Office of Technology Assessment (OTA), and the Prospective Payment Assessment Commission (ProPAC). The American Medical Association has also been an active player, as have medical specialty societies such as the American College of Physicians. Academic centers, hospitals, insurers, and some states have all taken an active role in the outcomes research movement. Private enterprises such as Dr. Paul Ellwood's Interstudy, Codman Research, and Value Health Sciences have a stake in this movement.

All of these groups have different agendas for their involvement; however, common to most is the goal of increasing the quality of care. Some are interested in protecting professional autonomy and reducing the risk of litigation. Minimizing practice variations and creating a document trail are important new considerations with the goal of generating evidence of effectiveness promoting efficiency. Finally, lowering health care costs, lowering insurance premiums, and reducing the federal deficit have been cited as goals worthy of the emerging emphasis on outcomes.

AHCPR was formerly the National Center for Health Services Research (NCHSR). In 1989, this new agency was funded in the amount of $32 million. In 1990, during a time of limited federal budget increases,

AHCPR received funding of $126 million.[27] As part of its mission, AHCPR has considerable contact with the National Library of Medicine, the National Institutes of Health, the Centers for Disease Control, the Health Care Financing Administration, the Department of Defense, and the Veterans Administration. A 17-member advisory council has been formed to guide the AHCPR.

Perhaps the most important work of the AHCPR concerns the Patient Outcomes Research Teams (PORTS). PORTS are empowered to consider the most effective means of treating disease entities and to recommend practice guidelines for the most effective treatment strategies. In effectiveness research, AHCPR has a clear mission: to evaluate what resulted from the application of health care goods and services as opposed to what was done. AHCPR has powerful support in Congress; however, the agency's task is formidable.

The pharmaceutical industry is well positioned to work within the emerging outcomes movement. For many years, the pharmaceutical industry has been required by law to prove the efficacy and safety of its products in well-controlled clinical trials. This has not been required for many other goods and services within the health care industry. However, many challenges remain to promote the efficiency of pharmaceuticals. Studies that evaluate lengths of stay, the costs of complications, the prevention of hospitalizations, and the improvement of outcomes are examples of future challenges for the pharmaceutical industry. The industry must focus on agents that improve therapeutic outcomes, offer greater effectiveness, offer more rapid response, offer less failure, and are safer. In the long run, dollar-for-dollar, pharmaceuticals will prove their competitive (with other goods and services) worth in the treatment of patients. Traditionally, the pharmaceutical industry has been required to prove the efficacy of a drug by assessing whether the drug works under optimal circumstances. In the future, we will have to prove the effectiveness of the drug by assessing whether the drug is a successful therapeutic intervention in practice, outside the confines of a tightly controlled protocol. Finally, it will be necessary to prove the efficiency of the drug and to measure its economic performance relative to other goods and services in the health care sector.

If we are successful in proving the efficiency of the drug, then the notion of value pricing may evolve. Historically, pharmaceutical pricing has been a function of the return on investment (ROI) philosophy (Table 23.7).[28] In the early 1980s, with formulary systems gaining power and influence in the pharmaceutical marketplace, pricing practices began to reflect these competitive pressures. Later in the 1980s, issues of cost-effectiveness (C/E) in selected situations influenced pricing behavior. The 1990s will probably be

TABLE 23.7. Pharmaceutical Pricing: The Influence of Reimbursement

Era	Reimbursement	Pricing
1960-1980	• Cost Plus	ROI
Early 1980s	• Cost Plus "But"	Drug-Drug
Late 1980s	• Prospective Payment	Drug-Drug
	• Early Managed Care	Some C/E
1990s	• Managed Care	Value:
	• "Outcomes"	• Society
	• Payer Influence	• Payers
		• Patient

characterized by proliferation of managed care systems, outcomes research, and payer influence. If pharmaceutical companies are successful in proving the worth of their products, value pricing practices could result (Figure 23.13).

The competitive merit of a product will have the primary influence on price. However, the movement from a cost-oriented approach based upon incremental changes to a value-oriented approach based upon the worth of a product could usher in a new era of pricing where free-market characteristics are dominant.

CONCLUSION

The pharmaceutical business is inherently risky. DiMasi has demonstrated that the greatest costs of average pretax pharmaceutical research and development occur in the preclinical period and account for approximately one-half of the cost of an approved NCE.[5] With more sophisticated measurement of outcomes, additional research will be necessary to prove the relative worth of an NCE in the marketplace. When pharmaceuticals are of proven value, their prices should be consistent with their value in a free-market setting.

FIGURE 23.13. Pricing and Product Positioning

As We Move into the 1990s a Variety of Perspectives Will Influence Price

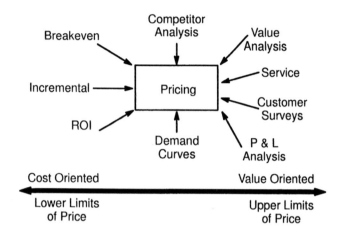

As the newly appointed editor of the *New England Journal of Medicine*, Dr. Jerome P. Kassirer, has commented: "Systemic reforms are needed . . ." in the health care sector.[29] However, Kassirer ". . . has strong reservations about a government-run national health insurance plan." The outcomes movement has the potential to shape the delivery of health care goods and services to benefit patient care. Under the influence of a pluralistic, free-enterprise system, this is possible; under a regulated, government-run system, innovation and value will be victims.

REFERENCES

1. Read JL. The new era of quality of life assessment. In: Walker SR, Rosser RM, eds. Quality of life: assessment and application. Lancaster, U.K.: MIP Press Limited, 1988.

2. Pharmaceutical Manufacturers Association. Facts at a glance, 1989.

3. Anon. The new world of drugs. Economist 1989;(Feb 4):63.

4. Redwood H. The price of health. London: Da Costa Print Company, 1989.

5. DiMasi J, Hansen R, Grabowski HG, Lasagna L. The cost of innovation in the pharmaceutical industry. J Health Econ: 1991;10:107-42.

6. Young FE. A new era in drug regulation and development. Unpublished.

7. Fuchs VR. The health sector's share of the gross national product. Science 1990;247:534-8.

8. Lazenby HC, Letsch SW. National health expenditures, 1989. Health Care Finan Rev 1990;12(2):1-26.

9. U.S. Bureau of the Census. America in transition: an aging society. Taueber CM. September 1983. (Current Population Report Series P-23, No. 128).

10. U.S. Bureau of the Census. Projections of the population of the United States, by age, sex and race: 1983 to 2080. Spencer G. May 1984. (Current Population Reports Series P-25, No. 952).

11. U.S. Congress. Office of Technology Assessment Health Program. Prescription drugs and elderly Americans: ambulatory use and approaches to coverage for Medicare. Solan G, Behney C, Herdman R. October 1987.

12. American Telephone and Telegraph. Flex Benefits '91 (benefits brochure).

13. Pear R. Against trend, health-care jobs rise. New York Times 1991 Jan 17:L19.

14. Samuels S. Net patient revenues lag behind increases in expenses. Hospitals 1991;(Feb 5):38-42.

15. Ginzberg E. High-tech medicine and rising health care costs. JAMA 1990;263:1820-2.

16. Anon. America's medical bill. New York Times 1991 Feb 3:F2.

17. Anon. Health care spending. Healthweek 1988;(Sept 19):3.

18. Gerry R. Moves to rational Medicaid healthcare spreading from Oregon to other states. Physicians Finan News 1990;8(13):2.

19. Garland SB, Freundlich N. Insurers vs. doctors: who knows best? Business Week 1991;(Feb 18):64-5.

20. Anon. Health costs. Washington Post 1991 Feb 16:D2.

21. Green J. Health benefits becomes a critical issue at the bargaining table. Am Hosp Assoc News 1990;26(12):8.

22. Winslow R. Patient data may reshape health care. Wall Street J 1989 Apr 17:B1.

23. Gonnella JS, Hornbrook MC, Louis DZ. Staging of disease: a case-mix measurement. JAMA 1984;251:637-44.

24. Markson LE, Nash DB, Louis DZ, Gonnella JS. Clinical outcomes management and disease staging. Evaluation Health Professions 1991;14(2):201-27.

25. Nash DB, Goldfarb NI. Exploring resource use in high-cost versus low-cost care: the pharmaceutical example. DRG Monitor 1987;8:1-8.

26. Woolf SH. Practice guidelines: a new reality in medicine. Arch Intern Med 1990;150:1811-8.

27. U.S. Department of Health and Human Services. Agency for Health Care Policy and Research. AHCPR program note; medical treatment effectiveness research. March 1990.

28. Thompson K. Personal communication.

29. Altman LK. Editor of journal envisions new directions and lighter tone. New York Times 1991 Feb 5:C3.

PART V:
ECONOMICS AND MARKETING

Economic changes and pressures affect marketing activities in many ways, with two of those being the effect on pricing policies and the use of economic principles in promotion. In this section we focus on the latter. Szeinbach et al. demonstrate appeals in promotion. Rubin provides insights into how promotion *can* be cost-effective, and Lovatt provides a worldwide perspective. Finally, Keith argues the economic benefits of promotion.

Chapter 24

Content Analysis
of Pharmacoeconomic Appeals
in Pharmaceutical
Drug Product Advertisements

Sheryl L. Szeinbach
John P. Juergens
Mickey C. Smith
Robert A. Freeman

INTRODUCTION

Organizations are affected by many environmental factors, including regulatory policies, competitive strategies, social changes, and technological advances. The market structure of the pharmaceutical industry, in particular, has been affected by governmental policies and competitive strategies designed to restructure the health care system. These policies, in general, will affect the market structure by altering barriers to entry, research and development activities, and promotional activities. As part of the exchange process, the function of promotional activities is to disseminate product information to physicians and other health care professionals, to create product loyalties, and to alter the conditions of entry to the market by potential competitors.[1] Promotional activities by the pharmaceutical industry include advertising, direct mailing, and professional detailing; all serve as major constituents in the resource exchange process. Without promotional activities, the loss of new products and product information could change the number of therapeutic alternatives and break-

Previously published in *Journal of Research in Pharmaceutical Economics*, Vol. 3(3), 1991.

through products available to patients. Promotional activities are an important component in ensuring the demand for a particular drug product by individuals and organizations in a dynamic environment. Thus, pharmaceutical firms are dependent upon elements in the task environment–such as physicians, wholesalers, and retailers–to distribute drug products.[2,3] Given the contingencies that exist in the task environment for pharmaceutical firms, promotional strategies must be revised continually to be effective in positioning a new product in the market.

The pharmaceutical industry has experienced the implementation of several health-related policies, from early statutes governing drug product safety and efficacy to statutes containing incentives to encourage cost containment and competition for drug products and medical services. Some of the policies implemented during the 1970s include the repeal of antisubstitution laws and the maximum allowable cost (MAC) program. This program limited the amount reimbursed by the federal government for drugs prescribed under federally subsidized health care programs to the lowest price at which a drug is generally available.

Of major interest for the present study is the Tax Equity and Fiscal Responsibility Act of 1983 (TEFRA). This policy change resulted in hospitals moving from a retrospective reimbursement system to a prospective pricing system for Medicare patients. Under the new system, hospitals were paid a flat fee based on each patient's classification into a given diagnosis-related group (DRG).[4] Shortly after TEFRA, the Drug Price Competition and Patent Term Restoration Act of 1984 was instituted. There were two reasons for this act. First, pioneer companies received an extension of patent life on new drugs to recapture market time lost during the lengthy drug development process. In exchange, generic drug companies were allowed greater market accessibility because the need for duplicative research procedures for post-1962 approved drugs was eliminated.[5] The Prescription Drug Marketing Act of 1987 was intended to reduce public health risks from adulterated, misbranded, and counterfeit drug products that enter the marketplace through drug diversion.[6] Despite the implementation of these policies, however, very few investigations in the area of pharmacy have addressed the indirect influence of regulatory activities on advertising appeals.

One way to examine the impact of these policies is to determine how pharmaceutical firms incorporate the changes mandated through various regulatory actions and policies into their promotional activities, including drug product advertising. The content of an advertisement, therefore, could be analyzed to investigate the possible impact of policies that result from governmental action. The purpose of this study was to investigate the impact of TEFRA on the content of drug product advertising for the years 1980, 1984, and 1988. Although several policies have influenced the pharmaceutical industry, TEFRA was selected for investigation because of its broad economic impact on health care.

RESEARCH METHOD

Content analysis is the study of words, signs, and symbols contained in a message without emphasizing the interpretational component imparted by the communicator.[7] Drug product advertisements contain information that is exchanged among physicians and other health care providers for educational and competitive purposes as related to pharmaceutical firms. Besides the importance of price, distribution, and advertisement placement, the content of the advertisement may be another important factor in establishing the drug product in the marketplace.

The method for content analysis first involves the selection of documents to be studied; a reasonable sample size for investigation; and an a prior unit of measurement which can be specific words, symbols, themes, or events. In the second phase of the methodology, individuals are trained to categorize the content of advertisements according to predetermined rules. Responses are usually coded on a form sheet specifically designed for the study.

The use of content analysis as a research technique for evaluating prescription drug product advertising is well documented in the literature. For example, prescription drug advertising has been investigated from the standpoint of market appeal, the pharmaceutical industry's role in advertising prescription drugs to pharmacists in professional journals, direct advertising of prescription drugs to consumers, and a historical perspective.[8-13]

Journals included for evaluation were selected based on Gagnon's national survey of the readership habits of pharmacists and awareness of scholarly journals in the area of pharmacy administration and hospital pharmacy.[14] The first category included two major medical journals intended for general circulation to various health care professionals. Several journals intended for mass circulation to the nation's pharmacists in all practice settings were included in the second category. The third category consisted of the hospital pharmacy journals targeted at pharmacists working in hospitals, clinics, long-term care facilities, and other specialty areas.

Using this approach for categorization, the first category was composed of the *New England Journal of Medicine* and the *Journal of the American Medical Association*. Included in the second category were *American*

Pharmacy, Drug Topics, American Druggist, Pharmacy Times, and *U.S. Pharmacist.* Chosen to represent the clinical pharmacy journals were *Drug Intelligence and Clinical Pharmacy,* the *American Journal of Hospital Pharmacy,* and *Hospital Formulary.*

The major purpose of this study was to assess the content of drug product advertisements for economic appeal. The year 1980 was selected as the baseline because the level of activity affecting health care policies was minimal. As mentioned previously, the prospective payment system was implemented through TEFRA. DRGs were expected to have their initial impact on the health care system during 1983 and 1984. As these policies affected the health care system, economic indicators should be observed in advertisements during 1984 and 1988. The year 1988 was selected as an equal interval.

Ten fourth-year pharmacy students were recruited into a training session specifically designed to familiarize students with content analysis and drug product advertising. Students were presented with several advertisements during the training session and asked to categorize each advertisement according to economic appeal. Preliminary evaluation of these advertisements also served as a qualitative assessment of validity by enabling the investigators to check the units of measurement, categories for economic appeal, and journals used in the study. Upon completion of the training session, students were given gridded audit forms and randomly assigned to journals and years. Statistical analysis was performed using the Statistical Package for the Social Sciences (SPSS).[15]

For the purposes of this study, an advertisement was operationally defined as any written or pictorial material within a promotional message. Only drug product advertisements bearing the prescription legend were included in this study; therefore, this definition excluded over-the-counter products, medical devices, self-diagnostic kits, and health and beauty aids. The specific objectives of this study were to: (1) characterize the number of pharmacoeconomic appeals encountered in the ten selected journals for the years 1980, 1984, and 1988; (2) evaluate the breakdown of the frequency of advertisements for 1980, 1984, and 1988 with respect to the type of economic appeal; (3) perform a statistical analysis of medical journals for 1980, 1984, and 1988 with respect to pharmacoeconomic appeal; and (4) perform a statistical analysis of hospital pharmacy journals for 1980, 1984, and 1988 with respect to pharmacoeconomic appeal. The chi-square test of statistical significance, Cramer's V, and Kendall's tau B were used to evaluate the third and fourth objectives.

Pharmacoeconomic Appeals in Drug Product Advertising

An appeal was defined as any statement, phrase, or word contained in drug product advertisements that related to cost-benefit, cost-effectiveness, quality of life, or compliance. Cost-benefit analysis studies were identified by the use of words and phrases such as money saved by decreased morbidity, decreased mortality, decreased cost of illness, or decreased cost of social benefits.[16] Advertisements were evaluated as cost-effectiveness appeals if they contained words or phrases such as dollars per life saved, increased life years, or quality adjusted life years (QALYs). Advertisements were considered an appeal for quality of life if they contained words or phrases such as improved quality of life, improved health status, or well-being.[17-19] Although quality adjusted life years is considered a measure of cost utility, it was thought that the distinction between the two techniques would not be evident in drug product advertisements; therefore, QALYs were included in the category of cost-effectiveness. Drug product compliance was considered as a separate category and included any assertion that influenced the patient's medication-taking behavior to produce a desired preventive or therapeutic result. The appeal was any assertion that could be classified into the designated categories.

RESULTS

A systematic random sampling technique was used to select 5% of the total advertisements to be evaluated for reliability. Intercoder reliability was assessed by calculating Cohen's kappa coefficient.[20,21] Intercoder agreement (expressed as a proportion) was .87 for the advertisements in 1980, .95 for 1984, and .97 for 1988. These reliability coefficients demonstrate a high level of agreement among the coders and are above the recommended .85 level suggested by Kassarjian.[7]

The two medical journals contained more than one-half of the pharmacoeconomic appeals identified for the years 1980, 1984, and 1988. The pharmacy journals targeted at mass circulation to pharmacists, on average, contained the lowest number of pharmacoeconomic appeals. Of the hospital pharmacy journals, both the *American Journal of Hospital Pharmacy* and *Hospital Formulary* displayed similar patterns for the number of pharmacoeconomic appeals, while *Drug Intelligence and Clinical Pharmacy* had the lowest number of appeals (Table 24.1). The total number of pharmacoeconomic appeals was about the same for each of the years.

The breakdown of advertisements by year with respect to the type of pharmacoeconomic appeal for the ten journals is shown in Table 24.2. The highest percentage of advertisements in 1980 used the pharmacoeconomic appeal of compliance (92%), while no advertisements contained an appeal for cost-benefit, and less than 10% of the advertisements contained appeals for cost-effectiveness and quality of life. A cross-sectional evaluation of advertisements indicates a decrease in the percentage of pharmacoeconomic appeals for compliance from 1980 to 1988, while the advertisements for cost-benefit,cost-effectiveness, and quality of life have increased from 1980 to 1988. The pharmacoeconomic appeal of cost-benefit was not identified in any of the advertisements for 1980, and only a small percentage of the advertisements contained a cost-effectiveness or quality of life appeal. The changes in the distribution of pharmacoeconomic appeals are particularly noticeable in 1984 and 1988, as these years followed TEFRA.

As noticeable patterns were identified for the number of pharmacoeconomic advertisements for these years, a chi-square analysis was performed to test the hypothesis of statistical independence between the observed and expected frequencies for the variables under investigation. As the chi-square test can be influenced by large sample sizes, Cramer's V and Kendall's tau B were also used to measure the degree of association among the variables.[22,23] Less than 5% of the advertisements in this study used cost-benefit appeals, and there were no cost-benefit appeals identified in the advertisements scanned in 1980; therefore, the categories containing appeals for cost-benefit and cost-effectiveness were combined.

Table 24.3 shows the results obtained from a statistical analysis of medical journal advertisements by year with respect to the type of pharmacoeconomic appeal. According to the results, the null hypothesis of statistical independence among the variables can be rejected. As a moderate level of association was observed in both cases, there is support for dependency among the variables. As displayed in this table, there is a decrease in the percentage of advertisements for compliance from 1984 to 1988, while the percentages of advertisements for cost-benefit, cost-effectiveness, and quality of life have increased from 1984 to 1988 (Kendall's tau B = $.528).

Shown in Table 24.4 are the results obtained from statistical analysis of hospital pharmacy journal advertisements by year with respect to the type of pharmacoeconomic appeal. The percentages obtained from contingency table analysis for the advertisements containing economic appeals changed considerably between 1984 and 1988, with a higher percentage of the economic appeals focusing on cost-benefit, cost-effectiveness, and quality of life than on compliance (Kendall's tau B = $.392). The results from statistical analysis demonstrate a consistent pattern for pharmacoeconomic advertisements, regardless of journal type, for the years 1980, 1984, and 1988.

TABLE 24.1. Number of Medication Advertisements by Journal and Year

Journal	Years			Total
	1980	1984	1988	
American Druggist	1	2	6	9
American Journal of Hospital Pharmacy	11	20	30	61
American Pharmacy	4	0	6	10
Drug Intelligence and Clinical Pharmacy	9	0	0	9
Drug Topics	9	13	10	32
Hospital Formulary	29	17	30	86
JAMA	68	74	78	220
New England Journal of Medicine	120	126	63	309
Pharmacy Times	11	22	25	58
U. S. Pharmacist	3	8	6	17
Total	265	292	254	811

TABLE 24.2. Frequency Distribution of Advertisements by Year with Respect to the Type of Pharmacoeconomic Appeal

Appeal	Year					
	1980		1984		1988	
	n	Percent	n	Percent	n	Percent
Cost-benefit	—		7	2.4%	16	6.3%
Cost-effectiveness	6	2.3%	42	14.4%	92	36.2%
Quality of life	15	5.7%	16	5.5%	29	11.4%
Compliance	244	92.0%	227	77.7%	117	46.1%
Total	265	100.0%	292	100.0%	254	100.0%

TABLE 24.3. Statistical Analysis of Medical Journal Advertisements by Year with Respect to the Type of Pharmacoeconomic Appeal*

Appeal	Year						Total
	1980		1984		1988		
	n	Percent	n	Percent	n	Percent	
Cost-benefit/ effectiveness	–	–	3	4.7%	61	95.3%	12.1%
Quality of life	–	–	11	32.4%	23	67.6%	6.4%
Compliance	188	43.6%	186	43.2%	57	13.2%	81.5%

*n = 529; chi-square = 228.62; Cramér's V = .465; d.f. = 4; p < .001

TABLE 24.4. Statistical Analysis of Clinical Pharmacy Journal Advertisements by Year with Respect to the Type of Pharmacoeconomic Appeal*

Appeal	Year						Total
	1980		1984		1988		
	n	Percent	n	Percent	n	Percent	
Cost-benefit/ effectiveness	6	7.1%	37	44.0%	41	48.8%	53.8%
Quality of life	10	58.8%	1	5.9%	6	35.3%	10.9%
Compliance	33	60.0%	9	16.4%	13	23.6%	35.3%

*$\underline{n}$ = 156; chi-square = 51.83; Cramér's $\underline{V}$ = .407; d.f. = 4f ; $\underline{p}$ < .001

DISCUSSION AND CONCLUSIONS

Governmental policies and regulations can have an impact on promotional strategies used by pharmaceutical firms. According to the results of this study, pharmaceutical firms have changed the content of prescription drug advertisements from 1980 to 1988. Although no causal link can be established between TEFRA and the type of appeal used in prescription drug product advertisements appearing in pharmacy and medical journals, several patterns of pharmacoeconomic appeal were identified in the content of advertisements analyzed in this study.

Of particular interest is the finding that the number of advertisements did not change greatly, but the content as related to pharmacoeconomic appeal did change. Similar patterns of change were observed in both the medical journals and the clinical pharmacy journals, with more pronounced changes observed in the medical journals. In both cases, there was a decrease in the percentage of advertisements targeted for compliance and an increase in the percentage of advertisements devoted to cost-benefit, cost-effectiveness, and quality of life.

A higher percentage of pharmacoeconomic appeals was identified in the medical journals. To a great extent, physicians serve as gatekeepers when they prescribe drug products. Not only do physicians play a role in controlling drug product costs, but dentists, nurses, pharmacists, and other health care professionals also have increased responsibility in this process. Many of these health care professionals also have become involved in drug use control, either directly or indirectly, as a result of third-party prescription programs, problems associated with therapy, and outpatient services. Because pharmacists, in general, participate actively in the process of drug use control, perhaps more pharmacoeconomic appeals should be directed toward pharmacists.

Governmental regulation is another environmental factor that influences the market structure of pharmaceutical firms; it influences both the supply- and demand-side economics of pharmaceutical firms. Supply-side regulation is associated with policies implemented by the Food and Drug Administration (FDA). These include the 1962 drug amendments to the 1938 federal Food, Drug, and Cosmetic Act. Studies have shown that the 1962 drug amendments had a significant negative impact on the research and development productivity of pharmaceutical firms.[24] Additional areas of involvement by the FDA include its role in regulating the content of prescription drug advertising and other promotional materials associated with a drug product.

Demand-side regulations are somewhat restricted in scope and affect the buyers of pharmaceutical products. Examples of demand-side regulations include state legislation to repeal the antisubstitution laws, the MAC program, TEFRA, formularies, and various efforts to increase the use of generic drugs. Because governmental policies constitute a dynamic element in the environment, marketing strategies must be revised to adjust for the impact of such policies on market structure. Drug product advertising, direct mailing, and other promotional strategies enable the pharmaceutical firm to manage the uncertainty in its task environment by increasing the demand for drug products.

Virts has identified one of the most significant aspects of demand-side regulation in the pharmaceutical industry: many of the effects of this type of regulation are long-run in nature.[25] Demand-side regulation may have some impact on short-term benefits, but the long-run benefits may also be jeopardized. For example, drug product innovation would be adversely affected in the long-run. This phenomenon is attributed to a reduction in cash flow that ultimately reduces the amount of funds available for research and development, thus slowing the production of new single-chemical entities.

Another interesting aspect of governmental policies is their impact on consumers. From a policy perspective, it would be interesting to assess the suggestion that patients may prefer to pay a higher price for medication if product information is provided by the physician.[26] Perhaps risk factors perceived by patients, such as the nature of their illness, possibility of side effects from the drug product, and the cost of therapy itself, may influence their desire for drug product information.

A time series design is frequently used to assess major changes in administrative policy.[27] One weakness of this design is failure to control for other events that may have influenced the observations. The other policy implemented during this time concerning pharmaceutical firms was the Drug Price Competition and Patent Term Restoration Act of 1984, which affected patent life and generic market accessibility. Despite efforts to control for the effects of history, one of the limitations of this study is the inability to separate the effects of other governmental policies instituted during this time period from those of TEFRA. Another limitation was the inability to control for the potential impact of cultural trends, as well as general concerns for cost containment through the use of another control group. In addition to the impact of governmental policies, socioeconomic forces in the environment could influence the content of prescription drug product advertising.

In summary, the economic task environment of pharmaceutical firms is dynamic. As discussed previously, the task environment constitutes that part of the environment defined by managers as relevant or potentially relevant for organizational decision making.[28] Economic factors such as governmental regulations and policies can have a profound impact on the market structure of pharmaceutical firms. Although the number of pharmacoeconomic appeals contained in drug product advertisements did not change considerably from 1980 to 1988, there was a change in promotional content. A noticeable increase in the percentage of advertisements containing pharmacoeconomic appeals, including cost-benefit, cost-effectiveness, and quality of life, was observed after the implementation of the Tax Equity and Fiscal Responsibility Act of 1983 while there was a decrease in the percentage of advertisements focusing on compliance.

REFERENCES

1. Hornbrook MC. Market structure and advertising in the U.S. pharmaceutical industry. Med Care 1978;16:90-109.

2. Dill WR. Environment as an influence on managerial autonomy. Adm Sci Q 1958;2:409-43.

3. Dess GG, Beard DW. Dimensions of organizational task environments. Adm Sci Q 1984;29:52-73.

4. Broyles RW, Rosko MD. A qualitative assessment of the Medicare prospective payment system. Soc Sci Med 1985;20:1185-90.

5. Flannery EJ, Hutt PB. Balancing competition and patient protection in the drug industry: the Drug Price Competition and Patent Restoration Act of 1984. Food Drug Cos Law J 1985;40:269-309.

6. Greenberg RB. The Prescription Drug Marketing Act of 1987. Am J Hosp Pharm 1987;45:2118-21.

7. Kassarjian HH. Content analysis in consumer research. J Consumer Res 1977;4:8-18.

8. Smith MC, Visconti JA. Appeals used in prescription drug advertising. Hosp Pharm 1968;3:5-13.

9. Freeman RA, Tonelli RJ. Trends in prescription drug advertising 1968-1976. Med Market Media 1979;14(2):44-7.

10. Freeman RA, Tonelli RJ. An overview of prescription drug advertising content. Med Market Media 1979;14(3):28-30.

11. Juergens JP. Advertising in the *American Journal of Hospital Pharmacy*. Am J Hosp Pharm 1987;44:1647-51.

12. Brinberg D, Morris LA. Advertising prescription drugs to consumers. Adv Mark Pub Pol 1987;1:1-40.

13. Neill JR. A social history of psychotropic drug advertisements. Soc Sci Med 1989;28:333-8.

14. Gagnon JP. Ratings of scholarly journals in five pharmacy disciplines. Am J Pharm Educ 1986;50:127-34.

15. Nie NH, Hull CH, Jenkins JG, Steinbrenner K, Bent DH. Statistical package for the social sciences. 2nd ed. New York: McGraw-Hill, 1975.

16. Warner KE, Luce BR. Cost-benefit and cost-effectiveness analysis in health care. Ann Arbor, MI: Health Administration Press, 1982.

17. Weinstein MC, Stason WB. Foundations of cost-effectiveness analysis for health and medical practices. N Engl J Med 1977;296:716-21.

18. Shepard DS, Thompson MS. First principles of cost-effectiveness analysis in health. Public Health Rep 1979;94:535-43.

19. Smith MC, Juergens JP, Jack W. Pharmaceutical differentiation through quality of life measurement. St. Louis, MO: Medstrat, Inc., 1989.

20. Cohen J. A coefficient of agreement for nominal scales. Educ Psychol Measurement 1960;21(1):37-46.

21. Fleiss J. Measuring nominal scale agreement among many raters. Psychol Bull 1971;76:378-82.

22. Kerlinger FH. Foundations of behavioral research. 3rd ed. New York: Holt, Rinehart and Winston, 1986.

23. Agresti A, Finlay B. Statistical methods for the social sciences. 2nd ed. San Francisco, CA: Dellen Publishing Company, 1986.

24. Cocks DL. Economic and competitive aspects of the pharmaceutical industry. In: Smith MC, ed. Principles of pharmaceutical marketing. 3rd ed. Philadelphia: Lea and Febiger, 1983:343-68.

25. Virts JR. Regulation of prescription drugs. In: Chien RI, ed. Issues in pharmaceutical economics. Lexington, MA: Lexington Books, 1979:195-209.

26. Fer MA, Smith MC. Advertising. In: Smith MC. Principles of pharmaceutical marketing. 3rd ed. Philadelphia: Lea and Febiger, 1983:369-99.

27. Campbell DT, Stanley JC. Experimental and quasi-experimental designs for research. Boston: Houghton Mifflin, 1963.

28. Duncan R. What is the right organization structure? Organizational Dynamics 1979;(Winter):59-76.

Chapter 25

Economics of Prescription Drug Advertising

Paul H. Rubin

INTRODUCTION

While at one time economists were somewhat hostile to advertising, in recent years most economic analysis has concluded that advertising is, by and large, informative and beneficial to consumers. Advertising provides information on product attributes and prices, including information about new product availability, and can make entry into a market of competing products easier than it would otherwise be. A negative effect of some advertising might be to insulate products from competition, perhaps leading to increased market power and higher prices. Overall, however, the benefits of advertising outweigh the disadvantages.

We must then ask, What would be the impact of restricting advertising and promotion of pharmaceuticals? Presumably, some costs and some benefits would result from increased regulation.

ADVERTISING TO PHYSICIANS

Advertising of prescription drugs facilitates entry of some new products and provides information regarding their benefits. On the other hand, some

This chapter was originally prepared for presentation at the Drug Information Association Seminar, "New Perspectives on Pharmaceutical Marketing and Promotion," March 14-15, 1991, New York. While accepting responsibility for errors, the author would like to thank Alison Keith and two referees for helpful comments.

Previously published in *Journal of Research in Pharmaceutical Economics*, Vol. 3(4), 1991.

advertising may entrench established products in their positions and thus make entry and price competition more difficult. However, research indicates that advertising tends to make entry by new, innovative products easier and entry by products with less innovative characteristics more difficult.[1] This indicates that competition by quality of product is in some sense more effective in the pharmaceutical industry than competition by price. Of course, higher returns earned by producers of innovative products are a stimulus for more spending on research and development, so even if advertising makes prices somewhat higher for some products than otherwise, the welfare implications are at best ambiguous.

Benefits of Advertising

Economic analysis of promotion expenditures for pharmaceuticals indicates that for a new drug, promotion is initially largely through detailing. This type of promotion is most effective for "brands that are the first to offer and promote some new therapeutic advantage," rather than for "brands that merely duplicate existing therapies."[1] Companies spend resources on detailing to inform physicians of the attributes of their products. Advertising to physicians serves a similar informative function and helps physicians recall the information presented through detailing.

In addition, advertising of some products helps physicians recall the name of the advertised product and thus make entry by new, competing products more difficult. (For a summary of economic research on the benefits and cost of prescription drug advertising, see References 2-4.) This is why the first product in an area tends to retain an advantage even as new products enter. Because the first product is by definition innovative, the major benefits of promotion are for new products, which are, of course, likely to be therapeutically most important.

Firms will use detailing and advertising in combination to maximize their profits. This approach is based on informing physicians about new products by brand name and helping physicians recall this information. Firms will spend more on advertising and promotion of some products than on others. Economic research has indicated that it generally pays to spend more on advertising of relatively better products.[5,6] Advertising can induce a consumer to try a product or induce the physician to prescribe the product. If the consumer or the physician is unhappy with the product, then he will not continue to use it, so the advertising gains the firm a relatively small return. Thus, a given level of advertising expenditure is more likely to be productive for a better product, and advertisers can be expected to spend more on promoting and advertising better products.

Consumers are implicitly aware of this relationship. Advertising that seems uninformative (such as product endorsements by famous people) will still convey information. The information is that the advertiser considers this product to be worth spending money on and, therefore, thinks that if the consumer tries the product, the consumer will like it. A similar analysis would apply to spending by pharmaceutical companies on expensive promotions such as seminars or symposia for physicians. if the company did not think that the product being promoted would be useful, it would not find the promotion worthwhile. Thus, a fear that these programs will induce physicians to prescribe inferior or inappropriate products is misplaced. It is much more likely that the seminar itself serves as a signal to physicians that the company thinks highly of its product.

In addition, of course, there is direct information about product characteristics conveyed by such seminars. As indicated above, information about new, innovative products is more likely to have an effect than information about less original products. This further indicates that drug companies would be more willing to spend large sums for promoting better products.

Firms also have incentives to promote their own corporate name. This will increase the value of the firm's reputation.[7] To the extent that physicians have satisfactory therapeutic experiences with a particular drug company, they will be more likely to prescribe its products in the future. Thus, promotion of the corporate name is also useful for consumers.

Costs of Advertising

Disadvantages of advertising might be of two kinds. First, there might be deception through ads that convey untrue information. Second, there might be economic costs of advertising if advertising entrenches existing brands and thus leads to price increases. There has been no evidence that economists have worried about deception in pharmaceutical advertising. Those who have studied the issue generally conclude that FDA scrutiny of ads is sufficient to allay any fears of deception.[3]

On the other hand, firms may have an incentive to overspend somewhat (from a social point of view) on advertising. For example, once generics become available, spending by the manufacturer of the branded product may retard the penetration of the generic by maintaining the goodwill of the original product. Such first-mover advantages are common in all markets but may be particularly important in pharmaceuticals.[8] This is because the person selecting the product–the physician–does not pay for the product and therefore has less incentive to worry about price than the ultimate consumer.[9] As discussed below, restrictions on direct-to-consumer advertising exacerbate this problem. Moreover, as indicated below, evidence in many markets generally indicates that increased advertising leads to reduced prices.

Policy Implications

While economists recognize costs and benefits of pharmaceutical advertising, it is fair to say that most economists ultimately believe that a significant portion of promotional expenditures is helpful and useful. Virtually no economist would argue that there are not significant benefits from these expenditures. Moreover, it would be difficult to find an informed economist who would be willing to argue for severe public regulation or limitation of such expenditures.

Where does this leave us? Increased regulation would probably not reduce deception because there is no evidence of any deception in this market. Advertising, in general, provides useful information about new, innovative products. Advertisers are more likely to spend money on advertising and promoting such products because spending on better products earns a higher return. Thus, there would be relatively small gains from increasing regulation of these expenditures, and there would be potentially large costs in terms of reduced information to physicians about new, better products. Moreover, if firms expected increased difficulty in promoting new products, the incentive for investment in research to develop such products would also be reduced. The cost to society of this reduction could be quite large.

DIRECT-TO-CONSUMER ADVERTISING

An interesting application of this perspective is direct advertising of prescription drugs to consumers. Economists who have studied this issue agree that such advertising is beneficial to consumers. To my knowledge, however, only two economists, Alison Keith and I, have studied the issue.[10-13] We have identified several health benefits from such advertising. These benefits accrue because consumers and physicians have different pieces of information. The information held privately by consumers can sometimes be combined with information in pharmaceutical ads to better match patients and drugs. Direct advertising will also reduce prices of drugs.

The FDA is apparently considering increasing regulatory scrutiny of such ads due to fear of deception.[14,15] This would be a serious mistake. There is no evidence of any deception in existing ads. More important, deception is highly unlikely in this market. Consumers are not mere pawns;

they are aware of the source of information and treat the information with appropriate skepticism.[13] A fear of masses of consumers rushing blindly to pressure their physicians to prescribe worthless drugs is misplaced.* Moreover, because approval by a physician is required for purchase of a prescription drug, there is less chance of deception in this area than in almost any other. A consumer will of necessity have a second, informed opinion before acting on an advertisement.

The FDA seems concerned most with making sure that ads (whether to physicians or to consumers) provide a fair balance of information, and it views ads without such fair balance as deceptive. To the FDA, this means that ads should convey information about both positive and negative effects of products. However, this requirement is not justified. It is not correct to assume (as the FDA implicitly seems to) that each ad is freestanding and that consumers will learn only what is in the ad. There are alternative sources of information. Competing products can provide their own ads, and physicians themselves are an important source of information, particularly for prescription drugs. Requirements of fair balance in each ad, aimed at increasing the information available to consumers, actually mean that advertising is more expensive and that there will be less of it, thus reducing information available to consumers.

It would be foolish to forego the benefits of direct-to-consumer advertising because of a misplaced fear of deception. The benefits are improved health and reduced drug costs.[10-13]

Health Benefits

We may identify the following benefits from direct advertising:

1. A consumer may not be aware that a treatment exists for some condition. Two prominent examples are Upjohn's Rogaine®, a treatment for some conditions of baldness, and Marion Merrell Dow's Nicorette® gum, a smoking cessation aid. In both cases, consumers may not be aware that there are prescription remedies for the conditions unless they are informed by advertising. Nicorette is particularly interesting because cigarettes can be advertised with only a brief, one-line mention of health risks, but a remedy requires the usual lengthy "brief summary."

---

*Sidney Wolfe of Public Citizen Health Research Group: "They encourage patients to pound on the doctor's door and demand the new miracle treatment" (as quoted in Rosenthal.[16]) Wolfe apparently views the ability of consumers to make rational judgments with some disdain.

The case of Rogaine points out another disadvantage of limiting advertising. After news reports began to indicate that there was a prescription remedy for some cases of baldness, producers of some OTC "remedies" began to advertise their products, implying in various ways that they were the prescription medication. Upjohn, the producer of Rogaine, was limited in its ability to respond by the FDA regulations.

2. A consumer may suffer some symptoms (e.g., thirst) without realizing that these are symptoms of a disease (e.g., diabetes). A consumer who does not realize that symptoms indicate a disease will not consult a physician and therefore cannot learn in this way that he or she has a treatable disease.

3. A consumer may have been previously diagnosed with some then untreatable disease for which a new treatment has since become available. Because the consumer believes that the disease is not treatable, he or she will not contact a physician and therefore will not learn about the new therapy. Advertisements can inform him or her, thereby leading to treatment. A similar analysis applies to the creation of a new vaccine for a condition to which some consumers may know themselves to be susceptible. An example is a vaccine for hepatitis B, a disease to which homosexuals are particularly susceptible.

4. A new remedy with reduced side effects may become available. Advertising can provide benefits in two cases. Consumers who do not know that symptoms they are experiencing are side effects, and so would not ask a physician about them, may learn from ads that there are alternatives without these side effects. Consumers who have ceased treatment because of side effects, and thus are not seeing a physician, may begin treatment again if they learn of therapies that do not impose the same side effects. An example is impotence caused by some antihypertensives. Some consumers may not know that the condition is drug related; others may have stopped therapy because of the condition. Either class of consumers can benefit from ads indicating that a treatment with reduced side effects is available.

Price Effects

Direct-to-consumer advertising may also be expected to lead to price reductions for pharmaceuticals. As indicated above, price is currently less effective as a competitive tool in pharmaceuticals than in many other lines of commerce because the physician chooses the product but does not pay for it. Therefore, providing consumers with information that would enable them to more easily compare prices would be expected to have a larger than average effect on price. There is evidence from many markets that increased advertising leads to lower prices.[16-21] (For a summary, see Reference 22.) Indeed, this evidence was cited by the Supreme Court in decisions overturning state bans on advertising of attorney services and of eyeglasses. In the pharmaceutical market, we would expect an even greater reduction in price from increased advertising because this advertising would provide information to the party actually paying for the product.

There are several mechanisms through which advertising can lead to lower prices. Advertising can inform consumers that two brands of the same drug are, in fact, equivalent. Consumers can also learn that two drugs are effectively equivalent and that one is cheaper, then ask physicians to prescribe the lower priced drug. Increased competition brought about by increased advertising can lead manufacturers to reduce prices for drugs. If one ad can simultaneously list the use, the price, and the name of a drug, then price competition between retail pharmacies can be increased.* Today, an ad cannot provide this information without including the brief summary.

Policy Implications

At present, there are severe restrictions on direct advertising of prescription drugs. However, in contrast to past policy, such advertising is at least allowed, although the FDA may be considering changing this policy. If an ad mentions both the name of the product and its intended use, then the ad must include the brief summary. This brief summary is virtually worthless to consumers because it is written in technical language and will probably be read and understood by only a very small minority of consumers. Moreover, since a prescription will be needed for the drug, the physician will have access to the required information before prescribing the drug.

Because an informed intermediary must be used for purchase of a prescription, information is probably better in the pharmaceutical market than in almost any other consumer market, and the requirement of an expensive and worthless piece of information provides no benefits. The main effect of this requirement is to eliminate television as a source of prescription drug advertising. Since television is a very effective medium for communication, this effect may be very costly.

---

*A recent study has found that only 36.4% of consumers "Never" use the price of a prescription product as a basis for choosing a pharmacy [see Wolfgang AP, Perri M III. Consumer price sensitivity toward prescriptions. J Res Pharm Econ 1989;1(4):51-60]. Greater provision of information would facilitate such price shopping between pharmacies, and more information would also allow price shopping between brands and drugs.

There would be definite advantages in being able to advertise more cheaply (i.e., without the brief summary) the name and function of a drug simultaneously. Firms are more likely to advertise if they can mention brand names because this diminishes the "free rider" problem and enables the advertising firm to capture the benefits of its ad. Moreover, advertising the name and function of a drug can increase the downward pressure on prices created by advertising. Ads containing both the brand name and the uses of a drug convey more information, thus providing all of the beneficial functions mentioned above.

There is little to fear from reducing regulatory stringency of ads because deception is not a real fear in this market. There are potentially large benefits from informing consumers about products that would lead to improved health. Any effort to increase regulation here would generate no benefits and *would* generate substantial costs; thus, further regulation should be avoided.

SUMMARY

In sum, current views by economists focus largely on the information effects of advertising. Advertising and promotion of prescription drugs is beneficial to consumers because of the information provided. Deception in this market–of physicians or consumers–is particularly improbable. If there is any harmful effect of advertising to professionals, it is that such advertising might lead to increased market power and thus increased prices. The most efficient way to reduce this effect is to allow increased direct advertising because consumers have the strongest interest in price reductions. Increasing regulation of advertising to professionals would be harmful and would not generate benefits.

A major weakness of the current regulatory system is the severe limitation of direct-to-consumer advertising. This advertising would provide health benefits and lead to price reductions. The FDA imposed an absolute ban on such advertising from 1983 to 1985. It then sensibly relaxed this ban. It is now time to take the next step and eliminate the costly and pointless requirement of a brief summary in ads that name the product and its use. A return to the system that severely limited direct advertising of prescription drugs would make consumers both less healthy and less wealthy, and this should not be a goal of sound public policy.

REFERENCES

1. Bond RS, Lean DF. Sales, promotion, and product differentiation in two prescription drug markets. Staff report to the Federal Trade Commission. Washington, DC: 1977.

2. Comanor WS. The political economy of the pharmaceutical industry. J Econ Lit 1986;24:1178-1217.

3. Leffler K. Persuasion or information: the economics of prescription drug advertising. J Law Econ 1981;24:45-74.

4. Hurwitz MA, Caves RE. Persuasion or information? Promotion and the share of brand name and generic pharmaceuticals. J Law Econ 1988;26:299-320.

5. Nelson P. Information and consumer behavior. J Political Economy 1970; 78:311-29.

6. Nelson P. Advertising as information. J Political Economy 1974;82:729-54.

7. Rubin PH. Managing business transactions: controlling the costs of coordinating, communicating, and decision making. New York: Free Press, 1990: Ch. 8.

8. Schmalensee R. Product differentiation advantages of pioneering brands. Am Econ Rev 1982;72:349-65.

9. Masson A, Steiner R. Generic substitution and prescription drug prices. Washington, DC: Federal Trade Commission, 1985.

10. Masson A, Rubin PH. Matching prescription drugs and consumers. N Engl J Med 1985;313:513.

11. Masson A, Rubin PH. Plugs for drugs. Regulation 1986;(Sept):37. Reprinted in J Pharm Market Manage 1986;1(2):29-43.

12. Masson A. Direct to consumer advertising. In: Mayer RN, ed. Enhancing consumer choice. Columbia, MO: American Council on Consumer Interests, 1991.

13. Rubin PH. The economics of regulating deception. Cato J (in press).

14. Gladwell M. New FDA chief promises crackdown on misleading ads by drug firms. Washington Post 1991 Mar 1:A13.

15. Rosenthal E. Drug makers set off a bitter debate with ads aimed directly at patients. New York Times 1991 Mar 3:34.

16. Benham L. The effect of advertising on the price of eyeglasses. J Law Econ 1972;15:337.

17. Steiner R. Does advertising lower consumer prices? J Market 1973;37:19.

18. Marvel H. The economics of information and retail gasoline price behavior. J Political Economy 1976;84:1033.

19. Farris P, Albion M. The impact of advertising on the price of consumer products. J Market 1980;44(Summer):17.

20. Kwoka J. Advertising and the price and quality of optometric services. Am Econ Rev 1984;74:211.

21. Haas-Wilson D. The effect of commercial practice restrictions: the case of optometry. J Law Econ 1986;29:165.

22. Albion M, Farris PW. The advertising controversy: evidence on the economic effects of advertising. Boston: Auburn House, 1981.

Chapter 26

The Role of Health Economics in Marketing New Pharmaceuticals Worldwide

Brian Lovatt

INTRODUCTION

Recent coverage in the media regarding concerns over the rising costs of health care and the price of pharmaceutical products is creating considerable public awareness of the potential impact of cost control measures that may be applied to the provision of health care.

What is often missing with regard to pharmaceutical products is balanced coverage of the significant advances in treatment that have occurred in a wide range of diseases and the relief of the suffering of many patients that has resulted from the development and marketing of new medicines. Since some $7-9 billion will be spent in the U.S. alone this year to produce significant new medicines for the future, it is important that the public come to appreciate the benefits new medicines can bring. Perhaps improved communication should be a major agenda item for the industry at present. Health economics is well placed to assist in the objective demonstration of the benefits that are brought to society by new and innovative medicines.

A good example of the health economics benefits that advances in treatment could bring comes from the areas of coronary heart disease and cerebrovascular disease. Health economists and other experts from Battelle Institute recently estimated that if current trends continue, by the year 2015 there will be 30 million people in the U.S. suffering from coronary

Previously published in *Journal of Research in Pharmaceutical Economics*, Vol. 4(4), 1992.

heart disease and four million suffering from cerebrovascular disease.[1] Lost productivity due to premature deaths in these groups would total some $1.5 trillion. However, the researchers went on to predict a two-thirds reduction in that number, with 50% of this benefit coming from behavioral changes (e.g., dietary improvements), 10% from various biomedical advances (e.g., surgical plaque-removing technology) and 40% from pharmaceutical advances (e.g., antihypertensives and lipid-lowering agents). In more tangible terms, this means that pharmaceutical advances in these disease areas are predicted to save 5.3 million people from premature death and $211 billion in indirect costs in the U.S. by 2015.

THE ROLE OF HEALTH ECONOMICS

Before considering the role of health economics from a pharmaceutical company's perspective, it is valid to review the environmental factors that have necessitated this specific response by the industry.

Spiraling health care costs worldwide have placed considerable pressure upon governments and third-party payers. There has been an explosion of new technology resulting in dramatic improvements in our ability to keep many people alive, people who only a few years ago would have died prematurely. We have the ability to operate in utero, control pain, replace worn joints, and control many diseases that in the recent past would have crippled a large percentage of the population. The proportion of the population that is elderly is increasing significantly, bringing a consequential higher utilization of services (Figure 26.1). These factors are all increasing the pressure on health care systems to control costs. There is also a high level of public expectation of the medical profession to cure at any cost and of "magic bullets" to treat all complaints.

Governments generally find themselves in the middle. On one hand, they desire to improve both the standards and availability of health care. On the other hand, they also must allocate the nation's taxes in an equitable way among the different programs competing for central resources (e.g., housing, education, defense, health). Major differences exist in the amount devoted to health care by different governments (ruling bodies, national administrations), both as a percentage of GDP (gross domestic product) and as the actual amount per capita (Figure 26.2). In response to the pressures on financing health care provision, we see a continual reorganization of health care systems worldwide, some minor, others major (e.g., National Health Service reforms in the U.K.). Yet there is no consensus on the best way to deliver health care or on the level of funding that is appropriate or necessary to ensure adequate services.

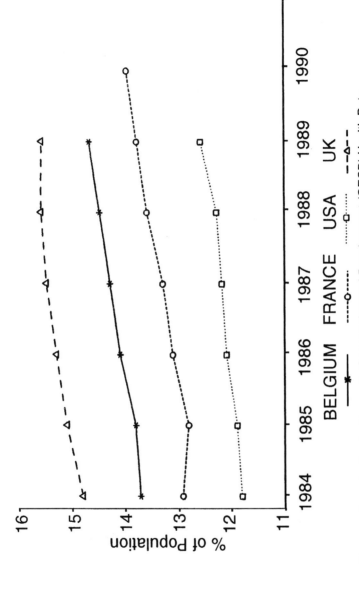

FIGURE 26.1. Populaton 65 Years and Over as a Percentage of the Population

BELGIUM   FRANCE   USA   UK

Source: Program Organization for Economic Cooperation and Development (OECD) Health Data
Data: OECD

FIGURE 26.2. Total Health Expenditure/GDP (%)

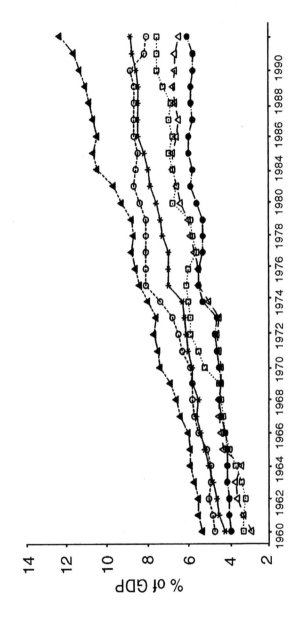

FRANCE GERMANY ITALY JAPAN UK USA

Source: Program OECD Health Data
Data: OECD

A common response to these financial pressures has been the devolution of responsibility for cost control to the various sectors of controlled health care systems. In turn, this has resulted in more rigorous monitoring of departmental budgets. Internationally, the trend is to change the focus from a purely clinical one to include financial and use of resource elements in decision making.

The pharmaceutical budget has become a common target for cost-containment measures despite the relatively small percentage that it contributes to a country's total health care costs (Figure 26.3). The reasons for this focus of attention would make a good topic for another chapter and will not be covered further here. Suffice it to say that pharmacy cost-containment programs are widespread and include comprehensive and relatively sophisticated mechanisms of control over both the availability and the use of products.

Pharmacy and therapeutics or formulary committees are charged with the responsibility of maintaining a list of appropriate agents to cover most requirements. These products should be safe and effective but also must demonstrate cost-effectiveness. There is no doubt that there is considerable expertise available in all markets to evaluate safety and efficacy, but this may not be so for cost-effectiveness. Why is this?

Historically, the industry has supplied information on the safety and efficacy of its products to regulatory authorities to obtain marketing approval and then subsequently supplied published information to two main customer groups, clinicians and pharmacists, to enable them to assess the profile of the product. Cost was not seen as the major factor in product choice. The next phase was that these customers demonstrated an increased awareness of cost. This factor, along with a more crowded marketplace, meant that they required information on the extra benefits they would obtain for the price.

Over the past few years, the financial pressures have grown, and a significant amount of health care reorganization has taken place that has resulted in many new decision makers becoming involved in new product adoption. These new decision makers represent new customers for the pharmaceutical industry, customers who are focusing on value for money and on quality of care. A new language is being used. Cost-effectiveness, cost-benefit, cost utility, and quality of life have become terms in regular use to compare different therapy options. Perhaps because this new language has come into use so suddenly, the incorrect use of these terms is widespread. The complexity of the new methodologies and a general lack of understanding of their meaning among certain customer groups in many countries is creating communication problems. In the current environ-

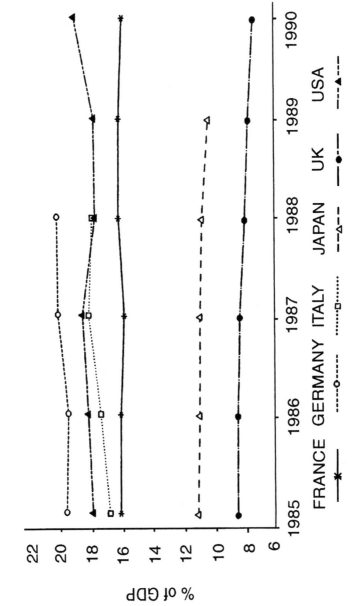

FIGURE 26.3. Medical Goods Expenditure: Total Exp. Pharmacy/Total Health Exp. (%)

Source: Program OECD Health Data
Data: OECD

420

ment, the industry will have to satisfy the needs of new customers if it is to flourish, but education must accompany the increased use of this type of information, both within the industry and with the various parties interested in using the information.

The industry is generally very good at communicating safety and efficacy and translating product features into benefits. However, many marketing executives now find themselves in an unfamiliar area as customers ask for resource utilization information relating to the use of products. As this information is not directly available from the traditional clinical trial data, marketing executives have to look to pharmacoeconomics to satisfy this need.

It is often said that people react to the new and unfamiliar in different ways, and this is no different for pharmacoeconomics. The fear of the unknown is causing some product managers to see pharmacoeconomics as a threat. They are concerned that in-depth analysis of the costs and outcomes created by their products might result in an unfavorable comparison with an emerging competitor. However, once these product managers gain a better understanding of the methodologies used, the vast majority will appreciate that pharmacoeconomics represents an opportunity for many products.

Understanding that an economic evaluation will look at the benefits of a product over a wider area than just the pharmacy budget and realizing that these studies will assist formulary (pharmacy and therapeutics) committees to assess the outcome and/or value in use of the product, without having to "best guess," helps product managers to see the benefits of well-conducted economic evaluations. These factors can result in a product's faster acceptance on the market with a resultant rapid product adoption curve that is more likely to be sustained (Figure 26.4).

Quality of life is a term that has been associated with pharmaceutical products for a long time; however, it was only in 1986 that the first major quality of life study was published in the *New England Journal of Medicine*.[2] Since then, a great number of publications have been used by the industry. While there still appears to be widespread difficulty in understanding, except in very broad terms, the true and full meaning of the results, the technology is refined enough at this time for the industry to obtain comprehensive information on the quality of life impact of treatments (and competitors). This will assist the product manager in differentiating a product from others and accurately targeting patient groups that stand to gain the maximum benefit from the product.

How else may this information be used? How will it be collected? The future role of pharmacoeconomics is bound to expand because by employing the methodology, one can gain an early understanding of the cost of a disease

FIGURE 26.4. Product Adoption Curve

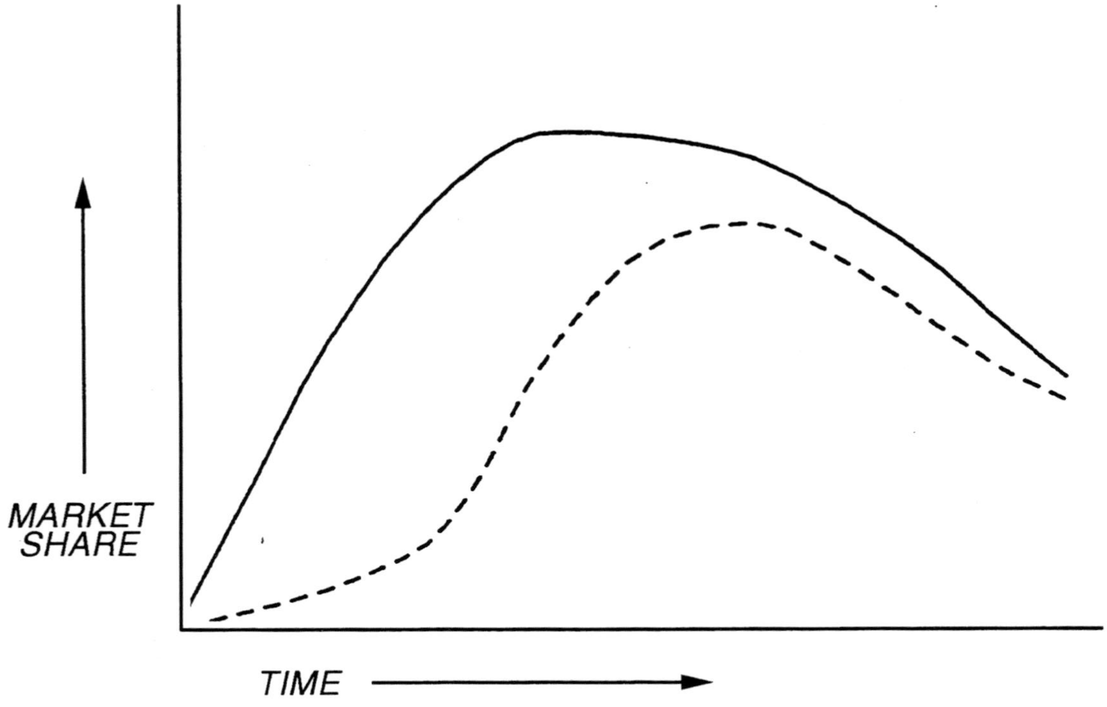

or illness and the likely impact that a development compound could have in these areas. This information will assist decision making during the early research and development stages. Also, forecasting can become more objective earlier in the life cycle of a product. Revisions of product forecasts can take place as more information becomes available during development, and through this increased knowledge, companies can improve their decision-making processes and gain a better understanding of a product's potential.

With today's expensive product development technology, seven out of every ten products will fail to pay back their investment and produce adequate profits. Therefore, it is easy to understand the requirement for improving the quality of information available early in a product's development. Companies will have to stop the development of some products and accelerate others if they want to improve the ratio of profitable products.

Pharmacoeconomic studies that are designed to produce data for an economic dossier to be used in pricing negotiations will have to be undertaken at an early development stage, perhaps mid-Phase III, as this information is often required prior to launch. Studies that are designed to assist in formulary listing will be comparative and have often been undertaken after the registration studies. However, for these studies to gain maximum effect, they must be available at or before launch. This means that in some cases the studies must start earlier and in other cases the launch date could be delayed.

An important factor to consider when planning economic studies is that although the majority of product safety and efficacy data is transferable internationally, other data must be collected on a local basis. This is because it is the way the product is used and the local costs and organization of the health care system that will determine the impact upon resource utilization. Local studies must be undertaken, and data outside the clinical trial program will require collection (e.g., costs of products, personnel). A central coordinating role is essential to maintain the quality and consistency of this activity.

As the focus of this chapter is to give a view as to the role of health economics in marketing new pharmaceutical products, no further discussion of the methodological challenges will be pursued. Those areas that are more controversial in the application of health economics studies will be addressed.

Is pharmacoeconomics science or marketing?* Pharmacoeconomics is a science. It employs well-tried and tested methodology taken from the

---

*"Science or Marketing" is the title of a discussion paper written by Professor Michael Drummond of the University of York, Department of Health Economics, which addresses the current stage of development of the methodology and can be highly recommended for further reading in this area.

discipline of economics, and although it may still be an unfamiliar methodology when applied to medicine, this does not make it any less valid. The marketing aspect comes in when this science is applied, ensuring that the information is seen as relevant to the particular customer and that it is communicated in a comprehensible way so that the product can be used appropriately.

When pharmacoeconomic studies are being planned, problems can occur in three main areas:

1. Defining the question the study should address. Attention must be paid to the following areas:

   • Which comparator is most appropriate?
   • What information does the customer need?
   • What should be measured?

   Many decision makers are indicating that they are willing to assist with guidance on what information they are looking for and which comparators would be most appropriate to include in a study. Some managed care groups have indicated that they are willing to share their comprehensive databases with companies. This provides an excellent opportunity to research the resource impact of a new agent within a real-life setting.
2. The analytical methodology to be used in a health economics study can be another area where decisions must be made. Including clinicians and other decision makers in exploratory discussions together with health economists will ensure that studies employ appropriate methodology to achieve results that will be perceived as relevant by the customer.
3. Reporting of results is not as clear-cut as it first appears. Simply presenting all of the data collected may seem to be the easy option. However, it is important that the information required by customers be presented in a clear and precise manner. Further, to avoid bias, it is important to state the assumptions that have been made and the type of methodology employed. This level of transparency in the reporting of results is important to the future acceptability of health economics studies conducted by the industry.

Without maintaining a professional approach to health economics, the industry will soon lose credibility and the benefits that can be gained from using this relatively new science. Promotional use of the data must be controlled in a way similar to the currently successful way that clinical data is approved for promotional use. Pharmacoeconomics is only a way of producing information to assist in decision making and is neither intended to, nor should it, replace individualized patient treatment decisions. Also, it should not be forgotten that good clinical information that demonstrates clear clinical benefits for a product is required before positive economic arguments can be made. Above all else, it should be appreciated that health economics will not provide benefits as if by magic for products that do not have a basically sound clinical profile.

REFERENCES

1. Battelle Institute. The value of pharmaceuticals: an assessment of future costs for selected conditions. Schering-Plough Corporation.

2. Croog SH, Levine S, Testa MA, Brown B, Bulpitt CJ, Jenkins CD. The effects of antihypertensive therapy on the quality of life. N Engl J Med 1986;314: 1657-64.

Chapter 27

The Benefits
of Pharmaceutical Promotion:
An Economic and Health Perspective

Alison Keith

Promotion conveys information, and information makes markets work better. In the context of prescription drugs, the benefits of promotion are better health and more vigorous competition, which, in turn, put downward pressure on prices.

The most direct informational effect of promotion, and the one easiest to see, is that it helps people sort through the array of available goods and services to choose those best suited to their needs and preferences, within the always-present constraint of ability to pay. With prescription pharmaceuticals, better information makes better matches of patients with drugs possible, leading to improvements in health.[1]*

Promotion has indirect effects as well-powerful effects. It enhances competition, putting downward pressure on prices. It makes it easier for new products to attract buyers and therefore, is an incentive for innovation. By facilitating the entry of new products and new firms, promotion further strengthens competition on quality and price.

This view of promotion is not unanimous, of course, yet whether promotion adds or subtracts from the well-being of society is less controversial among economists than among other observers. For example, many critics of promotion allege proliferation of misleading messages.

Previously published in *Journal of Pharmaceutical Marketing and Management*, Vol. 7(1), 1992.

*The term promotion is used here in a broad sense and includes such disparate forms of communication as pharmaceutical representatives' discussions with physicians, journal advertising, and health messages directed to consumers.

Many economists respond that even without taking government regulation into account, it is highly unlikely that most promotion would be misleading. Firms planning to stay in business for the long term have strong disincentives against misleading buyers; it is simply too costly to lose and then rebuild a good reputation. Moreover, modern economic theory emphasizes the importance of information in causing markets to perform well, but at the same time, generating and disseminating information is costly. Promotion is seen as a potentially valuable means of helping buyers make choices tailored to their preferences. Promotion is not dismissed as useful only to profit-hungry sellers. The debate among economists focuses instead on questions such as whether there is too much promotion and whether promotion by established firms hinders the entry of new firms.

In this chapter, I will explain the economic logic linking promotion with direct and indirect benefits. I will report the results of some economic studies of the effects of promotion in pharmaceutical markets and studies on some other markets as well. Finally, I will develop the implications for public policy of the view that promotion is valuable in making markets work better. Specifically, I argue that overrestrictive regulation of promotion can harm consumers by preventing them from getting useful information.

PROMOTION AIDS MATCHING
OF PATIENTS WITH DRUGS

It is easy to list a number of dimensions, such as indications and contraindications, on which a physician must have information to match a patient with a drug. Similarly, information on differences in side-effect profiles for therapeutic alternatives allows doctors and their patients to evaluate which side effects are clinically most important, which are most likely to influence compliance, and which the patient will find least distasteful. Another element of a good match is matching value to price. Many consumers still pay much of their prescription drug bills out of their own pockets. Some may be willing to accept some inconvenience, bad taste, or even an unpleasant but nonthreatening side effect if the price is lower, while others are willing to pay more for what they view as a better drug. Only with sufficient information can physicians working with their patients make the best choices among therapeutic alternatives, and more precise prescribing decisions translate into better health outcomes.

It is clear, then, that information is critical to the best use of prescription drugs. Indeed, the most useful way to view a prescription product may not be as a tablet or an ointment standing alone, but as a composite, a physical product bonded with information. Consider the physical product in isolation, stripped of information about it. If physicians were simply handed a pharmaceutical product without information on what it could accomplish and how it should be used, they would be at sea as to when and how to prescribe the product.

This situation is not entirely fanciful. In some less developed countries, where intellectual property rights are not acknowledged in the same way as in the U.S., generic products are sometimes approved even before the originator's product is approved. For example, Pfizer, the company that developed the antiarthritic Feldene® (piroxicam), was not the first company approved to sell piroxicam in Turkey. Another company, after obtaining first marketing rights, sold piroxicam without educating physicians about its use, perhaps because without being intimately involved in the development and testing of the drug, the company did not have sufficient information about it. Sales of the product were initially modest, then declined, even while Feldene was finding widespread acceptance in other countries. Later, when Pfizer also obtained approval to market Feldene in Turkey, it found the task of educating physicians about the drug more difficult because it had to overcome the negative attitudes toward piroxicam that physicians had developed when they, without adequate understanding, had tried the drug.

Indeed, information is formally the linchpin of the Food and Drug Administration's (FDA) entire regulatory system. A product is not simply deemed acceptable or unacceptable per se. Rather, it is approved for certain indications with specific directions for use. Only after the approval of the information–the information that makes the product useful–is a company allowed to market a new product.

While there can be no doubt that information is valuable, it is also costly to produce and disseminate. Promotion can be analyzed for its cost-effectiveness as a way of getting information to the person who makes the decision. I focus on promotion to physicians since it is the physician who has the authority to prescribe.

One way for information to get into the prescribing process is for each physician independently to seek a new information about prescription drugs by reading journals and consulting with professional colleagues. Economists speak of this process as "search." Search is not costless. The most costly component is typically time. The value of the time spent in search is measured by the value foregone, the value of the time had it been spent doing something else. For a physician, seeing patients is a high-value alternative use of the time spent in search. In light of the high opportunity cost of their time, physicians may find they cannot afford to spend many hours in searching out information on prescription drugs.

If self-initiated search is too expensive, the total amount of information physicians gather is likely to be less than if there is another, less expensive way for the information to reach them. One alternative method is through pharmaceutical companies' representatives, who visit doctors' offices to explain new evidence about disease processes, new therapeutic approaches, and new information about old products. If these representatives make it easier for doctors to receive information, doctors are likely to get more information and therefore, to be in a position to make even better prescribing decisions. This second information–dissemination technology may be cheaper than the first–cheaper for the doctor but perhaps also for society as a whole–in terms of total resources needed to effect the transfer of information, including the doctor's time. If this information delivery technology is indeed less expensive, it is likely to be used more, and more information will reach physicians.

If promotion were to do nothing but speed up the dissemination of information, it would benefit consumers. It is plausible that without company-generated promotion, doctors would eventually learn about a new product by reading about the new drug's approval in FDA publications or newspapers and by word of mouth. With promotion, however, more doctors hear about it quickly and start using the new product sooner, and more patients receive superior therapy right away. By generating appropriate use of the drug more rapidly, promotion provides health benefits.

EVIDENCE ON HEALTH EFFECTS
OF PROMOTION

The logic that promotion fosters health is upheld by statistical evidence. Even advertising severely attacked by critics has nevertheless had impressive health-promoting effects. Two examples, described below, are health claims for food and advertising for cigarettes. Evidence from a public service campaign provides a first example.

Television Advertising About Colon Cancer Risks

A four-market public service advertising program was recently conducted by the Advertising Research Foundation for the Advertising Council.[2] A single advertisement with the message that people should ask their doctors about colon cancer was shown over the period of one year. In the four viewing areas, the proportion of men aware of the usefulness of consulting a doctor about colon cancer jumped from about 6% to over 30% by the end of the year, and the number of men who did ask their doctors rose by more than 75%. The sponsors estimated that if the single commercial had been shown nationally, it would have persuaded 1.7 million to 2.7 million men over the age of 40 to consult physicians about colon cancer.

These television commercials clearly brought about substantial changes in health-seeking behavior. They happened to be public service messages, but information on the risk of colon cancer was also provided by producers trying to sell their own products.

Fiber Claims for Ready-to-Eat Cereal

Commercial messages highlighting the link between fiber and colon cancer, combined with emphasizing the fiber content of individual ready-to-eat cereals, led to increased fiber consumption through cereals and to the introduction of new high-fiber cereals. This began in 1984, when Kellogg began to promote its All-Bran® cereal as high in fiber. With the cooperation of the National Cancer Institute, Kellogg also emphasized the link between increased fiber consumption and lower risk of colon cancer. Other companies followed Kellogg's lead in emphasizing fiber content.

Ippolito and Mathios studied the effect of these health claims in the ready-to-eat cereal market.[3] Using survey data on actual food consumption, along with data on the composition of individual products, they showed that consumers changed their behavior and that advertising was an important source of information. The link between fiber and reduced risk of colon cancer was known before 1984, and that information was available through government publications and the media. Yet, the introduction of advertising made a dramatic difference in people's behavior. Before 1984, there had been no noticeable increase in fiber consumption through ready-to-eat cereals. In contrast, in the three years after Kellogg first introduced its health claim, the weighted average fiber content of cereals actually consumed rose by 7%.*

Producer health claims also led to significant product innovation. New cereals introduced in the advertising period were significantly higher in fiber (2.59 grams per ounce) than either the average cereal available prior to the advertising period (1.56 grams) or the new cereals introduced between 1978 and 1984 (1.70 grams).[3]

---

*The products were weighted by market shares.

Cigarette Advertising Led to Lower Tar Cigarettes

As a second example, cigarette advertising–perhaps even more controversial than health claims–also led to changes that were beneficial to health. Cigarette advertising does more than affect the number of cigarettes sold.* In particular, just as with ready-to-eat cereals, it changed the mix of cigarettes bought and the nature of products introduced into the market.

In the 1950s, there was a surge of advertising that featured tar and nicotine claims, termed the "tar derby." During that same time, and seemingly at least in part as a result of the tar derby, the average tar content of filter cigarettes declined by approximately 31% between 1957 and 1960, due in large part to the introduction of new products lower in tar.[4] In turn, later epidemiological evidence has shown that low-tar cigarettes have been a significant factor in reducing deaths from lung cancer. There was also a roughly 40% reduction in nicotine between 1956 and 1960, despite the fact that experts were saying, as late as 1951, that such reductions were technically impossible.

The rapid rate of improvement in the health characteristics of cigarettes–that is, in making them less unhealthy–slowed after 1960, when tar and nicotine claims were banned from advertising. In 1960, the Federal Trade Commission negotiated a voluntary agreement with the industry that eliminated all tar and nicotine claims in cigarette advertising because the agency believed there was no precise means of measuring tar and nicotine content.** The inability to make tar and nicotine claims reduced the incentive to make product changes by eliminating the opportunity to attract buyers by featuring lower tar.

---

*Indeed, statistical studies of advertising have not demonstrated a large demand-increasing effect. According to F. M. Scherer and David Ross, summarizing a series of studies, "The weight of evidence indicates that the long-run growth attributable to advertising has been modest." (Scherer FM, Ross D. Industrial market structure and economic performance. 3rd ed. Boston: Houghton Mifflin Company, 1990.)

**Only a few years earlier, many observers believed that there was no strong evidence that these characteristics even affected health. Calfee quotes from a Federal Trade Commission decision in 1950:

> The record shows . . . that the smoking of cigarettes, including Camel cigarettes [the target of R. J. Reynolds advertisements at issue in the case] in moderation by individuals . . . who are accustomed to smoking and who are in normal good health . . . is not appreciably harmful.[4]

PROMOTION'S ECONOMIC EFFECTS:
ENTRY, PRICES, AND INNOVATION

Promotion not only facilitates healthier behavior and encourages the introduction of healthier products, but it also powerfully affects more traditional economic measures of a market's performance: prices and the pace of innovation. The controversy over whether promotion improves or worsens the performance of markets–any market, not just the market for pharmaceutical products–has been vigorous. Although the controversy is not fully resolved, there is convincing evidence for the hypothesis that promotion leads to lower prices. It also strengthens competition by facilitating the entry of new products and new firms.

After summarizing the reasoning associated with two competing hypotheses, I report the results of some studies on retail advertising. I then describe briefly several studies on the effects of promotion by pharmaceutical companies.

Persuasion vs. Information

A shorthand for the controversy is whether advertising is primarily persuasive or primarily informational. Because ease or difficulty of entry by new competitors exerts such a powerful influence on a market, a principal criterion for judging whether promotion is beneficial is determining if it facilitates or hinders entry.

The hypothesis that promotion is primarily persuasive is built on the following line of reasoning: Advertising and other forms of promotion create strong brand loyalty. This strong brand loyalty allows sellers to charge higher prices because customers are less willing to switch to another product for any specific price difference. Promotion by established firms also makes it more difficult for new firms to enter the market or for existing firms to introduce new products because customers are more unwilling to switch to an unfamiliar product. Since the existence of more competitors puts downward pressure on prices, the absence of this competitive pressure–and indeed the absence of the threat of entry–keeps prices higher than if there were less promotion. This persuasion argument is associated with the term "barriers to entry," and those who argue or find that promotion erects such barriers infer that advertising is primarily a matter of persuasion.

The second hypothesis, that promotion is primarily informational, is that promotion leads to lower prices by making competition more vigorous. It does this by informing buyers about alternatives. When buyers compare alternatives, they compare on the basis of product characteristics and quality, but they also take price into account. Even if the promotion does not mention price, its effect is to make people consider whether the option to which promotion has directed attention is superior to the familiar choice, given the relative prices and product attributes. Proponents of the information hypothesis also argue that promotion facilitates the entry of new products and new firms. It does this by allowing a new seller to draw attention to the novel characteristics of the offering. New entry and awareness by established forms of the threat of entry put further downward pressure on prices. Research showing that promotion facilitates entry implies that promotion is primarily informational.

I do not pretend to provide in this chapter a full review of the many economic studies on these issues. I refer to two types of studies only: first, studies of retail advertising regulations showing that advertising has led to lower prices, and second, three recent studies of promotion by pharmaceutical manufacturers, all directly addressing the persuasion or information question.

Retail Advertising Prohibitions Raise Prices

Several studies on various products and services show that prices fell when advertising was introduced into retail markets. These studies took advantage of the presence of advertising in some states and its absence in other states due to state-to-state differences in advertising regulations. In some states, advertising of certain services was prohibited, while in other states, advertising was permitted and therefore used. A comparison of these sets of states, with appropriate statistical controls, showed differences in prices. The pioneer study, on optometry, was by Lee Benham.[5,6] In states where price advertising was permitted and in states where only nonprice advertising was permitted, prices for eyeglasses were lower than in states where advertising was prohibited. Other studies of retail markets have shown similar effects, including more recent studies of the market for eyeglasses and also studies of such disparate products as retail gasoline and lawyers' services.[7-12] John Cady published a similar study on retail pharmacy in which he found that retail prices of prescription drugs were, on average, 5% lower in states that permitted advertising of various pharmaceuticals.[13,14]

These studies stand in contradiction to those who argue that because advertising is costly, prices must be higher to cover those costs. Advertising was an added cost to retailers, yet prices fell. The reasonable explanation is that as consumers found it easier to identify and locate competing sources of products, they shopped more carefully, and retailers, in turn, found it necessary to lower prices to attract and keep customers.

Studies on Promotion by Pharmaceutical Companies Point to Its Procompetition Effect

Several studies have been done specifically on the effect of promotion by pharmaceutical companies. These studies have paid special attention to the effect of promotion on the success of newly introduced products.

In the first of this series of three studies, Leffler found that promotion of drugs already on the market made it more likely that entry of therapeutically important new drugs would be successful.[15] He inferred that promotion helps, rather than blocks, entry of new drugs and that this is evidence that promotion in informational. A paper in response by Hurwitz and Caves looked at the impact of promotion by pioneer brands when threatened by generic entry.[16] They found that such promotion boosted the ability of pioneer brands to maintain their market shares and fend off generic competition. This led them to conclude that the effect of promotion was, at least in part, persuasion, although they concurred in the paper that promotion was, in part, informational. These same authors, joined by a third author, Whinston, noted that for products whose patents expired during the 1970s and early 1980s, advertising by the pioneer brands dropped off before patent expiration and continued dropping before and after entry by generics.[17] They noted that total sales in the chemical entity dropped at the same time that advertising dropped. Based on this, they suggest that the advertising seems to have been for the purpose of expanding the market rather than for making it difficult for new products or firms–in this case, generics–to enter, and thus it protected market share and price.

Taken together, these studies point toward (although do not establish beyond doubt) the following conclusion: Promotion in pharmaceutical markets is informational and enhances competition, including through the entry of new products, which in turn can be expected to impose pricing discipline. The studies do not conclude that advertising is, in effect, anticompetitive, shielding sellers from competition and enabling them to keep their prices propped up.

This is consistent with common sense, which links promotion with innovation and thus with facilitating the entry of new products and new competitors. The evidence on ready-to-eat cereal and cigarette advertising reported above similarly links promotion with the introduction of new products. Advertisers are always looking for a new message to capture the attention of buyers. Looking at it another way, the incentive for innovation is increased, since income from the new product will be higher if diffusion is accelerated by promotion. Companies respond to this opportunity for higher income by investing more in developing and marketing new products. Advertising, then, can spur innovation.

PUBLIC POLICY IMPLICATIONS

The view that promotion, for the most part, does not hinder but rather contributes to the efficient functioning of markets has clear implications for public policy. In particular, the standards used by the FDA to judge the promotion of prescription drugs obviously influence—indeed control—the nature and content of advertising for prescription drugs and thus affect the performance of the market.

Since promotion conveys information, overly cautious standards as to what promotion is permitted can harm consumers by keeping valuable information from reaching purchasers or their agents. Two elements of regulation that can have this effect are: (1) too-stringent criteria as to what constitutes deceptive or misleading promotion; and (2) extensive disclosure requirements.

Decisions about what information should be permitted to be disseminated are not simple.* Policymakers and regulators must make decisions based on incomplete information since scientific evidence is always changing. However, much care and attentiveness to the public good must be exercised; any decision may well become outdated as subsequent studies shift the balance between "probably true" and "probably false," and hindsight is sure to show that some mistakes have been made. Policymakers should take into account the predictability that new information will emerge and that some policy decisions will be revealed as mistakes. There are two types of possible mistakes in regulating information flow:

Type I: Allowing a message that subsequently turns out to be (most probably) false.

Type II: Prohibiting a message that subsequently turns out to be (most probably) true.

It is not only misleading messages that harm consumers, but missing information as well.

---

*There is no place for deliberate falsity in advertising. If there is clear evidence that a claim is false, it should simply not be allowed.

For prescription pharmaceuticals, the paradigm of harm from inaction is familiar from discussion of the so-called drug lag, a term referring to earlier official approval of drugs abroad than in the U. S. Research in the 1970s emphasized the U. S. drug lag compared with the timing of drug approvals in Europe.[18] More recently, people with AIDS (Acquired Immunodeficiency Syndrome) and people active in seeking clearance for Alzheimer's treatments have been clamoring for early release of drugs. If approvals of valuable new therapies are unduly delayed, those who need those drugs are kept from health-improving therapy in the interim. In deciding whether or not to approve marketing of a new drug, the FDA must balance two types of possible errors: the harm that would be done by a drug that turned out to be unsafe or ineffective versus the harm that would be done if the drug turned out to be safe and effective and people had been deprived of its use for some time. The same dilemma that exists with respect to regulation of the marketing of drugs applies also to the dissemination of information.

My recommendation is very simple: compare the harm from and likelihood of a Type I error with the harm from a Type II error, with its likelihood also taken into account. It is necessary to look at the likelihood that the weight of the evidence will shift and show something that seemed probably true to be probably false, or vice versa, as well as the harm that will have occurred if such a shift takes place.[19]

Instead, the standard too often appears to overweigh Type I errors. Regulators and policymakers appear to focus only on the possible harm from misleading claims while disregarding the chance that further evidence may underscore the validity of the information–information that, if disseminated, would have influenced consumer and marketer choices toward better health. An unbalanced list of criteria can mean that too little information is disseminated, with harmful consequences.

It is understandable, of course, that regulators and policymakers have tended to put more weight on preventing errors of commission rather than errors of omission since errors of commission tend to be so much more visible. Moreover, as long as promotion is viewed primarily as an unavoidable nuisance, policymakers may not even consider the possibility that (over) restrictive regulation poses any possibility of social harm by suppressing information and has economic consequences. Overrestrictive policies may initially seem innocuous, but they are not.

If, instead, promotion is recognized as a valuable and productive means of disseminating information that in turn enhances competition, encourages innovation, puts downward pressure on prices, and ultimately leads to better health outcomes, then regulatory restrictions do not come free. They are costly, and those potential costs, in public policy terms, should be weighed carefully against the possible costs of errors of commission.

It is not only the standard by which deception is judged or, alternatively, by which substantiation of a claim is found acceptable that makes a difference. The same arguments apply to required disclosures, presumably required to avert deception. Disclosures are costly for the advertiser to include since they take time or space or both. With a higher cost per advertisement, the advertiser is likely to provide fewer advertisements. If so, the main advertising message reaches fewer people in the target audience. Ironically, then, imposing disclosure requirements may lead to less information being disseminated, not more. If the social value of the original promotion is recognized, any gain from the addition of the disclosure must be weighed against the harm due to diminishing the frequency or reach of the advertising. Imposition of a disclosure requirement may have serious and negative consequences for the quality of purchase decisions.

CONCLUSION

Promotion generally improves the functioning of the market. This is true for pharmaceuticals just as for other products and services. Promotion conveys information, making possible improved matching of patients with drugs. Promotion enhances competition, putting downward pressure on prices, and facilitates entry of new products, thereby encouraging innovation and further strengthening competition.

Regulatory standards, and public policy generally, should take into account this valuable informational function of promotion. Policymakers should weigh the harm done to consumers from suppressing useful information rather than focus too single-mindedly on the prevention of deception.

REFERENCES

1. Masson A, Rubin PH. Matching prescription drugs and consumers. N Engl J Med 1985;313:513-5.

2. Advertising Research Foundation for The Advertising Council. Establishing accountability: a strategic research approach to measuring advertising effectiveness. 1991.

3. Ippolito PM, Mathios AD. Information, advertising and health choices: a study of the cereal market. RAND J Econ 1990;21(Autumn).

4. Calfee JE. The ghost of cigarette advertising past. Regulation 1986; (Nov/Dec).

5. Benham LK. An estimate of the price effects of restrictions on drug price advertising on the price of eyeglasses. J Law Econ 1972;15(Oct).

6. Benham LK, Benham A. Regulating through the professions: a perspective on information control. J Law Econ 1975;18.

7. Kwoka JE Jr. Advertising and the price and quality of optometric services. Am Econ Rev 1984;74(Mar).

8. Bond R et al. Effects of restrictions on advertising and commercial practice in the professions: the case of optometry. Federal Trade Commission staff report. Washington, DC: Government Printing Office, 1980.

9. Marvel HP. Gasoline price signs and price behavior: comment. Econ Inquiry 1979;17.

10. Maurizi AR. The effect of laws against price advertising: the case of retail gasoline. Western Econ J 1972;10(Sept).

11. Porter WR, Jacobs WW et al. Report of the staff to the Federal Trade Commission. Improving consumer access to legal services: the case for removing restrictions on truthful advertising. November 1984.

12. Schroeter JR, Smith SL, Cox SR. Advertising and competition in routine legal service markets. J Industrial Econ 1987;36(Sept).

13. Cady JF. An estimate of the price effects of restrictions on drug price advertising. Econ Inquiry 1976;14.

14. Cady JF. A statement to the Federal Trade Commission regarding the proposed rules concerning prescription drug price disclosure. January 1976.

15. Leffler KB. Persuasion or information? The economics of prescription drug advertising. J Law Econ 1981.

16. Hurwitz MA, Caves RE. Persuasion or information? Promotion and the shares of brand name and generic pharmaceuticals. J Law Econ 1988;31(Oct).

17. Caves RE, Whinston MD, Hurwitz MA. Patent expiration, entry, and competition in the U. S. pharmaceutical industry: an exploratory analysis. Unpublished.

18. Lasagna L, Wardell WW. The rate of new drug discovery. Drug development and marketing. Washington, DC: American Enterprise Institute, 1975.

19. Federal Trade Commission. Bureau of Economics. How should health claims for foods be regulated? An economic perspective. Economic Issues Paper. By Calfee JE, Pappalardo JK. September 1989.

PART VI:
ECONOMICS OF NONCOMPLIANCE

One of the paradoxes in pharmaceutical economics is the simultaneous wish to limit consumption of costly pharmaceuticals and to assure that patients receive the medication they need to avoid unnecessary expenditures for other medical servicing. The first of the two chapters in this section reviews the economic consequences of *initial* noncompliance, i.e., failure to claim new prescriptions. The second chapter focuses on the consequences of noncompliance in terms of unnecessary hospitalization. Both studies find the economic implications to be enormous for payers, patients, manufacturers, and pharmacists.

Chapter 28

The Financial Implications of Initial Noncompliance: An Investigation of Unclaimed Prescriptions in Community Pharmacies

David J. McCaffrey III
Mickey C. Smith
Benjamin F. Banahan III
John P. Juergens
Sheryl L. Szeinbach

INTRODUCTION

Estimates of the economic costs of noncompliance amount to approximately 20 million lost working days per year and about $1.5 billion in lost income. In addition, there are approximately 140 million prescriptions that remain unfilled per year.[1] Using the *1991 Lilly Digest* estimate of approximately $21 for an average prescription, pharmacies in the United States are failing to realize some $2.8 billion in annual revenue.[2] Realizing this, health care professionals such as pharmacists must do all within their power to shape patient outcomes so that the patients will adopt proper health-seeking and compliance behaviors.

For a patient to assess fully a particular illness episode or condition, several decisions must be made. For example, if a patient develops a sore

The authors acknowledge the efforts of Cynthia Alderman and other members of the Research Institute of Pharmaceutical Sciences on this project and thank The Upjohn Company for generous contribution of the research grant.

Previously published in *Journal of Research in Pharmaceutical Economics*, Vol. 6(1), 1995.

throat and recognizes that he or she is in a state of "nonhealth," the patient behavior decisions for a typical path through the health care system might include the following:

1. Seek medical care
2. Receive prescription
3. Have prescription filled
4. Pick up prescription
5. Take medication as directed

In fact, the last decision, No. 5, must be repeated for every dose of medication taken. If the patient fails to recognize the need to continue the therapeutic treatment regimen for the full intended course and stops taking the medication prematurely, then he or she is noncompliant. This type of behavior represents the traditional type of noncompliance frequently addressed in the literature.

Another form of noncompliance is initial noncompliance. This would occur in either No. 3 or No. 4 identified above. If a patient fails to present a prescription or fails to pick up a prescription that has been presented to a pharmacy, initial noncompliance occurs. Initial noncompliance is defined as any prescription issued to a patient for which no medication was received. Initial noncompliance can be divided into two categories: unpresented prescriptions and unclaimed prescriptions. Unpresented prescriptions (also called unfilled prescriptions) are those prescriptions that are never received in a pharmacy for dispensing. Unclaimed prescriptions, however, arrive at the pharmacy to be filled but are never retrieved by the patient or a representative of the patient. Figure 28.1 illustrates how initial noncompliance relates to noncompliance as a whole.

In spite of the importance of this issue, no attempt has been made to investigate initial noncompliance using a national sample of retail pharmacies. The specific objectives of this study were to:

- Assess the overall monthly incidence of unclaimed prescriptions as reported by pharmacists
- Assess pharmacy-related characteristics of unclaimed prescriptions as reported by pharmacists
- Assess patient-related characteristics of unclaimed prescriptions as reported by pharmacists
- Assess product-related characteristics of unclaimed prescriptions as reported by pharmacists
- Determine the origins of unclaimed prescriptions as reported by pharmacists

- Determine how pharmacists are dealing with unclaimed prescriptions through policies and/or procedures

RELEVANT LITERATURE

Previous studies addressing initial noncompliance have concentrated on the unpresented prescription. Although unpresented prescriptions do have an impact on industry profits, the unclaimed prescription has the additional effects of lost pharmacist time, lost opportunity costs, and potentially higher stock costs.

Unclaimed prescriptions and unpresented prescriptions also have different characteristics with respect to addressing noncompliant behaviors. If a pharmacist is unaware of noncompliant behavior, as in the case of

FIGURE 28.1. Initial Noncompliance and Its Components

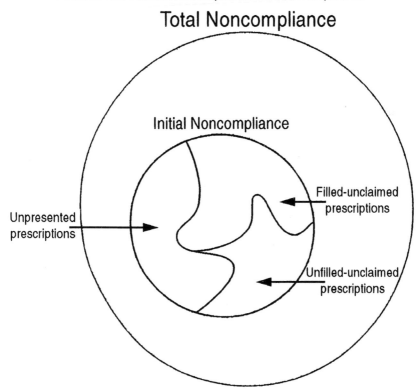

unpresented prescriptions, he or she is extremely limited in efforts to correct the behavior. The responsibility of recognizing and changing initial noncompliant behavior, as it relates to unpresented prescriptions, must lie with the physician at the time the prescription is written. In contrast, however, once the pharmacy receives a prescription, the pharmacist should and can become the major player in correcting initially noncompliant behavior.

The first known research in the area of unclaimed prescriptions was performed by Katz and Segal at the University of Toronto. They found that approximately 0.5% of all prescriptions went unclaimed.[3] Additionally, the authors found that anti-infectives (21.3%) and central nervous system agents (18.1%) made up the largest percentage of unclaimed prescriptions. More recently, Fincham and Wertheimer have investigated initial noncompliance in the elderly. In 1986, they found an unclaimed prescription rate of 0.28% for elderly patients enrolled in a large midwestern health maintenance organization (HMO).[4] In 1988, the same authors attempted to elicit the reasons the elderly failed to comply initially with their medications. Fincham and Wertheimer surveyed those elderly who had unclaimed prescriptions in the previous study and found that acute disease states and convenience items (cost, proximity to pharmacy, long waits, special trip, and possession of a supply of the medication) were most frequently mentioned.[5]

Craghead and Wartski conducted a study to investigate the effect an integrated hospital computer system would have on the number of unclaimed prescriptions in an outpatient pharmacy. The baseline rate of unclaimed prescriptions was reported to be 1.5%.[6] Following implementation of the computer system, they found that the rate of unclaimed prescriptions increased to 1.85%. Additionally, they found the rate of unpresented prescriptions to decline approximately the same percentage. To summarize, the implementation of an integrated computer system had no net effect on initial noncompliance. Although the system successfully reduced the number of unpresented prescriptions, it increased the number of unclaimed prescriptions, thus placing an additional burden on the pharmacy department. In a subsequent study, the authors reported that the rates of unclaimed prescriptions within general drug categories per total unclaimed prescriptions were: anti-inflammatories (17.5%), prenatal care (13.0%), antibiotics (9.2%), and cough and cold products (5.2%).[7]

Farmer and Gumbhir, auditing the prescription files of 21 pharmacies in and around Kansas City, Missouri, found that the mean age for *all* prescriptions was 45.62 days.[8] Additionally, anti-infective agents (17%), cough and cold products (11%), topicals (9%), analgesics (8%), and nonsteroidal anti-inflammatory agents (7%) made up over half of all un-claimed prescriptions.

Kirking and Kirking investigated the rate and composition of un-claimed prescriptions at the University of Michigan Ambulatory Care Pharmacy. Overall, they found that 1.2% of all prescriptions remained unclaimed seven to 13 days following receipt by the pharmacy.[9] Addition-ally, they found that topicals, central nervous system products, and anti-infectives were the most represented drug classifications among the ranks of the unclaimed. Interestingly, 64% of all unclaimed prescriptions were picked up within 30 days, leaving a final rate of unclaimed prescriptions after 30 days of only 0.5%.

The literature suggests many reasons for initial noncompliance. Much of the literature is based on audits and convenience sample surveys. The studies show the incidence of unclaimed prescriptions to be as low as 0.5% and as high as 3%. Reliance on convenience samples, however, does not allow us to make generalizations about the unclaimed prescription phenomenon other than in those areas and/or specific sites where the studies were conducted. To assess the magnitude of the problem, a survey was conducted using a national sample of retail pharmacies.

METHODOLOGY

A survey questionnaire was developed that consisted of pharmacy char-acteristics and respondent demographics and incidence and characteristics of unclaimed prescriptions as reported by pharmacy managers. Questions for the instrument were developed based upon the results of prior research as well as the past research experience of the investigators.

The pharmacy characteristics and respondent demographics section was placed at the beginning of the questionnaire to build rapport with the respondents prior to their answering the questions concerning unclaimed prescriptions. Respondents were then introduced to the phenomenon of unclaimed prescriptions and provided the following definition that was to be used when completing the remainder of the questionnaire:

> For the remainder of this questionnaire, an unclaimed prescription will be defined as any prescription, whether filled or unfilled, that is not picked up or delivered within seven days after it was received. This will include refills ordered by physicians, patients, or patient representatives.

The stipulation that a prescription remain in the pharmacy seven days was determined by combining a strict clinical argument that states that any prescription not picked up or delivered within 24 hours constitutes non-compliance with the tendency for pharmacies to allow a prescription to remain unclaimed for up to 30 days, or sometimes longer, before it warrants attention. In addition, the literature revealed that five to ten days was the cutoff for the definition of initial noncompliance in most of the existing research on unpresented and unclaimed prescriptions. Furthermore, using the aforementioned cutoff for defining an unclaimed prescription allowed for the greatest comparison to the research previously performed in the area of unclaimed prescriptions. However, using seven days as the time limit for defining unclaimed prescriptions could have resulted in an overestimation of what pharmacists would *normally* consider to be unclaimed prescriptions, or if this time limit was not adhered to by the respondents, it could have resulted in an underestimate of the magnitude of the phenomenon.

The sampling frame for the project was retail pharmacies in the United States. The minimum number of responses necessary, based on calculations using $z = 1.96$ for a 95% confidence interval and a power estimate of 0.05, was 384 usable responses.[10,11] On the basis of a conservative estimate of the effective response rate (25%), the minimum sample size needed to achieve the desired power and confidence level was calculated to be 1,536.[11] A geographically stratified random sample of 1,742 retail pharmacies was used for the survey. Pharmacy names and addresses were obtained from the 1991 Hayes Chain and Independent Pharmacy Database Guide. Each pharmacy received a four-page questionnaire accompanied by a cover letter explaining the purpose of the study and asking for participation. The envelopes were addressed to the attention of the pharmacy manager at each store. All questionnaires were coded with a unique identification number so nonrespondents could be identified for a follow-up mailing. Approximately four weeks after the initial questionnaire was mailed, a second questionnaire and cover letter were sent to all nonrespondent pharmacies.

RESULTS

A total of 545 (31.3%) responses were received, and one questionnaire was returned as undeliverable. Of the 545 responses received, a total of 23 responses were excluded from subsequent analysis. Eight questionnaires were excluded for arriving more than four weeks after the second mailing. Nine responses were excluded for incomplete response. An additional five responses became suspect based on the uncomplimentary remarks included on the survey instrument by the respondents. Those five responses were subsequently removed. Finally, one duplicate response was identified and removed. Overall, 522 (30.0%) usable responses were received.

For purposes of assessing nonresponse bias, the time trends extrapolation test was performed.[11] The assumption underlying this test is that nonrespondents more closely resemble late respondents than early respondents. The first 10% of responses (52) were coded to identify them as such, as were the last 10% of responses. *T* tests and chi-square tests were utilized to evaluate whether any significant differences existed between the groups or if group membership was associated with a difference in the studied variables. The two response groups were compared using eight demographic and experimental variables, and no significant differences were identified. Table 28.1 presents the monthly incidence of unclaimed prescriptions, rate per 1,000 prescriptions, and the pharmacists' perceptions of whether the number of unclaimed prescriptions had increased, decreased, or remained constant in the year prior to survey administration. The average incidence of unclaimed prescriptions was 30 per month. If extrapolated to the approximately 60,100 retail outlets nationwide, there are potentially 21,636,000 prescriptions that remain unclaimed each year.[11] Using the *1991 Lilly Digest* estimate of average prescription price, $21, retail pharmacies in the United States are failing to realize some $454,356,000 in revenue per year.

An unclaimed prescription rate was calculated to achieve two goals. First, expressing unclaimed prescriptions as a rate per thousand total prescriptions is a more meaningful measure for retail pharmacists and academicians as opposed to the mean monthly incidence. Secondly, the rate measure allows for control of the significant covariate effects exerted by both daily prescription volume and days the pharmacy is open per week. The rate measure was calculated using the following equation:

rate = [(number of monthly unclaimed prescriptions)(daily prescription volume*)(days open)(4)] 1,000

*daily prescription volume consists of both new and refill prescriptions

Table 28.1 shows the overall rate of unclaimed prescriptions per 1,000 total prescriptions to be 8.74 prescriptions. Using this rate and the *1991 Lilly Digest* average of 32,638 prescriptions per year, the average retail pharmacy would be expected to have approximately 285 unclaimed prescriptions at a retail loss of just over $5,990. Extrapolated to the 60,100 retail outlets in the United States, the number of unclaimed prescriptions per year could be expected to be 17,128,500 prescriptions at a retail loss of approximately $359,698,500. By controlling for prescription volume and

TABLE 28.1. Unclaimed Prescriptions: Monthly Incidence, Rate, and Net Change Over Past Year

	Mean # Rx	Std. Error	Median	Mode
Monthly Incidence	30.0	1.70	20.0	10.0
Rate*	8.74	0.31	6.94	7.14

In the past year, has the number of unclaimed prescriptions...

increased	71(13.7%)
decreased	53(10.2%)
remained constant	395(76.1%)

* Rate is expressed as the number of unclaimed prescriptions per 1,000 total prescriptions.

days open, the rate measure produces a much more conservative estimate of the influence that unclaimed prescriptions can have on retail pharmacy and the pharmaceutical industry. Regardless of whether one chooses to use the unclaimed prescription rate or the monthly incidence of unclaimed prescriptions, this phenomenon can and does have a dramatic influence on the profits of the pharmaceutical industry, on community pharmacy practice, and possibly on the health of the United States population.

Pharmacists were also asked to report whether they believed that the phenomenon of unclaimed prescriptions had increased, decreased, or remained constant. Almost 90% of the respondents thought that the number of unclaimed prescriptions had either increased or remained unchanged. Only 10% of the respondents stated that the number of unclaimed prescriptions had decreased in the year prior to survey administration.

Table 28.2 presents the results of the analysis of variance for the rate of unclaimed prescriptions based on pharmacy practice setting. The results show that the number of unclaimed prescriptions differs significantly across the five pharmacy practice settings.

The results of the analysis of variance indicated that there were significant differences in the rate of unclaimed prescriptions across the various pharmacy practice settings. Scheffé test results for pharmacy practice setting indicate that single-store independent pharmacies had the lowest reported rate of unclaimed prescriptions. Single-store independent pharmacies had a significantly lower rate of unclaimed prescriptions than chain

TABLE 28.2. ANOVA (Analysis of variance) Results for the Number of Unclaimed Prescriptions per 1,000 Total Prescriptions by Pharmacy Practice Setting

	D.F.	Mean Squares	F-Ratio	F-Probability
Between Groups	4	1000.40	18.73	0.0000
Within Groups	495	53.43		
Total	499			

Scheffé Results

Group	1 Single Indep.	2 Multistore Indep.	3 Drugstore Chain	4 Discount Store	5 Grocery Store	Sig. Differences ($p < 0.05$)
Mean # Rx	6.34	7.93	12.20	13.90	11.09	(1, 3), (1, 4), (1, 5), (2, 3), (2, 4)

drugstores and the pharmacy departments of both mass merchandisers and grocery stores; however, the rate was not significantly different from the multistore independent pharmacies. Additionally, multistore independent pharmacies were reported to have a significantly lower rate of unclaimed prescriptions than the chain drugstores and discount store pharmacies. These results are supported in Table 28.3, which shows the rate of unclaimed prescriptions by pharmacy type. The results of the *t* test show that chain pharmacies had nearly double the rate (11.6) of unclaimed prescriptions of independent pharmacies (6.59).

Table 28.4 presents the results of the analysis of variance for community population and the mean number of unclaimed prescriptions per 1,000 total prescriptions. Community population was categorized into three groups on the basis of distribution of the responses. The lowest third of the distribution, one to 14,000 residents, was coded as 1. The middle third of the distribution, 14,001 to 50,000 residents, was coded 2, and the highest third, 50,001 residents and above, was coded 3. The results of the analysis of variance show that the number of unclaimed prescriptions per 1,000 prescriptions differed significantly based on community population. As might be expected, the low population community pharmacies had a significantly lower rate of unclaimed prescriptions than the middle and high population area pharmacies.

Table 28.5 presents the results of the analysis of variance for prescription concentration. Prescription concentration is defined as the percentage of the pharmacy's total sales as prescription sales. The prescription concentration was also divided into categories based on distribution of the responses. The four quantities were: 1% to 53%, 54% to 72%, 73% to 85%, and 86% to 100%. The results of the analysis of variance show that the rate of unclaimed prescriptions differs significantly based on prescription concentration. Results of the Scheffé test show that low concentration pharmacies had the highest rate of unclaimed prescriptions (11.46). These low concentration pharmacies were reported to have significantly higher

TABLE 28.3. Number of Unclaimed Prescriptions per 1,000 Total Prescriptions by Pharmacy Type				
	Mean # Rx	Std. Error	*T*-value	Significance
Pharmacy Type			−8.35	*p* = 0.000
Independent	6.59	0.358		
Chain	11.60	0.482		

TABLE 28.4. ANOVA Results for the Number of Unclaimed Prescriptions per 1,000 Total Prescriptions by Community Population

	D.F.	Mean Squares	F-Ratio	F-Probability
Between Groups	2	443.97	17.42	0.0007
Within Groups	467	59.86		
Total	469			

Scheffé Results

Group	1	2	3	
	1-14,000.	14,001-50,000	50,001-highest value	sig. differences ($p < 0.05$)
Mean # Rx	7.12	10.39	9.47	(1, 2), (1,3)

453

TABLE 28.5. ANOVA Results for the Number of Unclaimed Prescriptions per 1,000 Total Prescriptions by Prescription Concentration

	D.F.	Mean Squares	F-Ratio	F-Probability
Between Groups	3	476.30	7.99	0.0000
Within Groups	482	59.56		
Total	485			

Scheffé Results

Group	1 1-53% Rx	2 54-72% Rx	3 73-85% Rx	4 86-100% Rx	
Mean # Rx	11.46	9.85	6.97	8.17	sig. differences ($p < 0.05$) (1, 3), (2, 3), (1, 4)

454

rates of unclaimed prescriptions than the third quartile (73% to 85%) and the high concentration pharmacies. Additionally, it was found that the middle to low concentration pharmacies (54% to 72%) had a significantly higher rate of unclaimed prescriptions than the middle to high concentration pharmacies (quartile three).

Two-tailed *t* tests were used to investigate whether the presence of a delivery service and the presence of a delivery charge influenced the rate of unclaimed prescriptions reported in those pharmacies. Table 28.6 presents the results from these analyses. The pharmacies that were reported not to have a delivery service were reported to have a much higher rate of unclaimed prescriptions (11.07) than those pharmacies reported to have delivery service (7.03). Additionally, those pharmacies that had delivery service and charged for that service had a higher rate of unclaimed prescriptions than those pharmacies where delivery was free. For the pharmacies reported to have a fee for delivery service, the average delivery charge was $2.25, with the lowest reported fee being $1.00 and the highest fee $5.00.

Table 28.7 presents the method of payment, gender, and age distributions of unclaimed prescriptions as reported by pharmacists. Over 70% of all unclaimed prescriptions are believed to come from cash customers. Medicaid constituted just over 11% and other third-party payers, such as PAID and PCS, just over 16%. With respect to gender, the percentage of unclaimed prescriptions was fairly evenly distributed. Male patients were perceived to contribute 43.5% of the unclaimed prescriptions, and females 56.5%. Although females are perceived to contribute the larger share of unclaimed prescriptions, this might be due to their high medication utilization rate. As for age distribution, the young patient (18 and under) was perceived to contribute least to the unclaimed prescription phenomenon,

TABLE 28.6. Number of Unclaimed Prescriptions per 1,000 Total Prescriptions by Presence of Delivery Service and Charge for Delivery				
	Mean # Rx	Std. Error	*T*-value	Significance
Delivery Service			−6.57	$p = 0.000$
Yes	7.03	0.376		
No	11.07	0.483		
Charge for Delivery			1.97	$p = 0.063$
Yes	9.73	1.415		
No	6.84	0.391		

with just over 9% of unclaimed prescriptions. The elderly (65 and over) contributed just under 20%, while the middle-aged population (19-64) contributed over 70% of the total number of unclaimed prescriptions.

Respondents were asked to identify reasons they believe patients fail to claim their prescriptions. Up to three reasons were coded for each respondent. The number of mentions and the percentage of respondents indicating each reason are shown in Table 28.8. Cost was the most frequently mentioned reason (63%) pharmacists thought patients did not receive their medications. Knowing that private-pay patients account for over 70% of unclaimed prescriptions, it is no surprise that prescription price is the leading reason patients fail to claim their medications. Other financially related reasons pharmacists thought patients failed to claim their prescriptions were product not covered on insurance (10%) and change in prescription coverage. These findings suggest that if we continue to see a rise in prescription drug costs and a decline in prescription drug coverage, we will likely see a steady rise in the number of unclaimed prescriptions in community pharmacies. The next most frequently mentioned reasons patients fail to claim their prescriptions were forgetfulness (33.6%), condition improved (31.8%), patient did not want medication (24.1%), and lack of communication (17.3%). Unlike the cost issue, these items are actionable. The pharmacist must educate his or her patients about the importance

TABLE 28.7. Method of Payment, Gender Distribution, and Age Distribution of Unclaimed Prescriptions		
	Mean Percentage	Std. Error
Method of Payment		
Private Pay	72.1	1.21
Medicaid	11.4	0.71
Other Third Party	16.1	0.84
Gender		
Male	43.5	0.72
Female	56.5	0.79
Age		
18 and Under	9.1	0.53
19 to 40	39.4	1.13
41 to 64	31.8	0.91
65 and Over	19.3	0.91

TABLE 28.8. Reasons for Patients' Failure to Claim Prescriptions as Perceived by Pharmacists

Reason	Count	Percentage of Respondents
Cost	313	63.0
Forgetfulness	167	33.6
Condition Improved	158	31.8
Did Not Want Medicine	120	24.1
Lack of Communication	86	17.3
Phoned-In to Wrong Pharmacy	31	6.2
Patient Disagrees with Physician	13	2.6
Patient Apathy	11	2.2
Not Covered on Insurance	10	2.0
Medicine Discontinued	10	2.0
Patient Expected Different Medication	9	1.8
Went to Different Pharmacy	8	1.6
Duplicate Prescription	5	1.0
Physician Gave Samples	5	1.0
Inconvenience	4	0.8
Patient Neglect	3	0.6
Patient Ignorance	2	0.4
Store Closed (Inconvenient Hours)	2	0.4
No Transportation	2	0.4
Changed Physician	2	0.4
Not Enough Time	2	0.4
Inconvenient Location	1	0.2
Change in Insurance	1	0.2
Change in Medication	1	0.2

Note: Each respondent was allowed up to three responses; therefore, the percentages will not total 100%.

of compliance and do anything within his or her power to assist patients' efforts to comply with their medication regimens.

Pharmacists reported that over 70% (71.35%) of unclaimed prescriptions are new prescriptions. The likelihood of having subsequent authorized refills dispensed is very low, thus leading to an even more dangerous possibility.

Pharmacists were asked if there were some product categories that appeared more frequently as unclaimed prescriptions. Just over 48% of the respondents stated that some product categories appeared more frequently as unclaimed prescriptions. These respondents were asked to identify the product categories that appeared often as unclaimed prescriptions. Up to three product categories were coded for each respondent. The number of mentions and the percentage of respondents indicating each category are shown in Table 28.9. Almost 80% of the pharmacists mentioned antibiotics as a product category frequently appearing as unclaimed prescriptions. In addition, analgesics (23.9%), cough/cold products (16.2%), and dermatologicals (13.0%) were frequently mentioned as product categories appearing as unclaimed. Somewhat surprisingly, oral contraceptives were mentioned by over 10% of those pharmacists reporting. Oral contraceptives have, in the past, been used as a model for compliant behavior. Based on these results, it is possible that oral contraceptives suffer from the same compliance pitfalls as other product categories even though noncompliance with this drug regimen can have serious implications for patients.

Overall, respondents estimated that just over 81% of unclaimed prescriptions are phoned into the pharmacy. This includes new and refill prescriptions phoned in by a physician, an agent of the physician, a patient, or a representative of the patient. The high percentage of unclaimed prescriptions coming from phoned-in prescriptions might be due to the patients' lack of involvement in the process of filling the prescription. By not having any physical "evidence," such as a written prescription or an empty bottle, the patient may be more likely to forget about the prescription. The next largest percentage (16.6%) of unclaimed prescriptions originated by some type of personal delivery. The remaining unclaimed prescriptions came from mail delivery, facsimile, and electronic transfer. Although these avenues are not suspect in the phenomenon of unclaimed prescriptions today, with increased use and the patient separation problems previously mentioned, these avenues might significantly contribute to the unclaimed prescription problem in the future.

DISCUSSION

Results showed that just over eight prescriptions for every 1,000 filled will not be claimed. Although these numbers may seem small, when

TABLE 28.9. Most Frequently Mentioned Product Categories Appearing as Unclaimed Prescriptions, as Reported by Pharmacists

Category	Count	Percentage
Antibiotics	196	79.4
Analgesics	59	23.9
Cough/Cold	40	16.2
Dermatologicals	32	13.0
Oral Contraceptives	26	10.5
Antihypertensives	21	8.5
NSAIDs	18	7.3
Antihistamines	10	4.0
Decongestant/Antihistamine	8	3.2
Smoking Deterrents	7	2.8
Vitamins	5	2.0
H_2 Antagonists	5	2.0
Antiemetics	3	1.2
Acne Preparations	3	1.2
Estrogens	3	1.2
Tranquilizers-Sedatives	2	0.8
Psychotropics	1	0.4
Ear Preparations	1	0.4
Antidiarrheals	1	0.4
Thyroid Preparations	1	0.4
Muscle Relaxants	1	0.4
Antiasthmatics	1	0.4
Antihyperlipidemics	1	0.4
OTC (Over the Counter) Drugs	1	0.4

Note: Each respondent was allowed up to three responses; therefore, the percentages will not total 100%.

extrapolated to a total of prescriptions at an average retail prescription price of $21, the costs to pharmacies are enormous. The amount of revenue pharmacies can expect to lose, nationally, as a result of unclaimed prescriptions is between $350 million and $450 million annually. These results show that unclaimed prescriptions significantly affect the financial health of both community pharmacies and the pharmaceutical industry, but these amounts may be grossly underestimated. Table 28.8 shows that prescription cost was the most frequently mentioned reason that patients fail to claim their prescriptions. Knowing this, one might conclude that the average retail price of an unclaimed prescription is greater than the $21 Lilly average. This seems to be supported by the results presented in Table 28.9. Many of the product categories mentioned contain products that would sell at a retail price at or above the $21 Lilly average; therefore, the financial implications of unclaimed prescriptions on community pharmacy could be much greater than the estimates presented in this manuscript.[13] Further, nearly 90% of those responding thought that the number of unclaimed prescriptions had remained unchanged or had increased in the year prior to survey administration. Additionally, results show that chain pharmacies reported a much higher rate of unclaimed prescriptions (11.60) than independent pharmacies (6.60). Not only do chain pharmacies accumulate unclaimed prescriptions at a rate almost double their independent counterparts, but chain pharmacies, on average, fill more prescriptions per outlet than independent pharmacies (Table 28.10) thus increasing the disparity between the two groups. Knowing this, pharmacy management, especially chain pharmacy management, must establish appropriate policies and procedures to deal effectively with the phenomenon of unclaimed prescriptions.

Additionally, results show that the rate of unclaimed prescriptions was related to prescription concentration. As the ratio of prescription sales to total store sales increased, a lower rate of unclaimed prescriptions was found. It seems logical that those pharmacies that depend highly on prescription sales for profits will concentrate more efforts on this portion of the business; this would include unclaimed prescriptions. What does not appear logical is that any business would let potential revenue languish without attempting to intervene. Those businesses that operate on such a scale that prescription sales make up only a relatively small percentage of

TABLE 28.10. Daily Prescription Volume by Pharmacy Type				
	Mean # Rx	Std. Error	*T*-value	Significance
Independent	104.34	4.14	−6.08	*p* = 0.0000
Chain	147.86	4.78		

total store sales should place additional emphasis on the prescription department. By recapturing some of the lost revenue caused by initial noncompliance, the pharmacy department, and thus the overall store, can become more profitable.

Results also showed that the population of the community surrounding the pharmacy was significantly related to the rate of unclaimed prescriptions experienced by pharmacies. Those pharmacies located in smaller communities reported a much lower rate of unclaimed prescriptions than the pharmacies located in more populous areas. A more personal relationship between pharmacist and patient in the smaller communities could be one of the reasons that the small community pharmacies experience a lower rate of unclaimed prescriptions. This does not imply that the smaller community pharmacy can ignore unclaimed prescriptions altogether; all pharmacies can benefit from added attention to unclaimed prescriptions.

An interesting finding was that those pharmacies offering a delivery service had a much lower rate of unclaimed prescriptions than pharmacies offering no such service. These results present an interesting opportunity for pharmacy. By offering a delivery service, a pharmacy can significantly reduce the number of unclaimed prescriptions by removing the inconvenience associated with picking up a prescription. By incorporating a policy in which all unclaimed prescriptions would be arranged to be delivered, the pharmacy could offset the increased cost of the delivery service with the revenue generated by "reviving" those prescriptions that would have normally gone unclaimed.

Although unclaimed prescription rates were found to be lower in those pharmacies having a delivery service, it seems that any benefit from a decline in unclaimed prescriptions was lost when pharmacies charged a delivery fee. Pharmacies charging for delivery service were more likely to have unclaimed prescriptions than those delivering at no charge. In an effort to boost profits or to cover the costs incurred by having a delivery service, pharmacies choosing to charge for delivery service might actually be experiencing a net loss. Not only did they not receive the $1-$5 charge for delivery, but they also did not realize the profit from the sale of the prescription. These results show that delivery is a viable means of reducing unclaimed prescriptions, but that charging for delivery may greatly reduce its effectiveness in this capacity.

Pharmacists were asked to report reasons they thought patients failed to claim their prescriptions. Overall, 63% of the respondents stated that cost was a reason prescriptions remain unclaimed. Other than contacting the physician for a less expensive alternative, cost and other financial reasons (e.g., not covered on insurance, lost insurance) are largely unactionable by pharmacists. The second most frequently mentioned reason for patients' failure to claim their prescriptions was forgetfulness (33.6%). The fact that this appeared as a reason for initial noncompliance is disappointing, but that it was reported with such frequency is inexcusable. All that is required to overcome this problem is for the pharmacist or support staff to contact the patients who forget to pick up their prescriptions. Another related and frequently mentioned item was lack of communication. This lack of communication was reported to have occurred between the physician and the patient, the physician and the pharmacist, the patient and the pharmacist, or a combination of the three. As with forgetfulness, lack of communication can be remedied by pharmacist action. Informing a patient that a prescription is waiting in the pharmacy is the first step to resolving initial noncompliance.

Pharmacists reported several items that could be influenced by patient education. Patient ignorance, neglect, and apathy—in addition to patients not wanting medications—are all amenable to educational efforts by the pharmacist. Counseling on proper medication use as well as the benefits of prescription drug therapy can go a long way in reducing initial noncompliance in those populations less knowledgeable about pharmaceuticals.

In addition to the reasons mentioned above, several convenience and accessibility items appeared in the responses (e.g., general inconvenience, store closed, lack of transportation, inconvenient location, time constraints). Many of these reasons are amenable to delivery and longer hours. These solutions must be evaluated to determine whether they are appropriate and whether the increase in revenue from unclaimed prescriptions can help justify their implementation.

As a percentage of total unclaimed prescriptions, just over 70% were perceived to be new prescriptions. Although the data would indicate that new prescriptions are a greater problem when considering unclaimed prescriptions, a "new" unclaimed prescription can, in fact, be more than just one unclaimed prescription. If a new prescription goes unclaimed, it is likely that all authorized refills are also lost. If all new prescriptions remaining unclaimed have a full year's worth of refills authorized, then the financial implications of unclaimed prescriptions would be, in those cases, 11 times greater than initially estimated. Refill prescriptions made up over 28% of the unclaimed prescriptions as reported by pharmacists. Although refill prescriptions do not seem to weigh as heavily in terms of unclaimed prescriptions, as unpresented prescriptions (authorized refills not used), refill prescriptions can have a significant influence on the profits of a pharmacy.

Pharmacists were asked to report whether some product categories more frequently appeared as unclaimed prescriptions. Almost half (48.6%) of the respondents stated that some product categories appeared more frequently among the ranks of the unclaimed. Almost 80% stated that antibiotics frequently appeared as unclaimed prescriptions. The remaining top five were analgesics (23.9%), cough/cold products (16.2%), dermatologicals (13.0%), and oral contraceptives (10.0%). These results show that prescriptions for self-limiting illnesses would need the most attention with regard to unclaimed prescriptions. Overall, pharmacists stated that almost 82% of unclaimed prescriptions came from phoned-in prescriptions. An additional 16% came from personally delivered prescriptions while a negligible number (< 1%) came from facsimile, mail, and electronic transfer combined. The lack of patient personal involvement in the phoned-in prescription process might be the reason phoned-in prescriptions appeared more frequently as unclaimed prescriptions. If phoned-in prescriptions are utilized to increase patient convenience, then the increase in convenience has the potential to be detrimental to a patient's health. One solution might be to limit the number of phoned-in prescriptions that a pharmacy ·will accept. If limiting the number of phoned-in prescriptions allowed is not feasible, then a procedure for contacting the patients to inform them of the arrival of a phoned-in prescription could help to reduce the overall rate of unclaimed prescriptions in that pharmacy.

For the purposes of the study, an unclaimed prescription was defined as any prescription remaining unclaimed after seven days. Pharmacists were asked to report in spite of this definition how many days a prescription must remain in the pharmacy before it is considered unclaimed. Overall, approximately 23 days elapsed before a prescription was considered unclaimed. When comparing chain and independent pharmacies, chain pharmacies (21.28 days) took action regarding unclaimed prescriptions significantly earlier than independent pharmacies (23.59 days). Although this comparison reveals a statistically significant difference, for practical purposes it has little meaning, for after three weeks the only practical action that should be taken is to return the product to stock and, in the case of a third-party prescription, credit the third-party payer.

This investigation, like all studies, is not without its limitations. Regardless of the appropriateness of the design and execution of a study, there are limitations to the generalizations that can be made from the results. The value for unclaimed prescriptions and the characteristics of the prescriptions come from pharmacists' perceptions, not audit data. By relying on pharmacists' perceptions, there is a chance that the data are biased in some fashion, but neither the literature nor the investigator's intuition revealed what direction this bias might take. However, it should be noted that the results obtained closely resemble those found in audits previously performed. In addition, the operational definition of unclaimed prescription limited the number of days elapsed to seven days. The results of the study show the average number of days elapsed before a prescription was considered unclaimed was nearly 23 days. Using seven days as the time limit for defining unclaimed prescriptions could have resulted in an overestimation of what pharmacies *consider* to be unclaimed prescriptions, or if this time limit was not adhered to by the respondents, it could have resulted in an underestimate of the magnitude of the phenomenon. Nevertheless, with consideration given to these limitations, the investigation provided information helpful in understanding the phenomenon of unclaimed prescriptions.

This chapter addressed many issues involving unclaimed prescriptions. The results showed that unclaimed prescriptions can and do have an impact on the pharmaceutical industry, especially community pharmacy. It is hoped that these results will provide information to pharmacy management and pharmaceutical executives regarding the far-reaching implications of unclaimed prescriptions. By ignoring unclaimed prescriptions, community pharmacy practitioners and the pharmaceutical industry are ignoring potential profit. Additionally, by ignoring unclaimed prescriptions, community pharmacy and the pharmaceutical industry are forgetting their primary concern: proper medical care for patients. The pharmaceutical industry has many opportunities to affect the health behaviors of patients. Attentiveness to patients' health care needs will allow the pharmaceutical industry to improve the physical health of its patients and in the case of patient noncompliance, improve the financial health of the industry. Initial noncompliance is an area where both community pharmacy and the pharmaceutical industry can "do well by doing good."

REFERENCES

1. Schering report XIV. Improving patient compliance: is there a pharmacist in the house? Kenilworth, NJ: Schering Pharmaceutical Corporation, 1992.

2. 1991 Lilly digest. Indianapolis, IN: Eli Lilly and Company, 1992.

3. Katz EF, Segal HJ. Unclaimed prescriptions. Hosp Admin Canada 1971;(Nov):51.

4. Fincham JE, Wertheimer AI. Initial drug noncompliance in the elderly. J Geriatr Drug Ther 1986;1(1):23.

5. Fincham JE, Wertheimer AI. Elderly patient initial noncompliance: the drugs and reasons. J Geriatr Drug Ther 1988;2(4):58.

6. Craghead R, Wartski D. Effect of automated prescription transmittal on number of unclaimed prescriptions. Am J Hosp Pharm 1989;46:311.

7. Craghead R, Wartski D. An evaluative study of unclaimed prescriptions. Hosp Pharm 1991;26:617.

8. Farmer KC, Gumbhir AK. Unclaimed prescriptions: an overlooked opportunity. Am Pharm 1992;NS32(10):55-7.

9. Kirking M, Kirking D. Evaluation of unclaimed prescriptions in an ambulatory care pharmacy. Unpublished.

10. Levy PS, Lemeshow S. Sampling for health professionals. Belmont, CA: Lifetime Learning Publications, 1980.

11. Aday LA. Designing and conducting health surveys. San Francisco, CA: Jossey-Bass Publishers, 1989.

12. Powis R. Retail pharmacy in the 1990's. Unpublished.

13. Regional prescription price survey. Indianapolis, IN: Medi-Span, Inc., 2nd quarter 1992.

Chapter 29

Noncompliance with Medication Regimens and Subsequent Hospitalizations: A Literature Analysis and Cost of Hospitalization Estimate

Sean D. Sullivan
David H. Kreling
Thomas K. Hazlet

INTRODUCTION

More than 35.2 million U.S. hospital inpatient admissions occurred in 1986, producing revenues to hospitals of approximately $179.6 billion.[1,2] Hospital inpatient expenditures comprise the largest and fastest growing component of all expenditures on health care services. In a cost-conscious era, it is important to ask how these admissions and related expenditures might be reduced without adversely affecting the quality of and access to medical care. One approach to this issue is to explore the factors leading to hospital admission. In this chapter, we evaluate and quantify drug therapy noncompliance as a small yet significant cause of preventable inpatient admission.

There are many factors contributing to preventable hospital admissions. One such factor is patient noncompliance with medication regimens. Pa-

This chapter was presented at the Drug Policy and Pharmaceutical Services Session at the 116th Annual Meeting of the American Public Health Association, Boston, November 1988.

The authors wish to thank Laura Gardner, Lisa Bero, Earle Lingle, and two anonymous reviewers for their helpful comments and suggestions.

Previously published in *Journal of Research in Pharmaceutical Economics,* Vol. 2(2), 1990.

tient noncompliance with drug treatment is one of the most important problems in clinical medical practice.[3] With treatment regimens becoming increasingly complex, the inability of patients to manage their medication regimens has economic as well as clinical implications.

Estimates of the scope of this problem are diverse. Binkley projected that more than 225 million unnecessary hazardous situations are created annually as a result of poor compliance with health care treatments.[4] He describes various consequences leading to costly unnecessary treatment, including recurrence of illness; risk of transmitting a communicable disease; increased hospital, doctor, and pharmacy visits; and economic costs to society and the individual. Levine calculated the cost of drug regimen noncompliance related to cardiovascular disease and estimated that in 1984 such noncompliance resulted in more than 125,000 deaths and several thousand hospitalizations per year.[5] He derived a societal cost of 20 million lost work days resulting in $1.5 billion in lost earnings. What he did not calculate, however, were the equally important costs of preventable hospital stays, doctor visits, laboratory tests, and other health care expenditures resulting from noncompliant patients.

Much research has been directed on the causes, consequences, and factors affecting noncompliance. Some of this work has focused on patients requiring institutionalization as a consequence of noncompliance. Strandberg investigated the effects of noncompliance on nursing home admissions by studying elderly nursing home patients in Oregon.[6] He found the single most important reason elderly patients were in nursing homes was their inability to manage complex drug therapies. Overall, 23% of the elderly persons in his study had no serious impairment other than an inability to manage their own medications. Evidence from the Medicare social HMO (health maintenance organization) demonstration projects indicates that 4.3% of the elderly HMO population required assistance with administration of medications.[7]

Given such findings, it is understandable that noncompliance with drug therapy is of interest to practitioners, health policy decision makers, and health insurance and benefit administrators. In this article, our attention is focused on hospitalization as a sequela of noncompliance. Our objective is to quantify the extent and direct cost of this phenomenon using published data from a variety of studies.

METHODOLOGY

Light and Pillemer and others have developed meta-analysis as a method for synthesizing the results of independent research.[8-10] Meta-analysis is a technique for combining two or more independent studies to yield a single summary statistic. We used a meta-analytic approach to systematically search, compile, and summarize the existing literature on hospitalization related to noncompliance with drug regimens. A summary measure of the number of hospitalizations due to drug therapy noncompliance was derived from the selected studies. Estimates of the direct costs of these hospitalizations were projected from the summary measure.

The phenomenon of patient drug therapy noncompliance includes a wide range of behaviors that can lead to difficulties in designing, evaluating, and reviewing compliance research.[11-13] Four categories of noncompliant behavior are commonly differentiated: overuse, underuse, erratic use, and abuse. This study included evaluations of the first three behaviors as they influence hospitalization. Although it is recognized that drug abuse is a substantial problem that can lead to hospitalization and even death, an attempt to study drug abuse behavior exceeds the scope of this study. Only literature that identified and presented quantifiable evidence of drug overuse, drug underuse, and erratic use was included in our analysis.

The major focus of our inquiry was literature describing inpatient hospital admissions related to drug therapy noncompliance. Much of the empirical evidence, however, is found within the results of more general research on nonspecific drug-induced hospitalizations. Therefore, an extensive review of the literature on this topic was undertaken.

Studies reporting primary data were identified using several literature search technologies. Computer retrieval data bases included *Medline, Hospital Literature Index*, and *International Pharmaceutical Abstracts*. Computer search outcomes were verified by manually searching *Index Medicus* and *International Pharmaceutical Abstracts* for 1985 and 1986 and comparing results. Bibliographies from key articles were examined to identify additional studies. To locate unpublished work, a contemporary researcher in the field, Professor Robert Maronde, MD, was contacted. His group recently completed a study quantifying hospitalizations associated with California Medicaid patients' noncompliance with antihypertensive drug regimens.[14] His preliminary results indicate a strong association between the underuse of prescription antihypertensive drugs and increased hospitalizations. Finally, we distributed a copy of this analysis to a contemporary researcher with some knowledge of the noncompliance literature. She was able to direct us to additional citations.

Research reports identified by the literature search were compared and criteria were applied to determine which studies had acceptable results from synthesis and development of the cost estimate. Four methodological criteria were used to screen and select acceptable studies:

1. *A priori* definitions in research design, as identified in the study methodology, were used to identify suspected drug-induced illness.
2. The probable causes of drug-induced admissions were determined through patient interview by the investigating team.
3. Specific interview questions were employed to evaluate noncompliance as a probable cause of the drug-induced admission.
4. Admissions of noncompliant patients were quantitatively measured by the investigating team.

Strict adherence to these criteria assured a valid summary measure of hospitalizations due to drug therapy noncompliance. Each study's methodology had to include consistent definitions of drug-induced illness and noncompliance. A rigorous protocol of inpatient questioning by a health professional was considered the acceptable standard for inclusion in the analysis. This included the use of physicians or pharmacists to investigate the reasons for admission. Once drug-induced illness was substantiated, the patient's drug compliance had to be evaluated as a causative factor. Although not a criterion for study inclusion, some studies included the use of drug blood level assessment on admission. Finally, studies were included if the rate of noncompliant admissions was provided by the authors, or if the rate could be determined indirectly by calculation of the author's results. Research reports failing these criteria were not included in the sample even though they may provide useful information. We thought that strict adherence to these criteria allowed us to calculate, with confidence, a generalizable summary statistic.

Inpatient hospital cost data from the American Hospital Association were applied to this summary measure of the rate of hospitalization due to noncompliance. This yielded an estimate of the direct costs of these hospitalizations.

The literature search resulted in identification of 24 research reports.[15-21] Applying the meta-analysis methodological criteria described above produced a subsample of seven studies. Characteristics of these studies are shown in Table 29.1. The other 17 studies were excluded from further analysis.[22-38] The number of studies excluded is large because the literature search used a broad list of key words to identify research reports and because the inclusion criteria were rigorous. The most common violation was lack of quantifiable measurement of noncompliance admissions; all 17 rejected studies failed this test. For example, many studies examined adverse drug reactions leading to hospital admissions rather than noncompliance per se. Other studies were excluded because they violated two or more of the four inclusion criteria. As an example, Caranasos, Stewart, and Cluff studied 6,063 consecutive admissions to a Florida teaching hospital. They concluded that

TABLE 29.1. Sample of Noncompliance-Induced Hospitalization Studies and Weighted Average Results*

Authors	Year	Total Admissions	Drug-Induced Admissions	Noncompliant Admissions N	%
McKenney and Harrison	1976	216	59	23	10.6%
Bergman and Wiholm	1981	285	45	21	7.4%
Levy, Mermelstein, and Hemo	1982	1,184	NA	34	2.9%
Salem, Keane, and Williams	1984	41	22	8	19.5%
Stewart, Springer, and Adams	1986	60	25	5	8.3%
Ives, Bentz, and Gwyther	1987	293	45	10	3.4%
Grymonpre et al.	1988	863	162	62	8.6%
Weighted Average		2,942	358	163	5.5%
Weighted Average without Psych. Studies		2,841	311	150	5.3%

* It is not meaningful to calculate a sample variance or confidence interval with these secondary data.

177 admissions were associated with drug-induced illness. They made no attempt, however, to differentiate admissions with respect to causation, and they did not calculate a specific measure of noncompliance admissions.

EMPIRICAL RESULTS
OF THE SEVEN RETAINED STUDIES

Number 1

McKenney and Harrison evaluated 216 consecutive admissions to a large teaching hospital. They found that 23 of 59 drug-induced admissions were attributable to patient noncompliance with prescribed drug regimens. Their results indicated that all noncompliant patients were on long-term maintenance drug therapies. Over the study period, five patients on anticonvulsant therapy were admitted to the hospital because of seizures. Blood level analysis confirmed noncompliance due to underuse of proper drug treatments. The results were used to assess the direct cost of these admissions under the assumption that all documented drug-induced admissions were preventable. The 59 patients admitted used 590 hospital days at a 1976 cost of approximately $60,000.

Number 2

Bergman and Wiholm, as part of a drug epidemiology study, assessed 285 consecutively admitted patients over 3.5 months. Noncompliance was assessed by interview and verified by serum level analysis. Results revealed that noncompliance was the primary cause of admission for 21 out of 45 drug-related admissions. The authors noted that an additional eight patients were admitted because of inadequate drug effect.

Number 3

Levy, Mermelstein, and Hemo completed the only study to date specifically focused on noncompliance. They reported that 34 of 1,184 medical admissions monitored at a large hospital in Jerusalem were caused primarily by drug therapy noncompliance. In this study, as in the study of McKenney and Harrison, all cases involved long-term maintenance drug therapy for chronic disease.

Number 4

Salem, Keane, and Williams documented drug-related admissions to a Veterans Administration psychiatric ward. Over a four-month period, researchers monitored a total of 41 consecutive referral admissions. Analysis revealed that eight of 22 drug-related admissions were attributable to patient noncompliance. Admittedly, psychiatric patients are different from those admitted to general medical-surgical wards. In some aspects, however, their long-term drug therapy profiles are similar to other chronically ill patients, and similar noncompliance rates and problems would be expected. An additional finding was a significantly longer length of stay for patients in the drug-related admissions group than for the control group (37.7 days and 17.2 days, respectively).

Number 5

Stewart, Springer, and Adams monitored 60 consecutive admissions to an inpatient psychiatric ward using methodology similar to that of Salem, Keane, and Williams (Number 4). Their results indicated that five of 25 drug-related admissions were due to therapy noncompliance.

Number 6

Ives, Bentzer, and Gwyther found that ten of 45 drug-related admissions were due to noncompliance. They followed 293 admissions to a large North Carolina hospital over a 12-month period and were able to show that patients in their sixth and eighth decades of life were at highest risk for drug-induced hospitalization.

Number 7

Grymonpre et al. studied 863 admissions of patients age 50 years and older to a Canadian health sciences hospital. The four-month study found one or more adverse drug reactions in 162 admissions. Data on intentional noncompliance and medication error (defined as accidental or unintentional non-adherence to a therapeutic program) included 62 hospital admissions (8.6%) that were a direct result of noncompliance with drug therapy.

In both the McKenney and the Levy studies, all patients hospitalized due to drug therapy noncompliance were on long-term maintenance drug regimens. Patients with such regimens have been shown to have noncompliance problems. In 1975 and 1976, Hulka et al. found that 42% of diabetic and congestive heart failure patients on long-term maintenance therapy deviated significantly from prescribed drug regimens.[39] In a chapter in *Compliance in Health Care,* Sackett and Snow tabulated the results from 14 studies of long-term drug therapy compliance and found the average compliance rate for 16,703 patients to be 46%.[11] Thus, patients with long-term drug regimens are particularly at risk for hospitalization related to noncompliance.

Another characteristic that may be associated with hospitalization due to noncompliance is patient age. Ives, Bentz, and Gwyther found that elderly patients were at the highest risk for drug-induced hospitalization. Haynes found similar associations. It seems likely that in some of these drug-induced hospitalizations, noncompliance played a role. Since long-term drug therapies are more probable among older patients, the contributions of these two factors may be confounding. The potential contribution of both factors to hospitalization should be recognized.

RESULTS

Clearly, the study populations, methods used, and subsequent rates of hospitalization varied among the seven studies. However, meta-analysis data aggregation techniques allowed us to combine the results from these studies to derive a composite number and rate of hospitalization due to drug therapy noncompliance. These results are included in Table 29.1. Overall, 5.5% of the hospital admissions evaluated were due to noncompliant patient behavior.

After excluding the two psychiatric studies, the percentage of admissions resulting from noncompliance dropped to 5.3%. We chose the more conservative rate for the cost estimates because these studies were based on a more homogeneous patient population with presumably similar compliance, hospitalization, and therapeutic outcome characteristics. Because the two psychiatric studies included small samples of patients, their overall impact on the data synthesis results is small.

We estimated the direct cost of hospitalizations using the aggregate rate of hospitalization and the formula shown in Figure 29.1. Analysis of 1986 AHA (American Health Association) hospital utilization and cost data from over 6,430 U.S. hospitals provided an annual direct cost of hospitalization due to drug therapy noncompliance of approximately $8.5 billion. In 1974, the Task Force on Prescription Drugs estimated $3 billion for all drug-related admissions.[40] Their $3 billion estimate represents $8.4 billion in 1986 dollars when inflated using the Hospital Room Index of the Medical Care component of

FIGURE 29.1. Formula Calculations for Estimating the Direct Cost of Hospitalization due to Noncompliance for 1986

PREVENTABLE HOSPITALIZATION	=	# PREVENTABLE HOSPITALIZATIONS	*	AVERAGE COST PER HOSPITALIZATION

PHC = (TOT ADMITS * % NONCOMPLIANCE) * (ALOS * ACPPD)

Where: TOT ADMITS = Total number of hospital admissions
           % NONCOMPLIANCE = Rate of hospitalizations due to
                             noncompliance with drug therapy
           ALOS = Average length of hospital stay
           ACPPD = Average cost per patient day

Thus:
           PHC = (35.2 million admissions * 5.3%) * (7.1 days * $639/day)
               = $8.5 billion

the Consumer Price Index, which is comparable to our finding of $8.5 billion for hospitalizations due to noncompliance.

DISCUSSION

Our study shows that over 5% of hospital admissions may be caused by noncompliance with medication regimens, which, when extrapolated to a national annual cost estimate exceeded $8 billion for 1986. This figure does not include indirect costs nor does it reflect the potentially high expense associated with strategies for promoting compliance. Calculating the total costs of drug therapy noncompliance can be difficult due to the complexity of factors involved. To produce an accurate assessment, one would need to look at a variety of economic and psychosocial direct and indirect costs, such as those in Table 29.2. The total economic cost of noncompliance includes both direct and indirect costs.

Indirect measures that calculate loss of productivity, morbidity, mortality, and other costs are noteworthy. The value of the loss of productivity due to morbidity and mortality have been projected in other cost-of-illness studies.[41-43] Such studies have shown that indirect costs are double or triple the direct costs. For example, this has been done with many disease states including, most recently, Acquired Immunodeficiency Syndrome (AIDS). The indirect cost of AIDS in 1986 is estimated to be, on average, three to four times greater than direct costs, largely due to the cost of mortality.[44] Noncompliance (especially underdosing) often leads to poor therapeutic control and outcomes similar to the debilitating effects of the illness itself. So, by extrapolating the results of the retained studies, we estimate an additional $17-25 billion in indirect costs related to drug therapy noncompliance.

Durant has illustrated most dramatically the indirect consequence of noncompliance.[45] He found that noncompliance with oral contraceptives appears

TABLE 29.2. Examples of Direct and Indirect Costs of Therapy Noncompliance

Direct Costs	Indirect Costs
Hospitalization	Loss of Productivity
Additional Physician Visits	Loss of Wages
Additional Pharmacy Visits	Economic Cost of Time
Emergency Room Visits	Other Opportunity Costs
Alternative Provider Visits	Unnecessary Therapies
Mortality	Mortality

to contribute to approximately 10% of all adolescent female pregnancies each year. Applying an estimated cost of $250,000 to rear a child to age 18 in a middle-class family yields sizeable indirect costs associated with this noncompliance.[46]

There are a number of limitations to the generalizability of this study. The estimate of noncompliant admissions is based on an international sample of 2,942 admissions from seven studies. By all measures, this is a relatively small sample from which to generate a national estimate. Also, our method assumes noncompliance behavior and subsequent outcomes are similar across countries and study populations. In addition, three of the studies not included in the aggregation sample reported adverse drug reaction (ADR) rates below our noncompliance estimate of 5.3%. This would suggest that if the researchers had measured noncompliance as a reason for admission, our weighted average would have been lower. While this information is useful in a qualitative way, it should be noted that these same three studies failed at least two of our inclusion criteria, and as a result, were not included in our final sample. Because of the rigorous criteria applied to these studies, the results represent the best attainable estimate from previously reported valid research.

An underlying purpose of the study was to highlight the obvious gaps in the literature that future researchers might address. In the context of other estimates used to make economic and policy forecasts, the criteria were especially strict.

Previous research indicates the average length of stay for drug-related admissions is greater than for normal admissions.[47] Analysis of the characteristics of noncompliant populations suggests that, on average, patients are older and are likely to require more costly services while in the hospital. If length of stay is longer and the intensity of care is greater for noncompliant admissions, the $8.5 billion figure is an underestimate of actual direct cost of hospitalization.

Finally, the hospital cost estimates were based on figures reported by responding AHA hospitals. Our estimates reflect the accuracy or inaccuracy of those data.

CONCLUSION AND RECOMMENDATIONS

An aggregate measure of the rate of hospitalization due to noncompliance with drug regimens was derived from published literature. Overall, it is estimated that noncompliance accounted for 5.3% of hospitalizations. The direct costs of these hospitalizations were estimated at over $8 billion.

This figure is comparable to the Task Force on Prescription Drugs estimate inflated to 1986 dollars.

The major policy issue raised by our results is the need to prevent costly hospitalizations resulting from drug therapy noncompliance. What approaches are best to enhance patient compliance, and which will be most cost effective? Should efforts be targeted toward specific populations? What are the effects of managed care delivery systems with utilization controls and targeted case management programs on therapy compliance? These and other questions deserve investigation.

Indeed, there is a need for better delineation of the problem and of potential solutions. Patient education, provider communication, and behavior modification efforts constitute psychosocial intervention strategies that need to be readdressed by the medical and pharmacy communities. Consistent drug therapy monitoring and concurrent drug use review programs also can enhance patient compliance, yet they are primarily restricted to managed care organizations. A universal drug coverage program would reduce the economic barrier of access to prescription drugs by the elderly and the indigent.

Given the extent and cost of this problem, strategies to enhance compliance and make more effective use of drug therapies deserve considerable attention from both the research and professional communities.

REFERENCES

1. Anon. Hospital statistics. Chicago, IL: American Hospital Association, 1987.

2. Division of National Cost Estimates, Office of the Actuary. National health expenditures 1986–2000. Health Care Fin Admin 1987;8:1-36.

3. Price D, Cook J, Singleton S, Feely M. Doctors' unawareness of the drugs their patients are taking: a major cause of over-prescribing. Br Med J 1986; 292:99-100.

4. Binkley HL. Economics of patient education. Address delivered at the Annual Conference of the National Council on Patient Information and Education, Alexandria, VA, 1983.

5. Levine D. Paper presented at the 33rd Pharmacy Conference, Improving Patient Compliance, Rutgers University, 1984.

6. Strandberg LR. Drugs as a reason for nursing home admissions. Am Health Care Assoc J 1984;10:20-3.

7. Greenberg J, Levtz W, Greenlick M, Malone J, Errin S, Kodner D. The social HMO demonstration: early experience. Health Affairs 1988;7:66.

8. Light RJ, Pillemer DB. Summing up: the science of reviewing research. Cambridge, MA: Harvard University Press, 1984.

9. Glass GV, McGaw B, Smith ML, eds. Meta-analysis of social research. Beverly Hills, CA: Sage Publications, 1981.

10. Drowns-Bangert RL. Review of developments in meta-analytic methods. Psychol Bull 1986;99:388-98.

11. Haynes RB, Taylor DW, Sackett DL, eds. Compliance in health care. Baltimore, MD: Johns Hopkins University Press, 1979.

12. Solomon DK, Baumgartner RP, Glascock LM, Glascock SA, Briscoe ME. Use of medication profiles to detect potential therapeutic problems in ambulatory patients. Am J Hosp Pharm 1974;31:348-54.

13. Inui TS, Carter WB, Pecoraro RE, Pearlman RA, Dohan JJ. Variations in patient compliance with common long-term drugs. Med Care 1980;18:986-93.

14. Maronde RF, Chan LS, Larsen FJ et al. Underutilization of antihypertensive drugs and associated hospitalizations. Unpublished.

15. McKenney JM, Harrison WL. Drug related hospital admissions. Am J Hosp Pharm 1976;22:792-5.

16. Bergman U, Wiholm BE. Drug-related problems causing admissions to a medical clinic. Eur J Clin Pharmacol 1981;20:193-200.

17. Levy M, Mermelstein L, Hemo D. Medical admissions due to noncompliance with drug therapy. Int J Clin Pharmacol Ther Toxicol 1982;20:600-4.

18. Salem RB, Keane TM, Williams JG. Drug-related admissions to a Veterans Administration psychiatric unit. Drug Intell Clin Pharm 1984;18:74-6.

19. Stewart RB, Springer PK, Adams JF. Drug-related admissions to an inpatient psychiatric unit. Am J Psychol 1980;137:1093-4.

20. Ives TJ, Bentz EJ, Gwyther RE. Drug-related admissions to a family medicine inpatient service. Arch Intern Med 1987;147:1117-20.

21. Grymonpre RB, Mitenko PA, Sitar DS, Aoki FY, Montgomery PR. Drug-associated hospital admissions in older medical patients. J Am Geriatr Soc 1988;36:1092-8.

22. Caranasos GJ, Stewart RB, Cluff LE. Drug-induced illness leading to hospitalization. JAMA 1974;228:713-7.

23. Bergman U, Wiholm BE. Patient medication on admission to a medical clinic. Eur J Clin Pharmacol 1981;20:1-7.

24. Black AJ, Somers K. Drug-related illness resulting in hospital admissions. J R Coll Physicians Lond 1984;18:40-1.

25. Burkholder DF. Adverse drug effects and their impact on patient care. Drug Intell Clin Pharm 1979;13:421-4.

26. Cooper JW. Home health care: drug related problems detected by consultant pharmacist participation. Hosp Form 1985;20:643-5.

27. Cooper JW, Love DW, Raffoul PR. Intentional prescription nonadherence by the elderly. J Am Geriatr Soc 1982;30:329-33.

28. Hulka B, Kupper L, Cassel J, Mayo F. Medication use and misuse: physician-patient discrepancies. J Chron Dis 1975;28:7-21.

29. Hurwitz N. Admissions to hospital due to drugs. Br Med J 1969;1:539-40.

30. Levy M, Kewitz H, Altwein W, Hillebrand J, Eliakim M. Hospital admissions due to adverse drug reactions: a comparative study from Jerusalem and Berlin. Eur J Clin Pharmacol 1980;17:25-31.

31. Levy M, Lipshitz M, Eliakim M. Hospital admissions due to adverse drug reactions. Am J Med Sci 1979;277:49-56.

32. Miller RR. Hospital admissions due to adverse drug reactions. Arch Intern Med 1974;134:219-23.

33. Ramsay LE, Freestone S, Silas JH. Drug-related acute medical admissions. Human Toxicol 1982;1:379-81.

34. Talley RB, Laventurier MF. Drug-induced illness. JAMA 1974;229:1043.

35. Trunet P, Borda IT, Rouget AV, Rapin M, Lhoste F. The role of drug-induced illness in admissions to an intensive care unit. Intensive Care Med 1986;12:43-6.

36. Hurwitz N, Wade OL. Intensive hospital monitoring of adverse reactions to drugs. Br Med J 1969;1:531-6.

37. Langman MJ. Did the drug do it? Br Med J 1986;293:219-20.

38. Perri GA, Biddle-Buoma R. Medication related hospitalization stays are target of new Medicaid program. Mich Med 1985;84:220-2.

39. Hulka B, Cassel J, Kupper L, Burdette JA. Communication, compliance and concordance between physicians and patients with prescribed medications. Am J Public Health 1976;66:847-53.

40. Task Force on Prescription Drugs. Final report. Washington, DC: U.S. Department of Health, Education, and Welfare, Office of the Secretary, 1974.

41. Scitovsky AA, Rice DP. Estimates of the direct and indirect costs of acquired immunodeficiency syndrome in the United States, 1985, 1986, 1991. Public Health Rep 1987;102:5-17.

42. Rice DP, Hodgson TA, Hopstein A. The economic cost of illness. A replication and update. Health Care Fin Rev 1985;7:61-80.

43. Rice DP. Estimating the cost of illness. Washington, DC: U.S. Department of Health, Education, and Welfare, 1966. DHEW Publication (PHS) No.947-6.

44. Scitovsky AA. The economic impact of AIDS. Health Affairs 1988;7 (Fall):32-45.

45. Durant RH. Influence of psychosocial factors on adolescent compliance with oral contraceptives. J Adolesc Health Care 1984;5:1-6.

46. Saxton L. The individual, marriage and the family. 5th ed. Belmont, CA: Wadsworth Publishing, 1983.

47. Chueng A, Kayne R. An application of clinical pharmacy services in extended care facilities. Calif Pharm 1975;23:22-8.

PART VII:
EFFECTS ON PHARMACY

Not since the early days of Medicaid drug programs has retail pharmacy faced such changes and challenges driven by economic forces. In this section we have an overview of the effects of managed care on pharmacy services along with some future projections by Curtiss. Huey, Jackson, and Pirl then provide some specific economic data on the impact of third-party programs on community pharmacy. McMillan, Carroll, and Kotzan illustrate one of the measures taken by pharmacies in response to economic pressures and the effect on private-pay patients. Finally, Raisch, Larson, and Bootman provide a methodology by which pharmacists could evaluate third-party contracts.

Chapter 30

Managed Care and Its Effects on Pharmacy Services

Frederic R. Curtiss

INTRODUCTION

In this article the following assertions will be discussed and defended:

1. The managed care industry is no longer comprised of only three market segments.
2. Many of today's HMOs (health maintenance organizations) show little resemblance to their predecessors.
3. A new market segment, "derivative models," showed the greatest magnitude of growth in the managed care industry in 1989 and 1990.
4. Public policy, notably the implementation of Medicare PPS in 1983, catalyzed the forces necessary to make managed care a reality and marked the shift in the balance of power from providers to payers.
5. Employers will use the purchasing power they wield to transfer financial risk to health care providers and managed care plans.
6. Access and convenience factors are already beginning to overtake price in relative importance in decision making in the design and operation of managed care plans.
7. Relative value scales and fee schedules are replacing discount pricing in both inpatient care and ambulatory care.
8. Utilization management in the managed care industry will be achieved through financial (price) incentives that affect beneficiaries as well as providers.

Previously published in *Journal of Research in Pharmaceutical Economics*, Vol. 1(4), 1989.

9. *Direct* capitation contracting will supplant price discounting in the management of ambulatory prescription drug benefits.
10. Success in controlling utilization *per case* will be the single most important factor in determining financial success in both hospital care and ambulatory care.

SEGMENTS OF THE INDUSTRY

In its infancy, the managed care industry was comprised of three distinct market segments: health maintenance organizations, preferred provider organizations (PPOs), and managed fee-for-service plans. Several forces conspired to blur the distinctions among these three segments and contributed to the creation of four market segments that can best be described as "derivative models" because their basic elements are common to the basic elements of HMOs and PPOs and, in fact, often involve HMOs as primary contractors.

Collectively, the managed care industry is projected to account for 85% of the private health insured population by 1992.[1] This represents phenomenal growth from a mere 11% of the population in 1984 to virtual market dominance in only a few years. Conversely, the statistics in Table 30.1 show that the antithesis of managed care, fee-for-service care, fell from 89% of the population in 1984 to 44% by 1987 and will account for 10% or less of the population by 1997. The data in Table 30.1 also show the relative distribution of the population across the three basic market segments. What is not reflected in these data are the large number of different models within each of these market segments and the recent growth of a category of models that does not fit the definitions of the three initial market segments.

TABLE 30.1. Managed Care Industry Enrollments*

	1984	1987	1992	1997
Fee-for-Service	89%	44%	15%	10%
Managed Care	11%	56%	85%	90%
HMO	7	13	28	50
PPO	1	15	47	30
Managed FFS	3	28	10	10

*Percentage of U. S. *private*-pay population enrolled in each segment. Statistics and estimates by Sanford C. Bernstein & Co., New York.

By 1988 there were HMOs that owned and operated PPOs, combination indemnity/HMO and indemnity/PPO plans, point-of-service HMOs, and open-end HMOs, shared-risk relationships that seemed to defy and transcend previous definitions of health insurance, and other health plans that can best be described as derived from the three initial managed care segments.

HMOs

HMOs comprise the most familiar segment of the managed care industry and have existed in various forms for more than 50 years. When first conceived, HMOs had five fundamental components: an enrolled (defined) population, prepayment (of premiums), coverage of a comprehensive scope of medical services, centralization in the delivery of medical and hospital services, and salaried (staff) physicians. In other words, HMOs combined prepayment with health care services *delivery* in one organization, without a third-party payer. Savings were expected from reduced utilization because physicians had no financial incentive to provide more services to generate income. Additional savings were expected from the commitment of HMOs to be health *maintenance* organizations through the provision of comprehensive services and expansion in coverage to wellness programs, such as smoking cessation, routine physical examinations, PAP smears, and other early detection programs.

After nearly 50 years of slow growth, the HMO industry showed phenomenal growth in the 1980s. Whereas much of the growth in enrollment in the HMO industry during its first 50 years was among staff model HMO plans in which members received medical services in centralized clinics from salaried physicians, during the 1980s much of the growth was in plans that did not use the staff model. Hence, the definition of HMO changed somewhat to include organizations that contracted with independent physicians, the so-called IPA or independent practice association, and the group model HMO that was structured around a group of physicians typically practicing in one major clinic. Often, the group model HMO is owned by the physicians. A fourth HMO model is the network model that contracts with IPA physicians and medical groups. The fifth type of HMO structure is a combination of these models, such as the staff/IPA model wherein some physicians are salaried and provide services in centralized clinics, and enrollees also have access to an IPA panel of physicians who have contracted with the HMO to provide services outside the designated clinics.

PPOs

A preferred provider organization is created for the express purpose of trading price discounts in return for a larger volume of services, achieved through the method of channeling patients. The participating providers in the PPO, the panel of providers, trades a price discount (e.g., 20%) in return for enrolled members using the panel of participating providers in preference to nonpanel providers. The typical PPO achieves the channeling phenomenon by making it less costly for the enrollee to use the panel of providers than to use nonpanel providers. For example, the PPO offers the 20% price discount to the buyer (e.g., employer), and the enrollee (employee or dependent) pays a 10% cost-share (i.e., co-insurance) for use of panel providers but a 30% cost-share for use of nonpanel providers. This channeling phenomenon can also be achieved through two-tier or differential copayments (e.g., $5 copayment for an office visit to a panel physician versus a $15 copayment for an office visit to a nonpanel physician) or differential deductibles (e.g., $150 annual deductible for use of nonpanel providers versus no annual deductible for use of panel providers). The basic elements that distinguish HMOs and PPOs are depicted in Figure 30.1.

Given these common characteristics, one might think that PPOs do not differ greatly one from another. However, one factor is particularly significant when analyzing PPOs and is of great importance when comparing PPOs with respect to provision of prescription drugs and pharmacy services: PPO sponsorship is a key factor in differentiating PPOs. The four

FIGURE 30.1. Outline of HMO and PPO Features

HMO Elements

1. Enrolled population
2. Comprehensive services
3. Prepayment
4. Centralization
5. Salaried staff physicians

PPO Elements

1. Enrolled population
2. Channeling through differential cost-sharing
3. Discounted fees for provider panel
   - % of U & C (usual and customary)
   - UCR (usual, customary, and reasonable)
   - RVS (relative value scale) and other fee schedules
4. Two-tier provider reimbursement structure
5. Selectivity in provider panel
6. Quality assurance and credentialing of providers
7. Utilization review

major categories of organizations that may sponsor PPOs (insurers, employers, providers, and brokers or independent agents) are discussed in detail elsewhere and described briefly below.[2]

One example of an *insurer*-sponsored PPO is a Blue Cross plan that solicits hospitals to participate in a PPO, usually through a formal process involving a request for proposal (RFP). A hospital response to an RFP will include a price discount. Blue Cross subscribers in the PPO are channeled to the PPO panel hospitals by a two-tier deductible structure (e.g., the member pays a hospital deductible of $200 for the first day in a PPO hospital compared to a $500 deductible for the first day in a nonpanel hospital). Insurers sponsored approximately 35% of all PPOs at the end of 1987, with 24% sponsored by commercial insurers and 10% sponsored by Blue Cross-Blue Shield plans.[3]

A variation of the insurer-sponsored PPO is the HMO-sponsored PPO. State regulation of HMOs falls under insurance statutes, and HMO-sponsored PPOs are therefore often classified as insurer-sponsored.[4] HMO-sponsored PPOs grew in number largely as part of a health insurance marketing effort to bring one-stop shopping to employers and other buyers. This one-stop product, usually referred to as "triple-option," combines three insurance products—an HMO, a PPO, and traditional indemnity insurance—that can be purchased from one vendor.*

While the success of HMO-sponsored PPOs and HMO-sponsored triple-option products is still in doubt, the market forces that gave rise to these products are clear and interesting. HMOs will be more acceptable to persons who do not have a regular source of health care or an established relationship with a particular physician. Those persons who do have a preference for a particular physician are likely to join the HMO that has a participation agreement with the physician. This otherwise objectionable feature of a closed panel HMO, in which coverage is essentially limited to the designated panel of providers, is removed by the PPO option or triple-option feature in which the enrollee encounters financial incentives to use panel providers but is not

---

*Triple-option is a menu of health insurance products presented to employers, unions, and other groups that allows the purchaser to select from among three health plan options—an HMO, PPO, or indemnity plan—from one insurance company. All major insurers such as CIGNA Corp. (Hartford, CT) and Metropolitan Insurance Co. (New York), as well as some large HMOs such as Maxicare Health Plans (Los Angeles), developed triple-option products in an effort to make the purchase of health insurance more convenient for buyers and to increase penetration (percentage enrollment) in a given group of beneficiaries. Most triple-option products include utilization review features in the traditional indemnity insurance option and may therefore be construed as managed fee-for-service indemnity options.

absolutely restricted to use of panel providers. Therefore, the HMO-sponsored PPO arose, at least in part, from the market demand for greater freedom of choice in the selection of health care providers.

The *provider*-sponsored PPO emerged as the most common type of PPO structure early in the growth of the PPO industry. Collectively, providers sponsored over 49% of all PPOs at the end of 1987, with 16% sponsored by physicians, 11% sponsored by hospitals, and 22% sponsored by joint ventures comprised of hospitals and physicians.

The provider-sponsored PPO is formed typically by a group of providers that has some common interest, such as participation in a buying group. The hospital PPO might market a product to local employers and insurers that offers a discount (e.g., 5%) of charges coupled with cost-sharing incentives.

An alternative structure is the *employer*-sponsored PPO, created when an employer or group of employers contracts directly with local providers to obtain a discount. The employer-sponsored PPO is possible whenever there is a sufficient number and concentration of employees in a given geographic area to represent market power in negotiating with providers. In a truly employer-sponsored PPO, the employer or employer coalition would write, negotiate, and maintain the provider participation agreements. An employer could initiate the PPO contracting process by sending a request for proposal (RFP) to all local providers asking for a bid from each provider. An employer-sponsored PPO is feasible for an employer that self-funds and self-administers the medical benefits of its employees.*

The fourth type of PPO structure is *independent* or broker sponsorship. For example, a medical claims third-party administrator (TPA) that performs medical claims administration under contract for employers, insurers, and other entities may form a PPO and elicit price discounts from providers in an effort to make the TPA more desirable than competing

---

*Self-funding of medical benefits by employers refers to a financing arrangement in which the employer assumes some or all of the financial risk arising from the cost of medical claims for the covered group of employees and dependents. Large employers may assume all financial risk while medium-size and smaller employers are more likely to reduce some of the financial risk by purchasing stop-loss coverage from an insurer. In stop-loss coverage, the employer pays all medical claims expenses up to some designated stop-loss amount per individual (e.g., $25,000 per year) or some aggregate amount for the group (e.g., medical expenses in excess of 110% of the projected claims expenses for the period). In self-administration, the employer assumes medical claims processing and administrative responsibilities as well as financial risk. A self-administered employer typically purchases or leases a computer software claims administration system and hires staff to perform the administrative functions.

TPAs.* A broker form of PPO may also be formed when an independent party organizes a network of providers, negotiates a package of medical benefits and prices with employers or other buyers, and subcontracts the claims processing and other paperwork to a TPA. The broker may be reimbursed for its services either by retaining a percentage of the monthly premium amount made by the employer, by retaining a negotiated amount per medical claim, or by simply accepting a monthly fee. Alternately, a broker form of PPO might be financed by a percentage of the savings obtained by the PPO.

Managed Fee-for-Service

The third segment of the managed health care industry is comprised of fee-for-service health plans that impose some management controls on the price, use, quality, or access of medical care services. Fee-for-service health plans have become "managed" most commonly through the imposition of a mandatory utilization review (UR) requirement. Therefore, managed FFS plans can be differentiated from HMOs and PPOs in the respect that HMOs and PPOs more commonly have the ability to achieve savings by controlling use and price factors, while managed FFS plans have more commonly, heretofore, sought savings by reducing the use of services.

Many FFS medical benefit plans were modified in the period from 1985 through 1988 by the addition of certain concurrent and prospective UR requirements; by the end of 1987, nearly 60% of major employers had implemented a preadmission certification requirement, and over 40% had a concurrent review program.[5]

For example, full coverage of a hospital admission for a nonemergency condition is conditioned on obtaining certification of medical necessity before the admission, hence the term preadmission certification. Another type of prospective review is the second surgical opinion program in which a proposal of surgery must be followed by an independent review of the medical necessity of the proposed surgery. Examples of concurrent UR programs include review of the medical necessity of additional days of hospitalization past some target length of stay for the particular diagnosis (known as continued stay review) and discharge planning programs in which post-hospital care is arranged, where necessary and appropriate, to enable a shorter hospital stay.

---

*TPA is a third-party administrator, an entity that assumes certain administrative functions for a health plan, most often eligibility determination, coverage decisions, claims processing, and provider payment.

Technically, of course, a managed fee-for-service plan would also exist whenever providers are reimbursed on a fee-for-service basis, but there is some management component, such as bundling of services into units for the purpose of establishing prospective prices, that attempts to identify higher quality providers and steer covered members to these providers.

In August 1988, Prudential Insurance Company of America became the first major insurer to channel organ transplant procedures to hospitals selected on the basis of price discounts in addition to quality factors. The first panel of 24 hospitals nationwide performed heart, kidney, and liver transplants and certain kidney stone treatments.[6] This initial panel of providers was later expanded to include hospitals specializing in coronary artery bypass grafts, allogenic bone marrow transplants, and trauma burn care. This Prudential program represents the principle of channeling applied to a fee-for-service insurance program, rather than a true PPO, since participation in the program by Prudential subscribers was entirely voluntary and without financial incentives for the subscribers.

Do managed fee-for-service plans represent a truly viable segment of the managed care industry? The performance data appear to be mixed, but most reports have shown savings for employers.[7] For example, General Motors was able to achieve sufficient savings to avoid shifting more of the costs of medical benefits to employees; Honeywell found savings in administering its own PPOs and negotiating directly with providers; Sun Company, an energy resource firm, achieved savings from UM (utilization management), benefit redesign, and direct negotiations with providers; Sunbeam Appliance Company produced savings through a comprehensive prenatal education program and avoidance of premature births; Milwaukee saved $1 million in 1987 through a mandatory UR program and per diem rate negotiations with area hospitals; and Xerox Corporation, Pacific Telesis, and other companies led employers in managing HMO premium rates through data collection, competitive bidding, and direct negotiations while simultaneously relying on private UR programs.[8-11]

EPOs and Derivative Models

At one time the managed care industry was packaged more easily into fairly distinct categories. At the beginning of the growth phase of the managed care industry, in 1985 and 1986, the distinction between an HMO and a PPO was relatively clear: HMOs restricted access to a defined panel of providers. If the HMO member used a provider outside of the panel, except in emergencies, the care received by the member was not covered by the HMO (i.e., the member paid for the care out-of-pocket). By contrast, the PPO segment of the industry grew, in part, by capitalizing on this restrictive feature of HMOs. PPOs typically had larger panels of providers than HMOs, but PPOs also covered care received outside the designated panel at a reduced rate (e.g., 70% coverage of the cost of the care versus 90% coverage of the care received from the panel).

By mid-1988 the distinction between the HMO segment and the PPO segment of the managed care industry had blurred considerably. In fact, the fastest growing segment of the HMO industry in 1988 was the open-end model HMO in which members could still enjoy coverage–at reduced levels–of care received outside of the HMO panel.[12] Second, PPOs were struggling with providers to establish financial-risk contract relationships that mimic HMO contracts in which providers become subject to incentives to control utilization as well as price.

There was also the exclusive provider organization, or EPO, a variation of the PPO model that preceded the growth of the open-end HMO. The EPO combined the elements of HMOs and PPOs. In the EPO model, the member receives no coverage of medical care services received outside of the designated panel of providers, hence the term exclusive. The California Medi-Cal Selective Provider Contracting Program, described in more detail below, operated on the basis of the EPO model since Medi-Cal recipients could receive hospital care only from contract hospitals, except in emergency situations. In contrast to the open-end HMO model, which grew out of market pressure brought by consumers for more access flexibility, the EPO model grew out of the interests of providers and third-party administrators. The EPO model offers providers the carrot of being the sole source of medical care for the enrolled members, and third-party administrators, such as the Medi-Cal agency in Medi-Cal SPCP, could use this aspect of the EPO model to negotiate the lowest possible prices from the providers because the EPO panel of providers was certain to experience an increased volume of services when covered members were restricted to a smaller number of contract (panel) providers.

Access and freedom of choice were, therefore, important factors in the development of alternative models in the managed care industry. EPOs have not been common due to the complete forfeiture of freedom of choice. Overall, it can be said that employees were a major factor in the development of the open-end HMO, and employers were a major factor in the change in PPOs that took place in the late 1980s. While employees wanted greater access and the flexibility to use a nonpanel provider when desired, employers found that some PPOs, perhaps most, were incapable of controlling total costs and that the PPOs saved them no money.[13]

At least two factors have contributed to elusive savings among PPOs: providers could negotiate discounted prices based on inflated charges, so the discount PPO fee was really no lower than previous actual charges; and PPO providers could usually influence the use of services to increase their total revenue because utilization management (UM) controls in most PPOs have been weak and limited in scope. Provider sponsorship of PPOs is an understandable market response and an alternative to the stricter use guidelines and (financial) risk contracts characteristic of HMOs and PPOs sponsored by payers and other entities.

Variations of the basic HMO and PPO models will continue to represent a large part of the growth of the managed care industry. Perhaps the greatest growth will occur in the derivation of managed care plans from self-funded employer and indemnity/managed FFS plans. This growth projection is supported by two factors. First, employee benefits managers have discovered that offering HMO plan options may result in adverse selection in which comparatively healthy employees join the HMO plan(s), leaving comparatively less healthy employees (and dependents) in the self-funded or insurance-based indemnity plan and thereby driving up *average* costs per employee covered by the indemnity plan. Additionally, since employers are required by federal law to make an equal contribution to HMO premiums on behalf of employees, the *total* costs of providing health benefits to employees can rise significantly when adverse selection occurs. For these reasons, at least some employers have experienced a growing need to control the costs of self-funded indemnity health plans when those plans are offered with HMO health plans.

The second factor that predicts rapid and significant growth in employer-based managed care plans has to do with the dichotomy between the desire of employers to control health benefits costs and the preference among employees for unrestrained access to health care services. Employers strive to offer welfare benefits, including health care, that are valuable and meaningful to employees in order to encourage and reward work performance and loyalty and to minimize turnover and retain employees. Because employees and dependents favor indemnity health plans that offer the greatest degree of freedom in choosing health providers, employers will search for the optimum combinations of elements of the managed care industry to meet the needs of employees while producing cost savings.

The conflict between price control and maximum access and freedom of choice has already precipitated significant changes in HMO plans. Two recent "derivative" models presage significant growth in the fourth segment of the managed care industry. Both models involve more direct sharing of financial risk by employers and HMOs or providers/insurers.

On March 1, 1988, a large employer with approximately 80,000 employees entered into a contractual relationship that can be described as a "hybrid risk" model[14,15] with the nation's largest triple-option insurer, CIGNA Corporation (Hartford, CT). This contract combined all three basic segments of managed care–HMO, PPO, and managed FFS–with a risk arrangement between the employer and the triple-option insurer. In return for designating CIGNA as the exclusive insurer/provider, the employer was guaranteed that its total insurance premiums would not rise more than a specified amount each year over the three-year period of the contract. The employees could enroll in only one plan, called "Health Care Connection," which consisted of CIGNA, HMO, and PPO providers and CIGNA indemnity claims processing services, with financial incentives for enrollees to use the HMO and PPO panel providers. This plan offers considerable freedom of choice for employees while controlling the potential problem of adverse selection and uncontrollable costs for the employer.

A more recent derivative model was developed for a smaller employer with approximately 30,000 employees and early retirees (under age 65) who are distributed over a large portion of the western United States. This derivative model, appropriately named "HealthSpan" was launched in early 1989.[16] HealthSpan bridged the employer's indemnity plan with an HMO option coordinated by one HMO plan. By selecting one HMO plan, the employer can negotiate a risk-sharing relationship, gain some control over the potential problem of adverse selection, and manage the administrative burden normally incurred by employers in interacting with a multitude of HMO plans.

HealthSpan was innovative in another aspect. Because the HMO assumed financial risk for all employees and not just HMO enrollees, HealthSpan could be designed to offer a greater degree of freedom of choice. The plan is called a "point-of-service" HMO because beneficiaries do not have to specify the use of panel providers, versus nonpanel providers, until medical services are actually sought and used. The POS-HMO plan is similar to an open-end HMO plan in that it combines the greater flexibility in access to many health care providers with a panel of HMO providers that have the potential to produce savings from a combination of price discounts and utilization controls, including financial incentives in risk-sharing relationships with providers or salaried (staff) physicians. What differentiates open-end HMOs from POS-HMOs is the degree of (financial) risk-sharing between the buyer (employer) and the HMO. An open-end HMO can simply offer a PPO panel of providers as an alternative and bill the employer for use of the panel at discounted prices, or the open-end HMO may assume financial risk by pricing all health care premiums of the employer. In this respect, an open-end HMO may differ little from a POS-HMO.

In both open-end HMOs and POS-HMOs, claims administration services are necessary to process claims from PPO and FFS providers. In HealthSpan, a third-party insurer (of the employer's former indemnity plan) assumed a three-part role as insurer, TPA, and contracts administrator. The insurer in HealthSpan was the primary contractor, in terms of financial risk, with the employer, and the HMO was the secondary contractor. The employer and insurer each agreed to assume 50% of the excess of health plan costs (medical claims) that exceeded the projected claims experience for the plan year (e.g., 1989); the employer agreed to assume 100% of costs in excess of 125% of the projected claims expense.

Derivative managed care plans include models that do not fit well into the three initial segments of the managed care industry, often because the derived model combines elements of more than one managed care market segment. The driving force behind future growth in this fourth segment of the managed care industry will be the desire among employers to control total health benefits costs by managing adverse selection and reducing the number of contractors.

THE TOOLS OF MANAGED CARE

The blurring of former distinctions among segments of the managed care industry begs the question of what constitutes "managed care." In a literal sense, managed care means that health care is "managed": one or more of the three fundamental parameters of health care (price, quality, or access) is affected by conscious decision making or predetermined courses of action. Eleven tools or components of managed care have been described in detail previously, but the most fundamental factor concerns shared decision making.[17] Decision making in fee-for-service plans is generally autonomous, involving only the primary physician and, often, little input from the patient. In managed care, however, the physician, patient, and third-party administrators share decision making.

The paradigm pictured in Figure 30.2 can be useful in analyzing health plans described as "managed care." A given health plan can be tentatively classified on the right side of the paradigm as a delivery vehicle, followed by analysis of the components of managed care that are inherent in the health plan and, ultimately, an evaluation of the degree to which one or more "parameters" of health care are directly influenced by the health plan.

The first three tools of managed care in the paradigm involve managing price per unit of service. The differentiation of these tools is important to predicting the degree of success in controlling the price of health care

FIGURE 30.2. Managed Care Paradigm

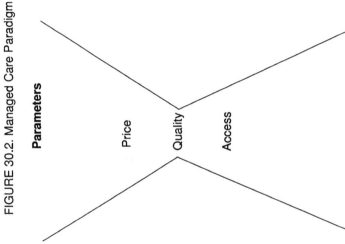

Managed Care Components

1. Prospective pricing
2. U and C price discounts
3. UCR pricing
4. Bundled services
5. Capitation reimbursement
6. Peer review
7. Mandatory UR
8. Benefit (re)design
9. Channeling
10. Quality criteria
11. Health promotion

Parameters

Price

Quality

Access

Delivery Vehicles

HMOs
- Staff
- IPA
- Group
- Network

PPOs
- Insurer/payer
- Provider
- Employer
- Independent

- Managed FFS
- Employer
- Insurer
- TPA

- Derivative Models
- Open-end HMO
- Hybrid-risk
- POS-HMO
- EPO

services. Discounts to usual and customary (U and C) prices are the least objectionable method of price control for providers because providers retain control over their own price setting, giving up only a percentage discount of their normal charges. When maximum U and C prices are identified, the method becomes a UCR ("reasonable") determination. This method results in reduction of the highest prices (e.g., the top 10%) for a given item or service and results in less variance in the actual amounts paid to providers. Conversely, prospective pricing involves the establishment of a specific price for a given item or service (i.e., the creation of a fee schedule). This method of pricing is the most objectionable to providers.

The method of bundling services for the purpose of tying health care outcomes more closely to resource inputs is the foundation of the Medicare Prospective Payment System and is now quite familiar to all health care providers. Medicare PPS combined (inpatient) services bundling with "prospective pricing."

Mandatory UR requirements have been used formerly to manage fee-for-service plans of employers and insurers, achieved through benefit (re)design in which beneficiaries are made price-conscious through cost-sharing requirements and sometimes channeling to certain providers who have agreed to price discounts. Peer review is a fundamental element in the quintessential HMO (staff) model and has been institutionalized in the Medicare Peer Review Organization (PRO). Specific criteria regarding quality of care (e.g., a low post-operative infection rate) are not yet common among health plans, hence the consideration of quality criteria as a tool for managing health care services. Because health promotion is once again being touted as a means to achieve savings in the use of health care services (in the range of $2.50 to $3.44 for every dollar spent), health promotion can be considered a tool of managed care when health benefit plans are revised to influence the behavior and lifestyles of beneficiaries.[18,19]

Capitation financing and reimbursement brings together price setting with incentives to control the utilization of medical services. Total spending for health care services is a function of volume as well as price (per unit of service) and is described by the following equation:

total spending = (price x utilization) + administrative costs

where price is a function of provider costs plus profits:

total spending = [(costs + profit) x utilization] +
administrative costs

Hence, health care *spending*, or the total expense of a given health care benefit, may not be truly managed or controlled in the absence of systems that manage utilization as well as price. Mandatory UR features may help to thwart unnecessary utilization, but capitation payment systems also remove the financial incentive for providers to render more services to patients. For example, a capitation payment amount of $30.00 per enrolled beneficiary might be paid to a primary care physician (PCP) each month. When this capitation amount covers the use of all ancillary services such as clinical laboratory testing as well as medical services that may be required, the PCP assumes financial risk for referrals to specialists and the use of all medical services by beneficiaries. From the payer perspective, capitation reimbursement obviates the need to establish and negotiate fee schedules and reduces the administrative cost and burden of conducting UR to detect and thwart fraud, abuse, and misuse of medical services.

Capitation reimbursement is the quintessential method of bringing together incentives for providers to perform *all* UR functions and the capability to accurately project total spending. Capitation reimbursement–the prepayment of a monthly defined dollar amount to health care providers for a given scope of services–differs from the HMO method of health care financing in the scope of services bundled into the prepayment amount. HMOs assume financial risk for a comprehensive scope of services, in contrast to a dental benefit, for example. A dental benefit might be financed by a given monthly premium and may be referred to as a "dental HMO," but it is not a comprehensive health plan.

Most observers equate HMOs with the capitation reimbursement method, but several factors conspire to limit the degree to which an HMO can use capitation reimbursement methods with providers. First, an HMO may not achieve sufficient market penetration and, hence, market strength to command capitation payment arrangements with providers, particularly hospitals and physicians. Financial risk arrangements between HMOs and hospitals are not common even in 1989, and hospital capitation arrangements are virtually nonexistent. Of the physicians who participated in HMOs in 1986, less than one-half were compensated on a capitation basis, 15% were salaried (i.e., primarily in staff model HMOs), and 39% were compensated on a fee-for-service basis.[20] Most HMOs in 1988 and 1989 attempted to share risk with physicians through FFS reimbursement modified by a method referred to as "withhold." In a withhold method, fee-for-service payments were made but an amount (e.g., 20%) was withheld to establish a "reserve" from which excess costs would be paid if claims were higher than expected and from which "profits" would be distributed if medical costs were less than projected. The important point is that an HMO must have sufficient size and market strength to cause physicians, particularly independent practitioners, to accept any financial risk, and the HMO or other managed care plan must have significant market power to implement the capitation reimbursement method.

Aside from staff models, which use predominantly salary compensation of physicians, IPA models are the least likely to have physician capitation arrangements (46%), compared to 68% of group model HMOs and 77% of network model HMOs that compensate physicians through capitation arrangements. IPA models were the fastest growing segment of the HMO industry in 1987 and 1988.[21] The age of the HMO plan is also important in determining the physician compensation method, with 60% of older HMOs (e.g., three to five years) using capitation compared to 45% of younger HMOs that use capitation, reflecting the greater size and market strength of more established HMOs and their ability to implement physician capitation arrangements.

Physician resistance to capitation reimbursement methods is well established, and the ability of managed care plans to bring more physicians under capitation arrangements will be an uphill battle, the outcome of which will be determined in large part by the purchasing power and market strength of the managed care plan. A 1988 study of physician capitation arrangements carried a warning that physician resistance to capitation would intensify if existing physician capitation methods were not changed. In an analysis of nine IPA-model HMOs, the authors of the report found that adequate methodology were not used to structure primary care physician (PCP) reimbursement systems, thereby creating the potential for some cost-conscious PCPs to terminate participation if they incurred personal financial losses resulting from factors beyond their control.[22]

Financial risk-sharing arrangements with providers are necessary for any managed care plan to attain true control over its service costs, including the ability to predict accurately its service costs in the future. Ultimate control of service costs would be attained by an HMO that is able to negotiate capitation payment agreements with *all* of its provider groups–including hospitals, physicians, pharmacies, and home care providers. Presumably, the monthly premium for that HMO would be calculated from the sum of the capitation payment amounts (e.g., $40 per member-month for hospital care, $30 per member-month for physician care and ambulatory care services, and $8 per member-month for prescription drugs) plus the administrative expenses and profit for the proprietary HMO plan.

Market supply can also influence the incidence of capitation reimbursement systems. Even though a given managed care plan may control only a small portion of the buyers' market (e.g., 10%), the managed care plan may be able to extract price concessions from providers if there is a sufficient supply of providers. An excess supply of hospital beds is now common in many market areas, and virtually every urban market has an abundant supply of community pharmacies.

FACTORS IN HEALTH BENEFITS FINANCING

The incessant rise in total spending for health care services has been the principal catalyst and fuel for the managed care industry. The birth and growth of this industry has also been influenced by a major change that has taken place in the financing of health benefits for employees. Over the last ten years, employers have adopted self-funding of health benefits as a means to avoid or reduce payment of risk charges and to enjoy the favorable cash-flow effects of paying medical claims when incurred, instead of prepaying in the form of health insurance premiums. Coincident with this trend, the functions of health insurance companies, including claims processing, provider payment, coverage determinations, and employee communications regarding benefits and coverage, have been assumed by a myriad of subcontractors. Third-party administrators process medical claims and pay providers; utilization review organizations (UROs) subcontract to detect and prevent waste caused by fraud, abuse, and misuse of services; other agents may negotiate price discounts with providers and manage PPOs; and other companies subcontract to provide a host of services related to the administration of health benefits.* There is even a niche in the URO industry for UROs that evaluate the performance of other UROs.[23] The proliferation of these subindustries has coincided with the componentization of once complete health benefits packages purchased from one insurer and has facilitated price competition in all aspects of health benefits.

EVOLUTION IN PROVIDER
REIMBURSEMENT METHODS

Some of the changes in provider reimbursement that are important to the managed care industry did not happen overnight. The still predominant

---

*Utilization review organizations (UROs) analyze and evaluate the medical necessity and appropriateness of health care services. UROs are generally private, for-profit, UR companies that contract to perform retrospective, concurrent, and prospective UR services for employers, third-party administrators, insurance companies, state Medicaid programs, and the federal government. UROs that perform UR services for the federal government (Medicare) are known as peer review organizations (PROs).

method of retrospective reimbursement, based on charges set by providers, was managed by some Blue Cross plans almost from their first days in business. Some Blue Cross plans were able to obtain price discounts (e.g., 92% of U and C charges) because of their size, market power, and political climate. Other Blue Cross plans attempted to manage hospital costs through budget review and other rate setting methods. Prospective pricing became a fact of life for hospital managers virtually overnight with the adoption and implementation of Medicare PPS in 1983.[24] Medicare PPS also incorporated services bundling in the form of 468 discrete groups based on the principal diagnosis of the patient and other patient-related factors. The concept of services bundling has also been applied to ambulatory care in the forms of ambulatory visit groups and ambulatory care groups.

Prospective pricing and services bundling were associated with other efforts in price discounting and negotiated fees, particularly among PPOs. Providers have become accustomed to signing contracts with PPO and HMO plans that reimbursed them at prices that are significantly discounted. For example, by the end of 1987, hospitals in California, a hotbed of PPO development, had an average of ten PPO contracts per hospital.[25] Greater sophistication in managing capitation reimbursement will propel significant growth in this aspect of managed care.

PROVIDER REIMBURSEMENT IN PUBLIC PROGRAMS

The significance of Medicare PPS to the growth of the managed care industry cannot be ignored. At the least, Medicare PPS caused the entire hospital industry to think in terms of producing a new product–patient discharges–in which the component services and costs must be managed. Second, Medicare PPS heralded a new era in which Congress and society mandated shared decision making in health care. Because Medicare accounts for almost 40% of hospital patients and total hospital revenues, PPS made it imperative that hospitals work with physicians to control the cost and use of services that go into the DRG bundles. And, as noted previously, Medicare PPS was implemented coincident to national peer review–the Medicare Peer Review Organization (PRO) program–before the end of the first year of Medicare PPS;[26] the PRO was designed to manage unnecessary utilization (hospital admissions). The combined effects of Medicare PPS and PROs were significant, causing the average length of hospital stay for Medicare admissions to decrease by 23% during the first two years of PPS (i.e., in 1984 and 1985) from an average of 10.0 days to 7.7 days, and a spill-over effect of Medicare PPS was evidenced by a corresponding decrease in the ALOS (average length of stay) for non-Medicare patients during this period.[27,28]

The Medicare PRO program and Medicare PPS had a two-fold depressant effect on the use of Medicare inpatient hospital services, and the depressant effect of the PRO program may have been as great as Medicare PPS itself. The effects of Medicare PPS were first felt in the hospital industry in 1983 and 1984. The Medicare PRO program probably had its greatest effect on suppressing the use of Medicare inpatient hospital services during 1985 and 1986; Medicare acute-care hospital admissions fell 5.2% during 1985 and declined further by 3.6% in 1986.[29,30] By 1990, Medicare PPS and the Medicare PRO program would save 20%, or about $18 billion in one year alone, over what would have been spent under the retrospective, cost-based method that preceded Medicare PPS.[31] One-third of these savings stem from fewer admissions, and two-thirds of the savings are created by the price component of Medicare PPS.

The principles of services bundling, prospective pricing, and peer review are now being contemplated for Medicare reimbursement of ambulatory care, particularly physician reimbursement. The initial efforts at suppressing price increases of physician fees have been unsuccessful. For example, Medicare Part B spending for physician services rose 30% (a 22% increase, when adjusted for inflation) from 1983 to 1986 despite a two-year freeze on physician fees because physicians were able to increase their Medicare revenues by increasing the utilization of services, such as surgery, lab tests, and office visits.[32] Subsequent efforts to restrain spending on physician services are now focused on developing a more equitable schedule of payment rates through imposition of a relative value scale (RVS), known as the Medicare Resource-Based Relative Value Scale (RBRVS), in which physician payment rates are based on input costs (such as amount of time required for the procedure or office visit) rather than on historical physician prices (fees).[33] Later Health Care Financing Administration (HCFA) will direct its attention to bundling physician services and hospital outpatient services into illness- or episode-based payment groups.

In home care HCFA has relied upon prospective pricing (at low rates) to control home health agency reimbursement and durable medical equipment (DME) spending (e.g., payment rates for home oxygen were reduced several times by HCFA during 1987 and 1988).[34] However, HCFA is also experimenting with demonstration projects in competitive bidding of durable medical equipment and with a prospective pricing method based on services bundling to contain home health services spending. In the Medicare hospice benefit, Congress and HCFA employed services bundling in the form of patient days and prospective pricing in the form of rates per diem to produce savings of as much as $3.7 million in 1985.[35]

Elsewhere, Congress and HCFA drew upon the cost-saving potential of capitation financing for the Medicare program in enacting and implementing risk contracts with health maintenance organizations and a new entity, competitive medical plans (CMPs–organizations in which physicians were not necessarily employees of the HMO) beginning in 1985.[36] By early 1988, HCFA had signed or was reviewing nearly 200 contracts with HMOs or CMPs, and over one million Medicare beneficiaries nationwide were enrolled in HMOs or CMPs.[37] Medicare savings from capitation have thus far been limited by the low percentage of Medicare beneficiaries enrolled in these risk contracts (less than 5% of the total Medicare population) and uncertainty regarding selection factors in beneficiary enrollment in these plans (i.e., to what extent have some HMOs and CMPs enrolled comparatively healthy Medicare beneficiaries).[38,39]

More recently, HCFA has designed and initiated PPO demonstration projects that are intended to produce savings through lower physician fees (price discounts) and by channeling beneficiaries to the contracting physicians through a differential in the coinsurance amount (e.g., 10% coinsurance for the use of panel physicians versus 30% coinsurance for the use of nonpanel physicians).[40] At the same time, HCFA has begun implementation of the Medicare Insured Group (MIG) demonstration project, prescribed by section 4015 of the Omnibus Budget Reconciliation Act of 1990 (OBRA), which creates the equivalent of an employer HMO or CMP for Medicare-eligible retirees. Three large employer health plans contracted with HCFA on a capitated basis for the care of Medicare-eligible retirees.[41] The MIG demonstration project combines public (Medicare) and private health plans in a financial risk (capitation) arrangement.

Medicaid program change was paced by reform that took place in four states during the period from 1980 to 1983.[42] Creation of the Arizona Health Care Cost Containment System (AHCCCS) marked a dramatic departure from other state Medicaid programs by employing competitive bidding to select primary care managed health plans. These plans functioned as HMOs, contracting with hospitals, physicians, and others to provide medical care services to the enrolled Medicaid recipients. AHCCCS was based on prepaid, capitated payments to providers; establishment of a "gatekeeper" system in which each Medicaid recipient was assigned to a primary care physician who had responsibility for monitoring, supervising, and directing the care of the Medicaid recipient; the use of nominal copayments or coinsurance to cause recipients to be sensitive to the need for services and the price of the services; and channeling recipients through reduced freedom of choice.

The California Medi-Cal Selective Provider Program included the creation of a new contracts office that analyzed hospital cost and price data and negotiated directly with hospitals to obtain per diem payment rates (i.e., bundled, prospective prices). Medi-Cal SPCP is credited with saving California more than $1 billion over four years, with $385 million in savings in fiscal year 1987 alone, without sacrificing access or quality of care for Medicaid recipients. In New York, an all-payer prospective per-diem rate setting method is credited with keeping adjusted hospital per diem rate increases below the national average. Pennsylvania Medicaid has employed a prospective hospital pricing method based on DRGs and, more recently, a physician gatekeeper method in which each Medicaid recipient selected or was assigned a primary care physician who had responsibility for monitoring and directing the recipient's medical care services.[43]

In all, 35 states had obtained a hospital reimbursement waiver by 1984, thereby permitting the use of prospective pricing of hospital services. A study published in early 1988 found that the hospital prospective pricing methods used in these states reduced the rate of growth in real spending per Medicaid recipient by 3.1% compared to the rate of spending growth in states without hospital prospective pricing.[44] This study also suggested that utilization review programs, particularly preadmission certification review programs, may produce additional Medicaid program savings over the long term that exceed the savings realized by prospective pricing.

In the context of managed care, Medicaid program initiatives have fallen into four categories: hospital prospective pricing and competitive bidding (e.g., California), utilization control programs, physician gatekeeper models, and enrollment of recipients in HMOs and prepaid health plans.

Enrollment of Medicaid recipients in HMOs and other prepaid health plans was undertaken with particular enthusiasm in a handful of states, including Arizona, whose program used prepaid health plans exclusively. In 1988, California, Illinois, Michigan, and Wisconsin led the nation in Medicaid enrollments in HMOs. Evaluation of the Wisconsin program produced estimated savings of $12.7 million for the period from 1985 through 1987.[45]

UTILIZATION MANAGEMENT

Managing utilization of medical care services is now possible. The passive-sounding utilization review has been replaced with the more ominous "utilization management." The retrospective review of the medical necessity and appropriateness of medical care services has been supplanted with more aggressive and obtrusive concurrent and prospective methods, including preadmission certification, second surgical opinions, and treatment protocols. A large measure of peer review completes the recipe for UM.

Private UR companies sprang up almost overnight during 1986 and 1987, propelled by promises of guaranteed reduction of as much as 20% in the number of hospital inpatient days.[46] An employer with a history of 800-900 hospital days per 1,000 members per year could experience as much as a 50% reduction in hospital use through preadmission certification and concurrent review services. The resultant level of 400-450 days per 1,000 members would rival hospital use rates among HMO plans. The Blue Cross and Blue Shield Association reported nearly $1.5 billion per year in hospital spending for the period from October 1, 1983 through the end of 1986 from reduced hospital admissions attributed to its preadmission certification programs and the use of in-house and contracted UROs.[47]

Today the term utilization review more commonly refers to retrospective review of the medical necessity and appropriateness of services rendered. If some action is taken when care is found to be inappropriate or unnecessary, such as communication of the findings to the provider, then retrospective utilization review might be described as utilization management. But management of utilization is more likely to be achieved when the medical necessity and appropriateness of services are assessed at the time that the services are being rendered (i.e., concurrent review) or before the services are rendered (i.e., prospective review).

Concurrent review programs are considered part of utilization management because the course and end point of care are generally affected. Concurrent UR (UM) would include continued stay review of hospital cases, discharge planning efforts to include proper and efficient placement of the hospital patient upon discharge, and case management. Case management entails monitoring the medical necessity, the appropriateness, and the proper site of care during the course of care. Patients (cases) who require intensive care, such as victims of trauma injuries (e.g., motor vehicle accidents), or extended care (e.g., spinal cord injuries and paralysis) are the principal targets of case management UR programs. Case management of mental health care, substance abuse, and rehabilitation (particularly of workmen's compensation patients) has grown in popularity since mid-1987 and marks the second growth phase of the private case management industry.[48]

The importance of UM to further development and success of the managed care industry cannot be overemphasized. Major targets of UM will evolve from the work of researchers in analyzing the medical necessity of care and the variation in the use of medical services and surgical procedures by geographic area. Retrospective analyses have found that up to 65% of some surgical procedures such as carotid endarterectomies are inappropriate or questionable, 44% of coronary bypass procedures are unnecessary or equivocal, 50% of spinal disk surgical procedures are unnecessary, and 20% to 35% of all hospitalizations may be unnecessary.[49-52] Similar unnecessary utilization and waste have been discovered in diagnostic and medical procedures and outpatient services.[53,54] A study by HCFA found that over 25% of hospital outpatient services for laboratory, radiology, emergency medicine, and physical therapy were unnecessary.[55] These findings complement other research in the variation of use of medical and surgical procedures among different areas of the country, creating a body of knowledge and literature referred to as "small-area" or "inter-area" variation analysis.[56,57] The implication from this research is that much medical care utilization has to do more with the supply of medical care providers, such as hospital beds and physician specialties (e.g., surgeons), than with the actual medical needs of the population.

Retrospective UR research suggests that physician practice style plays a role in medical care utilization. HMO physicians, for example, are more cost-effective in providing medical care services than FFS physicians.[58] The lower use of medical services among patients of HMO physicians may result from two factors: (1) financial incentives for physicians, in most HMO plans, to provide more medical care services have been eliminated; and (2) resource-conscious physicians are more likely to be attracted to the HMO practice model. There are some data to support this hypothesis, including a study which found that salaried HMO physicians were more likely to judge hospital admissions as inappropriate (nonacute) upon retrospective review than FFS physicians who reviewed the same patient medical records.[59]

The retrospective research has led to the development of treatment protocols (i.e., prospective UR) and will spur efforts to target prospective UM and concurrent UM services to certain medical and surgical procedures. For example, a change in hospital policy and guidelines for obstetricians in one teaching hospital, including mandatory second opinion for all nonemergency cesarean sections, was successful in reducing the C-section rate by 34%, from 17.5% in 1985 to 11.5% in 1987.[60]

Retrospective UR studies have also contributed to a body of literature that shows an unmistakable inverse relationship between the volume of services in a given facility and the incidence of morbidity and mortality.[61,62] Other research has shown that volume can be related to cost and efficiency for certain medical and surgical procedures.[63] Collectively, these findings suggest that both quality and price can be affected in a favorable manner if patients are channeled to higher quality or more cost-efficient providers.

UM has not been restricted to hospital inpatient services. The success of Medicare PPS, PROs, and private UR/UM programs in reducing inpatient hospital utilization was met with burgeoning use of ambulatory and alternate care services and the expansion of UR and UM activities to ambulatory care. While the number of inpatient hospital admissions nationwide declined by 2% in 1986 (to 33.8 million) and by 0.5% in 1987 (to 33.6 million), the number of ambulatory visits increased by 8.3% in 1986 (to 263.6 million visits) and by 5.8% in 1987 (to 278.9 million visits), and total health care expenditures rose by 8.4% in 1986 and in 1987 (to approximately $500 billion).[64] Both public and private programs focused on treatment patterns of physicians and, in some cases, tracked services received by individual patients and compared these cases with normative data by diagnosis and by groups of diagnoses analogous to DRGs.

EFFECTS OF MANAGED CARE
ON PHARMACY SERVICES

The managed care industry has already had profound effects on the delivery of prescription drugs and pharmacy services in hospitals and in the community. In hospital pharmacy practice, the effects are primarily related to Medicare PPS because managed care plans are still focusing on price discounting rather than services bundling. Hospitals in most areas have not yet been forced to accept per-case and DRG-based reimbursement from private payers. The most common price concession is a percentage discount of U and C charges, in some instances up to a maximum per diem price. These per diem limits do not always include ancillary services such as pharmacy and laboratory; therefore, aside from Medicare PPS, hospital pharmacy management is still concerned with revenue maximization through strategic pricing, with concerns regarding cost control taking on secondary importance. The situation produces conflicting incentives, and the pressures that prevail may differ from one hospital to another, depending on factors related to the payer mix in each hospital and the percentage of revenue accounted for by the Medicare program.

In contrast to hospital reimbursement, prescriptions and pharmacy services in the community have been financed predominantly through out-of-pocket payments by consumers (only about 25% of these bills are paid in some manner by a third party such as Medicaid or a major medical benefit of an insurance company), and, therefore, prescription services and pricing have been subject to a greater degree of price competition among suppliers (pharmacies).

The maturation of the managed care industry means that hospital pharmacy management will be increasingly concerned with cost management rather than revenue maximization. In the short term—and longer for some hospitals in markets without large managed care plans and buyers–strategic pricing of pharmacy products and services can enhance hospital revenues and operating margins. Longer term, more managed care plans will negotiate greater shared risk with hospitals in the form of per diem price caps that include all inpatient services, per case prices, and fee schedules based on DRGs. When services bundling is combined with prospective pricing, hospital pharmacy management assumes new responsibility for managing utilization of pharmacy services.[65,66] In per diem reimbursement, it is necessary to manage the input costs, including utilization, for each patient for each day of care. In per case reimbursement, input costs must be managed for each patient's entire stay, making shorter patient stays advantageous. Hospital pharmacists have employed measures such as drug formularies (to reduce inventory costs and to reduce the drug product cost per unit dispensed), analysis of staffing ratios, and improving productivity through changes in drug and intravenous admixture distribution systems to manage costs, and they have developed prescribing protocols to help manage utilization of inappropriate and expensive drug therapies.[67,68] Pharmacy department input costs have even been analyzed and managed per individual DRG category.[69]

The incentives for hospital pharmacists to engage in all aspects of drug and IV utilization management have never been greater and will become more important with the maturation of the managed care industry. The most significant research opportunities in hospital pharmacy finance and economics lie in examination of the effectiveness and efficiency of pharmacists in utilization management. Two particularly important research areas are determination of the magnitude of cost savings from prescribing protocols and the generation of prescribing profiles, by individual physician, and subsequent education efforts with outlier prescribers.

Managed care means case management, which is now expanding rapidly from its first generation of trauma-related cases into mental health and substance abuse, workmen's compensation, and rehabilitation.[70] Since case management programs generate the savings to justify their existence from patient placement in alternate care settings, hospital pharmacy managers may continue to find revenue opportunities in alternate care services such as home infusion therapy and from outpatient and nonhospital patient prescription services.[71,72]

Community pharmacists have found that managed care means a higher level of price competition. Managed care plans in some metropolitan markets have pushed prescription reimbursement down to as low as average wholesale price (AWP) less 15%, plus a $1.50 administrative and dispensing fee. HMOs, particularly IPA plans such as Maxicare Health Plans (Los Angeles), have also been successful in transferring financial risk to community pharmacy providers in the form of pooled capitation contracts in which the pool of providers is at risk for utilization of prescription drugs as well as the average prescription price.[73] Managed care plans can use competitive bidding to intensify price competition for prescription drug benefits due to the abundant supply of pharmacy providers in most markets.[72]

In comparison, community pharmacies in many areas of the country have assumed greater financial risk, in the form of pooled capitation contracting, associated with the managed care industry than hospitals have assumed. The need for utilization management, therefore, is sometimes more acute in the delivery of community pharmacy services than in the delivery of hospital pharmacy services. Provider-sponsored pharmacy PPOs have had to become more sophisticated in the design and development of meaningful drug utilization review (DUR) reports that can be used to educate and influence physician prescribing behavior and to reduce the incidence of fraud, abuse, and misuse among beneficiaries and providers.[74] Retrospective DUR was complemented by case management (concurrent DUR) of high-cost drug therapy cases and by prospective DUR, accomplished through drug prescribing protocols.

The financial need to develop effective DUR methods and truly manage drug utilization spawned innovative measures in ambulatory prescription drug benefits. As many as 17 cost-management methods have been described, including reduction of claims processing costs through the use of pharmacy third-party administrators (TPAs) that specialized in drug claims processing; generic dispensing incentives for pharmacists and generic-use incentives for members (e.g., a lower copayment amount for a generic drug); drug formularies and drug prescribing protocols; and starter or trial dose protocols for certain expensive, often wasted drugs such as nonsteroidal anti-inflammatory agents.[75] More recently, financial incentives and disincentives for prescribers have been added to better manage prescription utilization and to double or even triple the ratio of generic drugs dispensed, expressed as a percentage of total prescriptions in a prescription drug benefit.[76]

As with hospital pharmacy practice, a particularly fruitful avenue of economics research exists in prospective UR or prescribing protocols; prescribing protocols have the potential to favorably influence utilization as well as the average prescription price. Another poorly researched area in prescription drug benefits is the economic effects of a closed formulary versus an open formulary. Because most HMO plans that subcontract their prescription drug benefits are of the IPA model, these plans have not generally had the wherewithal to impose the restriction of a closed drug formulary on their provider panels comprised of independent physicians. Financial pressure on HMOs and the deteriorating balance sheets of many HMOs presage more aggressive action to manage the total costs of all covered benefits, including prescription drugs.[77]

The next generation of managed care applied to prescription drug benefits will involve more widespread use of direct capitation contracting, in which each pharmacy provider receives a monthly capitation amount for its roster of covered members. Direct capitation contracting has not been common in community pharmacy practice for two reasons. First, the method requires assignment of beneficiaries to one provider, as in the gatekeeper or primary care physician (PCP) model. This requirement may encounter some resistance from beneficiaries and is conceptually antithetical to access flexibility. Second, direct capitation contracting requires some degree of sophistication in data collection and risk management for individual pharmacy providers. Nevertheless, potential savings from concurrent DUR will propel expanded use of this reimbursement method among managed care prescription drug plans. And, at the least, the direct capitation method has the potential for favorable effects on the quality and safety of prescription drug use.

FUTURE DEVELOPMENTS IN MANAGED CARE

Some of the future directions of managed care have already been described, including growth outlook for derivative model health plans. The performance record of managed care is mixed, which should not be surprising for a young industry, but the accomplishments seem to outweigh the shortcomings. It seems likely that managed care will be with us until Congress imposes a regulatory system on health care, perhaps like the Canadian system, that focuses on price regulation and control over supply.

The accomplishments of managed care are paced by the performance record of Medicare PPS, which was successful in reducing the average length of hospital stays and the use of inpatient hospital services without sacrificing quality of care and in reducing the rate of growth of Medicare spending for inpatient hospital services.[78,79] The DRG method of bundling services into one payment rate (per diagnosis) caused a revolution in the management and delivery of hospital services. Medicare PPS was successful in driving some formerly inpatient hospital services to alternate care providers, such as ambulatory surgery centers and home health agencies, but a thorough examination of the data shows that Medicare Part A spending is 20% lower than it would have been under cost-based reimbursement.[80,81] The savings–about $18 billion next year–are contributed two-thirds by price savings (from the DRG method of prospective pricing combined with services bundling) and one-third from lower admission rates.[31]

HMOs and PPOs have been successful in using prospective pricing and competitive bidding to lower the prices they pay for certain hospital and medical services. In 1987 HMOs were paying an average of about $750 for each day of hospital care, 17% less than the $900 per day paid by fee-for-service plans and nearly 9% less than the $825 per day paid by PPOs.[1] This discount is projected to rise to an average of 39% by 1992, with HMOs paying an average of $1,100 per day of hospital care compared to an average of $1,800 per day among fee-for-service plans and 24% less than the $1,450 per day paid by PPOs.

Some HMOs have been successful in reducing the use of hospital services. In 1986, established HMOs (those over three years old) reported an average hospital utilization rate of 351 inpatient days per 1,000 enrollees under age 65, compared to a national average hospital utilization rate of 606 inpatient days per 1,000 persons. For both old and new HMOs, the hospital utilization rate was still 25% lower at 452 inpatient days per 1,000 enrollees.[82] Similar savings from reduced hospital utilization were achieved by HMOs among their elderly enrollees (those over 65): an average of 1,835 days per 1,000, or 41% less than the national average of 3,121 days per 1,000 persons. HMO proponents attribute these savings to effective utilization management and removal of the financial incentives for physicians to hospitalize patients by placing physicians on salary or capitation reimbursement. HMO critics, of course, attribute much of the lower hospital utilization to enrollee selection bias (favorable selection).

Medicare PPS, the PRO program, and private UR companies caused a reduction in the use of inpatient hospital services and drove some inpatient hospital care to alternate care providers. The use of inpatient hospital services declined, as measured by the number of inpatient days, the average length of stay, the number of admissions, and average hospital occupancy. Many managed fee-for-service plans of employers and insurers have reported savings estimates from managed care programs such as mandatory UR, benefit redesign (primarily to greater cost-sharing by the enrollee at the time of service through coinsurance and copayments), wellness promotion programs, director or provider contracting, competitive bidding, prospective pricing, HMO rate negotiations, and services bundling such as per diem contracting with area hospitals.

The jury is still out regarding the success of PPOs. Heretofore, many PPOs have been structured as little-modified fee-for-service plans, and the PPO industry has tremendous opportunity to document savings from provider risk contracting and effective utilization management. But the PPO model, unless combined in hybrid-risk arrangements, has the inherent shortcoming of not being able to lock-in beneficiaries, precluding effective control of use behavior and making savings determinations difficult.

On the down side, the managed care industry has found that health care is more a local or perhaps regional phenomenon and is not easily managed through megasystems and national corporations.[83] Second, managed care plans can expect continued resistance from hospitals and physicians to participation in risk contracting. As long as the financial incentives in managed health plans are largely fee-for-service, effective utilization management will be beyond reach. The alternative to arm twisting with providers regarding risk contracting is the formation of partnerships between managed care plans and physicians.

Third, much of the recent growth in the managed care industry has been achieved at a high price in advertising expenditures to gain entry to new markets and to increase the number of enrolled members. The competition for enrollment and premium revenues may, therefore, have the effect of increasing administrative costs, which may overwhelm the savings that are achieved through lower utilization of hospital and other medical care services.[84] In 1987, HMOs spent approximately $660 million, or about $1 million per plan, on marketing. Each HMO must obtain 13,000 new members at an individual premium of $77 per member-month to recover these marketing costs.[85] Because these (higher) costs incurred in marketing, advertising, and other administrative areas must ultimately be recouped, lower premiums that are offered by some managed care plans at the outset to gain market entry and build market share are necessarily followed at some point by higher premiums.

Competition for market share among the various segments of the managed care industry will be influenced by legislation and case law. At present, employer self-funded health plans escape state (insurance) regulation because of preemption provisions of the Employee Retirement Income Stability Act of 1974 (ERISA), and the PPO industry also remains largely unregulated. By contrast, the HMO industry is highly regulated. The HMO Amendments of 1988 (P.L. 100-517) will ultimately provide some additional regulatory flexibility to HMOs, but political pressure at the state level seems to be in the direction of increased regulatory requirements of minimum reserves and net worth and more financial guarantees, which will be most onerous for small HMO plans.[86]

In the legal arena, the evolving case law favors increased competition and supports the efforts of managed care plans to manage participating providers, including providers' exclusion when they are not cost-efficient in comparison to their peers.[87] Even managed care plans owned by physician-providers have been able to establish fee structures and risk-sharing arrangements intended to control costs when this is done without discrimination or intent to exclude competitors.[88] Innovation will continue in the legal structures that are devised to encourage risk-sharing relationships and more effective utilization management.

REFERENCES

1. Kenkel PJ. Managed care will dominate within a decade-experts. Mod Healthcare 1988;18(Jul 29):31.

2. Curtiss FR. Pharmacy preferred-provider organizations. Am J Hosp Pharm 1987;44:1797-801.

3. Anon. Directory of preferred provider organizations and the industry report on PPO developments. Bethesda, MD: American Medical Care and Review Association; Dec 1987.

4. Rolph ES, Rich JP, Ginsburg PB et al. State laws and regulations governing preferred provider organizations. Santa Monica, CA: Rand Corporation; Aug 1986.

5. Kittrell A. Cost-sharing plans are successful: study. Bus Insurance 1988;22(Sept 5):3, 32.

6. Anon. Insurer selects care facilities. Bus Insurance 1988;22(Aug 1):2.

7. Bradford M. Mandatory second opinions dropped by New York Life. Bus Insurance 1988;23(Mar 28):2, 35.

8. Anon. Smart buyers of health care: case studies of GM, Honeywell and Sun. PPO Newsl 1987;10:6, 7.

9. Anon. Prenatal care class trims firm's health bill. Bus Insurance 1987;21(Dec 14):14.

10. Hofmann M. City of Milwaukee cuts health costs in 1987 by 5%. Bus Insurance 1988;22(Apr 4):1, 18, 19.

11. DiBlase D. Benefit managers scrutinize HMOs. Bus Insurance 1988;22(Apr 25):1, 53, 54.

12. Interstudy. The Interstudy edge. Excelsior, MN;3:1988.

13. DiBlase D. Employers seek accountability from PPOs. Bus Insurance 1988;22(Dec 19):3.

14. Garcia BE. Cigna bets on "managed" health care. Wall Street J 1989 (Feb 16):B8.

15. DiBlase D. Allied-Signal health plan. Bus Insurance 1988;22(Feb 22):1.

16. DiBlase D. Bank blends HMO and indemnity plans. Bus Insurance 1989;23(Jan 2):3.

17. Curtiss FR. Managed health care. Am J Hosp Pharm 1989;46:742-63.

18. Schachner M. BC/BS reports health education savings. Bus Insurance 1989;23(7):6.

19. Kittrell A. Wellness plans can save money: survey. Bus Insurance 1988;22(Mar 28):3, 10.

20. Hillman AL. Financial incentives for physicians in HMOs? N Engl J Med 1987;317:1743-8.

21. Kittrell A. Provider payment in HMOs changing. Bus Insurance 1988;22 (Oct 10):88.

22. Fleming NS. Approaches to primary care physician capitation. GHAA J 1988;9(Fall):4.

23. Anon. Reviewing the health care reviewers. Med Benefits 1988;(Aug 15):8.

24. Medicare Program. Prospective payment for Medicare inpatient hospital services. Fed Regist 1984;49(Jan 3):233-340.

25. Arstein-Kerslake C. PPOs continue to grow. CAHHS Insight 1987; 11(Nov 30):1-(California Association of Hospitals and Health Systems, Sacramento).

26. Medicare. Utilization and quality control peer review organization (PRO) area designation and definitions of eligible organizations; proposed rule and notice. Fed Regist 1983;48(Aug 15):36969-77.

27. Health Care Financing Administration. Medicare prospective payment system monitoring activities. Washington, DC: DHHS; Apr 1985; HCFA background paper.

28. Office of Inspector General, Office of Analysis and Inspections. The utilization and quality control peer review organization (PRO) program: quality review activities. Aug 1988; OIG Report No. OAI-01-88-00570. In: Medicare and Medicaid guide. Chicago: Commerce Clearing House, para. 37, 450.

29. Health Care Financing Administration. Medicare prospective payment system monitoring activities. Washington, DC: DHHS; Jan 1986; HCFA background paper.

30. General Accounting Office. Effects of legislation on Medicare/Medicaid program and beneficiary costs. 26 Jul 1988; GAO report No. HRD-88-85. In: Medicare and Medicaid guide. Chicago: Commerce Clearing House, para. 37, 212.

31. Russell LB, Manning CL. The effect of prospective payment on Medicare expenditures. N Engl J Med 1989;320:439-44.

32. Anon. Fee freeze didn't faze doctor fees. Wash Rep Med Health 1988; (Aug 1):2.

33. Ruffenach G. Big changes proposed for doctors' fees. Wall Street J 1988 (Sept 9):17.

34. Curtiss FR. Recent developments in federal reimbursement for home health-care services and products. Am J Hosp Pharm 1988;45:1682-90.

35. Davis FA. Medicare hospice benefit: early program experiences. Health Care Fin Rev 1988;9(Summer):99-111.

36. Medicare Program. Payment to health maintenance organizations and competitive medical plans; final rule with comment period. Fed Regist 1985;50 (Jan 10):1313-418.

37. Fackelman KA, ed. Capitation: an uncertain future. Wash Rep Med Health: Perspectives 1988;42(Feb 29):1-4.

38. Simone BM, Lichenstein RL, Adams-Watson J. Enrollment in the TEFRA risk program: Interstudy's data differ markedly from HCFA's. GHAA J 1988;9(2): 4-12.

39. Kasper JD, Riley GF, McCombs JS, Stevenson MA. Beneficiary selection, use, and charges in two Medicare capitation demonstrations. Health Care Fin Rev 1988;10 (1):37-49.

40. Sorian R, ed. HCFA plans PPO experiments. Wash Rep Med Health 1988;42(Apr 4):1.

41. Medicare Program. Medicare: disclosure of information–new system of records. Fed Regist 1988;53(Nov 30):48314.

42. Bachman SS, Altman SH, Beatrice DF. What influences a state's approach to Medicaid reform? Inquiry 1988;25(Summer):243-50.

43. Anon. Pennsylvania medical assistance bulletin no. 99-86-01. Philadelphia: Pennsylvania Medical Assistance Program; 5 Feb 1986.

44. Zuckerman S. Medicaid hospital spending: effects of reimbursement and utilization control policies. Health Care Fin Rev 1987;9(2):65-77.

45. Anon. Wisconsin HMO enrollment savings. Wash Rep Med Health 1986;40 (Jun 2):2.

46. Curtiss FR. Recent developments in organizing and financing health-care services. Am J Hosp Pharm 1986;43:2436-44.

47. Anon. BC/BS saved $6 billion: study. Bus Insurance 1988;22(Aug 22):2.

48. Geisel J. Insurers, UR firms target rising outpatient claims. Bus Insurance 1989;23(Feb 20):3, 10.

49. Winslow CM, Solomon DH, Chassin MR, Kosecoff J, Merrick NJ, Brook RH. The appropriateness of carotid endarterectomy. N Engl J Med 1988;318:721-8.

50. Vibbert S, ed. Rand criticizing bypass surgeries. Med Util Rev 1988;16 (Jul 28):2.

51. Anon. Surgery on ruptured disks unnecessary half the time. Am Coll Util Rev Phys 1988;16(Sept):8.

52. Kemper KY. Medically inappropriate hospital use in a pediatric population. N Engl J Med 1988;318:1033-7.

53. Chassin MR, Kosecoff J, Park RE, Winslow CM, Kahn KL, Merrick NJ, Keesey J, Fink A, Solomon DH, Brook RH. Does inappropriate use explain geographic variations in the use of health care services? A study of three procedures. vJAMA 1987;258:2533-7.

54. Feldstein PJ, Wickizer TM, Wheeler JRC. The effects of utilization review programs on health care use and expenditures. N Engl J Med 1988;318:1310-4.

55. Health Care Financing Administration. National hospital outpatient study–1988. Program Memorandum (Intermediaries) No. A-88-22, October 1988. In: Medicare and Medicaid guide. Chicago: Commerce Clearing House; para. 37, 484.

56. Wennberg JE. Population illness rates do not explain population hospitalization rates. Med Care 1987;25:354-9.

57. Stano M, Folland S. Variations in the use of physician services by Medicare beneficiaries. Health Care Fin Rev 1988;9(Spring):51-8.

58. Hornbrook MC, Berki SE. Practice mode and payment method: effects on use, costs, quality, and access. Med Care 1985;23:484-511.

59. Strumwasser I, Paranjpe NV, McGinnis J et al. To hospitalize or not to hospitalize: HMO versus fee-for-service. GHAA J 1988;9(Fall):42-54.

60. Myers SA, Gleicher N. A successful program to lower cesarean-section rates. N Engl J Med 1988;319:1511-6.

61. Chassin MR, Kosecoff J, Park RE et al. Indications for selected medical and surgical procedures: a literature review and ratings of appropriateness. Santa Monica, CA: Rand Corporation; 1986.

62. Showstack JA, Rosenfeld KE, Garnick DW. Coronary artery bypass graft surgery in California, 1983: outcomes and charges. Discussion Paper Series. San Francisco, CA: Institute for Health Policy Studies, University of California; 1986.

63. McGregor M, Pelletier G. Planning of specialized health facilities: size vs. cost and effectiveness in heart surgery. N Engl J Med 1978;299:1979-81.

64. Kenkel PJ. New programs target outpatient utilization. Mod Healthcare 1988;18(Aug 26):37.

65. Curtiss FR. Deregulation of health-care financing. Am J Hosp Pharm 1985; 42:1136-43.

66. Curtiss FR. Current concepts in hospital reimbursement. Am J Hosp Pharm 1983;40:586-91.

67. Curtiss FR. Pharmacy management strategies for responding to hospital reimbursement changes. Am J Hosp Pharm 1983;40:1489-92.

68. Curtiss FR. Contract pharmacy services. In: Smith MC, Brown TR, eds. Handbook of institutional pharmacy practice. 2nd ed. Baltimore, MD: Williams and Wilkins; 1985:238-46.

69. Curtiss FR. Analysis of nationwide pharmacy charges per DRG. Am J Hosp Pharm 1985:42:2168-74.

70. Woolsey C. UR firms attempt to balance cost, quality of care. Bus Insurance 1989;23(Feb 20):3, 11.

71. Curtiss FR. Reimbursement dilemma regarding home health-care prodvucts and services. Am J Hosp Pharm 1984;41:1548-57.

72. Curtiss FR. Looking beyond DRGs: opportunities for hospital pharmacy. Am J Hosp Pharm 1984;41:721-3.

73. Curtiss FR. Methods of providing prescription drug benefits in health plans. Am J Hosp Pharm 1986;43:2428-35.

74. Curtiss FR. Pharmacy services and managed care: TPAs, PPOs, and DUM. Employee Benefits J 1987; 12(Dec):32-7.

75. Curtiss FR. Control costs of retiree prescription drug benefits. Personnel J 1988;67(6):92-100.

76. Curtiss FR, Tichon MJ. Cost and use management in prescription drug benefits. GHAA J 1988;9(Fall):97-104.

77. Kenkel PJ. For HMO firms, recovery complicated by skepticism of investors and regulators. Mod Healthcare 1988;18(Dec 16):43.

78. DesHarnais S, Kobrinski E, Chesney J, Lory M, Ament R, Fleming S. The early effects of the prospective payment system on inpatient utilization and the quality of care. Inquiry 1987;24(Spring):7-16.

79. Eggers PW. Prospective payment system and quality: early results and research strategy. Health Care Fin Rev 1987;S:29-37.

80. Prospective Payment Assessment Commission. Medicare prospective payment and the American health care system, report to Congress, June 1988. In: Medicare and Medicaid guide, extra edition no. 560. Chicago: Commerce Clearing House 26 Jul 1988.

81. Fisher CR. Trends in Medicare enrollee use of physician and supplier services, 1983-86. Health Care Fin Rev 1988;10(1):1-15.

82. Group Health Association of America. HMO industry profile. 2: Utilization patterns. Washington, DC: GHAA, Research and Analysis Department; 1988.

83. DiBlase D. Maxicare slims down to regain health. Bus Insurance 1988;22(Sept 5):1.

84. McLaughlin CG. Market responses to HMOs: price competition or rivalry? Inquiry 1988;25(Summer):207-18.

85. Goldberg A, Pallarito K. Investing in membership: a market strategy. GHAA Newsl 1989;30:2.

86. Health Maintenance Organization Amendments of 1988. Conference Report (Text of Law Amendments) No. 100-1056, 5 Oct 1988. In: Medicare and Medicaid guide. Chicago: Commerce Clearing House, para. 37, 512.

87. Burda D. Ruling defines price-fixing law's limits. Mod Healthcare 1988; 22(Nov 11):6.

88. Contributed paper. The ChoiceCare case: excerpts from the statement of claims and facts. Group Health Institute Proceedings. Washington, DC: Group Health Association of America; 1988.

Chapter 31

Analysis of the Impact of Third-Party Prescription Programs on Community Pharmacy

Cheryl Huey
Richard A. Jackson
Margaret A. Pirl

INTRODUCTION AND LITERATURE REVIEW

Third-party prescriptions accounted for 41.1% of total prescriptions filled in 1990, compared to 38.1% in 1989.[1] Indications are that this increasing trend will continue, and with it many aspects of community pharmacy will be affected, including pharmacy gross margins, the cost of dispensing prescriptions, and patronage motives and practices. A *Lilly Digest* analysis indicates that pharmacies with high (55% to 99%) versus low (2% to 15%) third-party prescription revenue had higher costs of goods sold, lower proprietors' salaries, lower net profits, and lower total incomes as a percentage of sales.[2]

Many pharmacy owners have traditionally encountered difficulties with third-party programs. A frequent complaint from providers is that the level of reimbursement from third-party programs is inadequate. Another major complaint has been that the third parties are slow in paying submitted claims. A major concern of providers is that third parties frequently present programs on a "take it or leave it" basis, thereby eliminating the possibility of negotiating the contract terms and forcing pharmacists to either accept or reject the entire contract, including its reimbursement provisions.

This research was funded through educational grants from the NARD Management Institute, the American College of Apothecaries, and The Upjohn Company.

Previously published in *Journal of Research in Pharmaceutical Economics*, Vol. 6(2), 1995.

In a recent survey concerning pharmacists' attitudes about third-party programs, it was reported that:

1. Over 85% of independent pharmacists stated that joining one or more third-party programs did not increase the profits of the prescription department in the past year. Thirty-five percent said that profits stayed the same, and 50.7% said that profits diminished.
2. Approximately 90% of independent pharmacists stated that the third-party payments were lower than their private-pay charges, with the majority answering that they were 11-20% lower.
3. Eighty-five percent of independent pharmacists said third-party plans have not contributed significantly to their front-end business.
4. Four-fifths of independent pharmacists said that third-party claims are taking some of the "joy" out of pharmacy.[3]

Third-party dispensing fees have not increased at the same rate as prescription cost of goods sold. From 1982-1988, the average cost of goods sold for Medicaid prescriptions increased by 86.5% (three times the consumer price index [CPI]), while the average dispensing fee increased only 15.2% (0.5 times the CPI).[4]

Other studies have shown the need for higher levels of reimbursement from third-party programs. A Purdue University assessment of chain pharmacies' costs of dispensing third-party prescriptions found that in 1988 the cost of dispensing a third-party prescription was $6.39 while the cost of dispensing a private-pay prescription was $5.14—a difference of $1.25.[5] The higher cost of dispensing a third-party prescription was due to higher personnel costs, delays in third-party reimbursement, denied claims, and other third-party claims transaction costs.

In a 1991 study of independently owned Virginia pharmacies, Carroll found that the average cost to dispense a third-party prescription was $1.55 higher than private-pay prescriptions.[6] Another study by the same author using differential analysis showed that the long-term effects of increased third-party reimbursement will be detrimental to independent community pharmacy profits.[7]

Some pharmacists may react to these problems by cost shifting. Cost shifting is the practice of charging more to one group of customers because another group of customers is not paying the full price for a particular product or service. A recent analysis of cost shifting revealed that private-pay patrons of independent community pharmacies pay, on average, an additional $0.31 per prescription due to inadequate third-party reimbursement rates.[8] It is anticipated that cost shifting will increase as the number of third-party prescriptions increases in the future, and the burden will fall on the private-pay customer. Unfortunately, many of the private-pay customers are elderly persons who cannot afford increased prescription prices.

A 1989 study of 300 Rite Aid customers revealed that only 36% of the patients having a third-party prescription filled made additional nonprescription purchases during the same visit.[9] These nonprescription sales averaged only $4.65. If all 300 customers who obtained prescriptions are taken into account, the average additional purchases totaled only $1.66 per customer. This prompted a Rite Aid CEO to conclude: "There is simply no truth to the claim that participating in third-party programs in some way attracts other meaningful business. . . . Our survey conclusively indicates that third-party prescription sales must stand on their own."

Until reforms are made within the pricing structure and reimbursement levels are raised, pharmacists must learn to evaluate third-party programs and accept or reject them with limited information about their financial impact on the pharmacy. The problems faced by pharmacy owners have created the necessity of documenting, analyzing, and validating these concerns and problems.

Many times, pharmacists accept a third-party prescription plan even though it offers low reimbursement. Several reasons have been suggested as to why this may occur. Pharmacists may feel that if only a few (for example, 5%) of their patients are covered with each plan, the financial impact on the pharmacy may not be of great significance. Also, pharmacists may feel that they will lose many of their customers if they refuse to honor the third-party plan. On the other hand, if they honor the insurance plan, they may gain new customers. Another reason may be that pharmacists are under the impression they will make up for the "loss" with increased nonprescription purchases. Whatever the reasons, accepting third-party plans with low reimbursements will have a financial impact on the pharmacy.

OBJECTIVES

This research endeavored to evaluate third-party reimbursement, the nonprescription purchase patterns of third-party customers, and the cost of dispensing third-party and private-pay prescriptions in independently owned community pharmacies. The specific objectives of the study were to:

1. Compare the cost of dispensing third-party and private-pay prescriptions.

2. Compare the gross margins of third-party and corresponding private-pay prescriptions.
3. Using typical third-party reimbursement plan terminology (i.e., AWP–average wholesale price–minus a certain percentage plus a fee), express a fee structure that would be equivalent to the pharmacies' average usual and customary prescription price.
4. Investigate the nonprescription purchasing habits of third-party prescription patrons, including:

   a. The dollar amount of nonprescription purchases necessary to offset the difference between third-party prescription reimbursement versus usual and customary pricing.
   b. The average nonprescription purchase per third-party prescription.
   c. The average nonprescription gross margin per third-party prescription.
   d. The average nonprescription purchase per third-party patron.
   e. A determination of what percentage of patrons visit the pharmacy only when they have prescriptions filled.
   f. A determination of the percentage of patrons who make nonprescription purchases from the pharmacy when they do not have prescriptions filled, how often they visit, and how much they usually purchase.
   g. A determination of how patrons' nonprescription purchases would be affected if the pharmacy ceased to honor their third-party plan.

METHODOLOGY

Letters were mailed to 150 independent community pharmacy owners in the metropolitan Atlanta area requesting their participation in the study that would involve a personal interview with the owner, analysis of financial data, and observation and interview with third-party prescription patrons in the pharmacy. Seventeen (11.3%) indicated they would be willing to participate in the study. A convenience sample of ten pharmacies was chosen from these 17 based upon their third-party prescription volume. Since patron interviews and other data were to be collected by a research assistant, those pharmacies with the highest third-party prescription volume (at least five to ten per day) were selected for the study to minimize the time required to collect data from third-party patrons.

Personal interviews with the pharmacy owners were conducted to collect the financial data. This was accomplished over an average of two to three days during which the research assistant was in the pharmacy conducting the desired number of third-party prescription patron interviews and collecting third-party prescription and nonprescription purchase data.

Third-party patron data were collected by personal interview and observation. Nonprescription purchases as well as the personal interview were recorded at the time of purchase. After the purchase, nonprescription and prescription cost data were collected. The research assistant interviewed and collected data on all third-party patrons at each pharmacy until the required number of 30 per pharmacy was obtained. This required a minimum of one to two days at each pharmacy. Each day of the week was equally represented in the data collection. The interviewer used a standard set of written questions to structure the interview.

Nonprescription purchases were recorded prior to the interview. Nonprescription and prescription cost data were collected from the pharmacy owner or manager through personal interview.

Cost of Dispensing

The cost to dispense prescriptions was determined for each of the ten pharmacies in the study using a methodology adopted from a study by Carroll.[6] This determination included an overall cost to dispense, the cost of dispensing a private-pay prescription, the cost of dispensing a third-party prescription, and the difference between these latter two. Financial data were obtained from the pharmacy owner by personal interview.

Determination of the Overall Operating Cost of the Prescription Department

Total operating cost in the pharmacy is made up of five components:

1. *Direct Expenses:* Those expenses incurred by the prescription department itself while operating and are 100% allocated to the prescription department. These include expenses for prescription containers and labels, prescription bags, prescription tape, prescription blanks, professional dues, publications, continuing education expenses, third-party claim forms, statement forms, and third-party enrollment and participation fees.

2. *Personnel Expense:* An expense calculated by multiplying salary by the percentage of time spent in prescription department activities. These data were obtained through personal interviews with each of the pharmacy owners. The pharmacy owner estimated the percentage of time each employee spent in the prescription department, and that portion of salary was allocated to the prescription department. In addition, that portion of the

owner's salary not allocated in this procedure was multiplied by the ratio of prescription sales to total sales. This amount was also allocated to the prescription department inasmuch as it represented the cost associated with the time he or she was not in the prescription department, but was performing activities associated with the prescription department, such as paying invoices, making orders, or talking with sales representatives.

3. *Housing Expense:* Expense that is determined by multiplying the expense for rent, utilities, repairs, and maintenance by the ratio of the size of the prescription department to the size of the entire pharmacy.

4. *Other Expenses:* Other expenses found on the income statement (taxes, insurance, computers, interest paid, miscellaneous, etc.) were allocated to the prescription department based upon the ratio of prescription sales to total sales.

5. *Opportunity Cost (accounts receivable carrying cost):* The opportunity costs associated with accounts receivable was determined by multiplying the average outstanding prescription accounts receivable by the estimated value of money. In this study, opportunity costs were operationally defined to be 10%.

The sum of the five categories above–direct cost, personnel, housing, other expenses, and opportunity cost attributable to the prescription department–was then divided by the total number of prescriptions filled during the last year to determine the overall cost of dispensing a prescription for each pharmacy individually.

$$\text{Sum} = \frac{\text{Overall Operation Expense of Pharmacy}}{\text{\# of Prescriptions Filled}} = \text{Overall COD}$$

Determination of the Cost of Dispensing a Third-Party and a Private-Pay Prescription

To determine the cost of dispensing (COD) a third-party versus private-pay prescription, the extra costs associated with filling a third-party prescription were determined and subtracted from the overall cost of operation of the prescription department for each pharmacy.

The extra cost associated with dispensing a third-party prescription is the sum of three components:

1. Claim forms, statement forms, etc., and third-party enrollment fees (if any).
2. Employee salary multiplied by an estimated amount of time spent on performing third-party functions besides filling prescriptions. This can include reconciling accounts, billing, filling out additional

forms, etc. These data were estimated by the owner and obtained from the owner in the personal interview in the pharmacy.

3. Opportunity cost for third-party prescriptions. If a percentage of the accounts receivable is due to third-party prescriptions, this opportunity cost can be figured by multiplying the accounts receivable due to prescriptions (found in the overall cost to dispense section) by the percentage of total third-party prescriptions. Ten percent of that figure would be opportunity cost associated with third-party prescriptions.

The sum of these three factors is equal to the additional cost of filling third-party prescriptions. If this is subtracted from the total operation expense of the prescription department (the sum of all expenses allocated to the prescription department), the result is the expense of the pharmacy to dispense private-pay prescriptions. Private-pay operation expense divided by the total number of private-pay prescriptions dispensed will yield the private-pay cost to dispense.

The third-party cost to dispense is the sum of private-pay cost to dispense and the additional expense per third-party prescription. Additional expense per third-party prescription was calculated by dividing the additional cost of participating in third-party programs by the number of third-party prescriptions filled.

RESULTS AND ANALYSIS

Comparison of Cost to Dispense
Private-Pay and Third-Party Prescriptions

The average overall cost to dispense a prescription in the ten pharmacies surveyed was $5.98 (see Table 31.1 for summary data). If this figure is separated into private-pay and third-party cost, the average cost to dispense a private-pay prescription was $5.75. The average cost to dispense a third-party prescription was $6.77. The difference, representing the additional cost to dispense a third-party prescription, was $1.02.

Comparison of Third-Party
and Private-Pay Gross Margin

For each of the ten pharmacies, an average gross margin using actual acquisition cost per third-party prescription was determined and compared

TABLE 31.1. Summary Data for Study Pharmacies

Annual Rx Volume	Mean
Private-pay	$22,901
Third-party	$8,928
Total	$31,829

Annual Sales	$888,063

Type of Rx Volume	
Private-pay	70.53%
Total third-party	29.47%
Private third-party	16.39%
Medicaid	9.08%

Cost to Dispense	
Overall cost to dispense	$5.97
Third-party cost to dispense	$6.77
Private-pay cost to dispense	$5.75
Additional third-party cost to dispense	$1.02

Prescription Data	
Average usual and customary Rx price	$27.73
Average third-party reimbursement	$25.02
Average acquistition cost (after earned discounts)	$18.08
Average AWP	$20.55
Average usual and customary gross margin per Rx	$9.65
Average third-party gross margin per Rx	$6.94

to the pharmacy's usual and customary gross margin. The third-party reimbursement was figured for each third-party prescription based on the particular third-party plan involved. The pharmacy managers were asked to price each of these prescriptions using their normal pricing procedure for private-pay patients to determine what the pharmacies' usual and customary prescription charge would be. The average private-pay gross margin was $9.65 compared to an average third-party gross margin of $6.94. Therefore, the difference between usual and customary gross margin and third-party gross margin was $2.71.

Total Difference Per Third-Party Prescription

The figure above represents the difference between third-party prescription reimbursement and private-pay. The additional cost to dispense a third-party prescription was determined to be $1.02. Therefore, the total difference based on less revenue and more expense is $2.71 + $1.02, or $3.73.

Third-Party Reimbursement Terms Equivalent to Usual and Customary Price

Most third-party reimbursement terms involve average wholesale price and/or the subtraction of a percentage plus a fee. To compare the surveyed pharmacies' usual and customary prescription prices to widely used third-party reimbursement terms, two common third-party reimbursement terms were used. One uses the format AWP $-$ 10% + Fee, and the other uses AWP + Fee. AWP was estimated to be actual acquisition cost divided by 0.88, resulting in acquisition cost being AWP minus 12%.

1. AWP $-$ 10% + Fee = Usual and Customary Price:
   ($20.55 $-$ 10%) + x = $27.73
   $18.50 + x = $27.73
   x = $9.23

Stating the surveyed pharmacies' usual and customary prices in terms of AWP $-$ 10% + Fee results in a fee of $9.23. This makes the comparison of the pharmacies' usual and customary prices to a third-party reimbursement of AWP $-$ 10% + Fee more meaningful.

2. AWP + Fee = Usual and Customary Price:
   $20.55 + x = $27.73
   x = $7.18

Using these reimbursement terms, the surveyed pharmacies' usual and customary prices were equal to AWP + a fee of $7.18.

Nonprescription Purchases

Nonprescription Purchases Per Third-Party Prescription. In the survey of ten pharmacies, the nonprescription purchases of the third-party patrons were recorded and analyzed. The average nonprescription purchase per third-party prescription (not per patron because some patrons received more than one prescription) was $1.24.

Increased Nonprescription Revenue Needed to Offset "Loss." The difference in reimbursement per third-party prescription compared to usual and customary price was determined to be $3.73 per prescription. The gross profit on nonprescription purchases made by third-party patrons was determined to assess the quantity of nonprescription purchases necessary to make up the difference between the third-party reimbursement and the pharmacies' usual and customary private-pay prescription prices. The gross profit of the nonprescription purchases made by third-party patrons was determined to be 33.1%. Since the average nonprescription purchase per third-party prescription was so small, it may be reasonably assumed that variable costs would not increase with this minuscule increase in sales of out-front merchandise. Therefore, the nonprescription purchases necessary to offset the $3.73 difference in third-party reimbursement and usual and customary private-pay prescription price may be determined as follows:

$$\frac{\$3.73}{x} = \frac{\$33.10}{\$100}$$

$$x = \$11.27$$

For every $100 spent on nonprescription items, $33.10 is the average gross margin or profit. Therefore, to replace the $3.73 difference with $3.73 profit, $11.27 in nonprescription sales must be made per third-party prescription.

Nonprescription Purchases Per Third-Party Patron. The average nonprescription purchase per third-party patron was $2.10.

Third-Party Patron Interviews. The 300 third-party patrons were asked specific questions to determine their purchasing habits when visiting the pharmacy (Table 31.2). Of those surveyed, 58% of the patrons indicated that they patronize the pharmacy only when they have a prescription to fill. The remaining 42% indicated that they patronize the pharmacy and purchase nonprescription items at the pharmacy even when they are not having a prescription filled.

Of the 58% who said they patronize the pharmacy only when they have a prescription filled, 75% purchased no nonprescription items. The other 25% of the patrons who patronize the pharmacy only when they have prescriptions filled purchased some nonprescription items, resulting in an average purchase of $5.84 per person.

Of the 42% who said they purchase nonprescription items at the pharmacy even when they are not having a prescription filled, 63% of these patrons purchased no nonprescription items. Thirty-seven percent of these

TABLE 31.2. Third-Party Patron Interviews

		Purchased Non-Rx	25% (44)
Patronize *only* when Rx filled	58% (174)	No Non-Rx Purchases	75% (120)
Patronize when *not* having Rx filled	42% (126)	Purchased Non-Rx	37% (47)
		No Non-Rx Purchases	63% (79)

patrons purchased nonprescription items, resulting in an average purchase of $9.08 per person and an average gross margin of $2.37 per person.

Those 42% above were queried about the times they come into the store when they are not having a prescription filled (Table 31.3). It was determined that the regular nonprescription patrons come into the store an average of 3.5 times a month and spend an average of $11.50 per visit on nonprescription purchases. Two-thirds of these customers would continue to purchase the same amount of nonprescription items if the store ceased to honor their third-party plan.

DISCUSSION

The results of this study illustrate the significant negative impact that third-party prescription programs may have on independent pharmacies. The cost of dispensing third-party prescriptions in the pharmacies surveyed was $1.02 more than private-pay prescriptions. Further, a comparison of the third-party reimbursement with the pharmacies' usual and customary private-pay prescription price revealed a $2.71 difference. Taking both these differences into consideration means that the pharmacy incurs a total difference of $3.73 for each third-party prescription compared to private-pay prescriptions. This has serious implications for the private-pay patrons inasmuch as the pharmacy may be forced to engage in significant cost shifting to make up the difference. If the cost shifting is not done, the impact on the pharmacy's profit will be significant. This can have serious implications for the elderly because a significant proportion of private-pay patrons are elderly persons who may not participate in third-party programs.

TABLE 31.3. Customers Who Patronize Pharmacy When *Not* Having Rx Filled

1. Patronize pharmacy average of 3.5 times/month.
2. Estimate spending average of $11.50 per visit.
3. Sixty-seven percent would continue to purchase same amount if pharmacy discontinued third-party plan.

Even though it costs more to fill third-party prescriptions and pharmacies receive lower fees, many third-party administrators would have pharmacy owners believe that this may be offset by third-party patron nonprescription purchases. This study revealed that nonprescription purchases of $13.66 per third-party prescription must be made by third-party patrons to offset the difference. Data indicate that the third-party patrons purchased far less than that amount, or $1.24. The gross margin garnered by the pharmacy per third-party prescription was determined to be $0.41. When this is compared to the difference per third-party prescription of $3.73, it becomes clear that the pharmacies are not making up for the difference on nonprescription purchases. This may account for the recent negative trends in profit levels and increases in the necessity for additional cost shifting.

Data concerning nonprescription purchases were collected only from patrons who made purchases when having a third-party prescription filled. The question may be raised as to whether the third-party patrons make nonprescription purchases in the pharmacy on other occasions when they do not have prescriptions filled. Over half indicated they patronize the pharmacy only when they have prescriptions filled. Of those who patronize the pharmacy when not having prescriptions filled, two-thirds indicated that they would continue to purchase the same nonprescription items if the pharmacy did not continue to honor their third-party plan. Results such as these provide further indication of the minimal impact of third-party plans on nonprescription purchases.

Since most third-party plans reimburse according to terms associated with the average wholesale price plus a fee, this study determined an equivalent third-party reimbursement that would yield the same results as the pharmacies' usual and customary prescription prices. These were determined to be (1) AWP plus a fee of $7.18 and (2) AWP minus 10% plus a fee of $9.23. Since most third-party fees in use today are in the neighborhood of AWP minus 10% plus $3-$4, it is obvious that the fees currently offered are grossly inadequate compared to the pharmacies' usual and customary prices and provide evidence of the significant negative financial impact of third-party programs on independent pharmacies.

In addition to the extremely low volume of nonprescription purchases made by third-party patrons, the data indicate that the third-party program has little impact on nonprescription purchases inasmuch as a majority (66%) of the patrons would continue to purchase the same amount of nonprescription items if the pharmacy ceased to honor their third-party plans. Further, among those third-party patrons (58%) who patronize the pharmacy only when having prescriptions filled, only 25% actually purchased nonprescription items.

No attempt is made in this study to generalize the results of the study beyond the group of urban pharmacies in which the data were collected. Nevertheless, the nature of the results has implications for the future financial status of independent retail pharmacies. Since a greater proportion of its sales volume is associated with the prescription department and there are fewer private-pay patrons to whom costs may be shifted, cost-shifting becomes more difficult for independent pharmacies. There may be some point wherein cost-shifting is not possible. Unless significant changes are made in third-party reimbursement practices, many pharmacies may simply be unable to continue to operate. This issue becomes one of public policy in some communities where a significant proportion of a pharmacy's volume is associated with one third party that provides inadequate reimbursement. If the pharmacy is the only one in a particular community or town and is forced to close, the community would be denied appropriate access to what may be the only health care provider in the area.

For pharmacy managers to evaluate third-party prescription programs effectively, it is essential that they have a clear understanding of the financial impact of these programs on their pharmacies. This study has quantified the seriousness of this problem for the independent pharmacy owner. It has also indicated that the claims by third-party administrators that losses on third-party prescriptions are offset by increased prescription volume and nonprescription purchases are unrealistic. The significant difference in third-party reimbursement versus usual and customary price indicates that considerable cost shifting must occur if profit levels continue to decrease.

REFERENCES

1. Anon. Third party takes the money. Am Druggist 1991;203:50-4.
2. 1990 Lilly Digest. Indianapolis: Eli Lilly & Company, 1990.
3. Anon. Survey: pharmacists speak out about third party programs. Am Druggist 1991;203(4):40-51.

4. Schondelmeyer SW. Pharmacist reimbursement. In: Proceedings: Medicaid pharmaceutical purchasing: a conference on implementation issues. Baltimore, MD: Center for Drugs and Public Policy, University of Maryland School of Pharmacy, 1991.

5. Schafermeyer KW, Schondelmeyer SW, Thomas J III. An assessment of chain pharmacies' costs of dispensing a third party prescription. West Lafayette, IN: Purdue University Pharmaceutical Economics Research Center, 1990.

6. Carroll NV. Costs of dispensing private-pay and third-party prescriptions in independent pharmacies. J Res Pharm Econ 1991;3(2):3-16.

7. Carroll NV. Forecasting the impact of participation in third-party prescription programs on pharmacy profits. J Res Pharm Econ 1991;3(3):3-23.

8. McMillan JA, Carroll NV, Kotzan JA. Third-party-associated cost-shift pricing in Georgia pharmacies. J Res Pharm Econ 1990;2(4):33-47.

9. Press release. Rite Aid Corporation. June 8, 1989.

Chapter 32

Third-Party Associated Cost-Shift Pricing in Georgia Pharmacies

John A. McMillan
Norman V. Carroll
Jeffrey A. Kotzan

INTRODUCTION

Third-party drug reimbursement programs represent a significant market force that accounted for roughly one-third of all prescriptions dispensed in 1987.[1] With the leverage of such a large share of the outpatient prescription market, third parties have been able to reduce their own costs by channeling patients to specific (low cost) providers and to set low reimbursement rates unilaterally.[2,3] Antitrust provisions severely limit the ability of pharmacists to counter such third-party market pressure through collective bargaining or competitive operation of pharmacist-controlled third-party plans.[3-5] Pharmacies are, therefore, constrained to negotiate third-party reimbursement rates from a position of weakness, resulting in frequent complaints of low third-party reimbursement rates, high third-party-associated administrative costs, payment delays, and claim rejections.[6-8] The individual pharmacy could refuse to participate as a third-party provider; however, the potential for lost market share and accompanying loss of nonprescription sales may necessitate acceptance of third-party terms in hopes of balancing depressed third-party revenues by charging higher prices to self-paying consumers, a practice termed cost shifting.[2,9,10]

In a 1982 study of the impact of third-party reimbursement, Pathak reported that Ohio's independent pharmacies would have to levy a cost

---

Previously published in *Journal of Research in Pharmaceutical Economics*, Vol. 2(4), 1990.

shift of $0.41 per private-pay prescription to recover lost revenues resulting from an existing 27% third-party market share and a shift of $0.62 per private-pay prescription if third-party market share increased to 36%.[11] Pathak cautioned that the reported estimates may overstate actual cost shifting since Ohio pharmacies may have absorbed a portion of the needed shift.[11]

Empirical attempts to quantify cost shifting in the hospital market have often defined the cost shift as the difference between the average price charged private-paying (uninsured) patrons and a hypothetical all-payer rate. The all-payer rate is the one price that, if charged to all consumer groups, would yield the same aggregate revenue as that produced by an existing differential pricing/reimbursement structure. First to analyze community pharmacy cost-shifting practices under an all-payer concept, Stone reported an average cost shift of $0.48 per prescription in independent stores and $0.17 per prescription in chain stores resulting from inadequate third-party reimbursement. Stone also reported a significant association between the magnitude of cost shifting and the percentage of volume attributable to third parties.[12]

Two important assumptions of an all-payer analytical framework are:

1. Pharmacies could meet target revenues under an all-payer pricing structure.

$$(QTP * APP) + (QPP * APP) = TR \qquad \text{(Eq. 1)}$$

Where:
QTP = The quantity of third-party prescriptions dispensed;
QPP = The quantity of private-pay prescriptions dispensed;
APP = The all-payer price–the single price that, if charged to all payers (third-party and private-pay), would generate the target revenue requirement; and
TR = The pharmacy's target revenue.

2. Pharmacies are meeting target revenues by setting private-pay prices that exceed the all-payer rate by an amount sufficient to balance (in aggregate) the revenue-reducing effects of third-party reimbursement rates below this all-payer price.

$$QTP(OTPP) + QPP * (APP + \frac{QTP(APP - OTPP)}{QPP}) = TR \qquad \text{(Eq. 2)}$$

Where: OTPP = The third-party reimbursement price observed in the market.

Under the all-payer approach, the existence of private-pay prices above an all-payer price has been considered evidence of cost-shifting activity. Although cost shifting will generate private-pay prices in excess of an all-payer rate, such differentials may also result from a simple lowering of third-party reimbursement rates in the absence of a cost-shifting response. Therefore, valid cost-shifting inferences depend upon evidence that private-pay prices rise with increasing third-party presence. As demonstrated below, the all-payer methodology implicitly characterizes this relationship. Equations 1 and 2 indicate that:

$$OPP = \frac{QTP}{QPP} * (APP - OTPP) + APP \qquad (Eq. 3)$$

Where: OPP   = The observed private-pay market price.

Rearranging Equation 3 into the more cogent gross margin form (which reflects the sales residual contributing toward operating cost and profit, thus providing control for variance in price due to differing acquisition cost categories) yields the following:

$$OPP - AC = \frac{QTP}{QPP} * (APP - TPP) + APP - AC \qquad (Eq. 4)$$

Where: AC   = Ingredient acquisition cost.

Based upon the assumptions of the all-payer model, Equation 4 indicates that the average gross margin generated from a private-pay prescription by cost-shifting pharmacies is a linear function of the ratio of third-party to private-pay prescription volume, with a slope representing the degree by which average third-party reimbursement falls below an average all-payer prescription price, an intercept equal to the average all-payer prescription margin. The cost-shift premium assessed each private-pay prescription is represented as:

$$\frac{QTP * (APP - TPP)}{QPP} \qquad (Eq. 5)$$

The implicit linear relationship described above is consistent with the significant relationship between cost-shift magnitude and percentage of third-party volume also reported by Stone.[12]

OBJECTIVES AND HYPOTHESES

The goal of this study was to quantify third-party-related cost-shift pricing practices through empirical application of Equation 4. The specific analytical objective was to determine if private-pay gross margins were positively related to the ratio of third-party to private-pay prescription volume within the pharmacy and to employ this relationship in quantifying the average cost shift.

Because differences in magnitude of reimbursement and administrative considerations could promote plan-dependent cost-shift responses, Medicaid and private third-party categories were considered separately within the analyses. The appropriate alternate hypotheses for the objective were:

Alternate Hypothesis 1

Private-pay gross margins are positively related to the ratio of Medicaid to private-pay prescription volume within the pharmacy.

Alternate Hypothesis 2

Private-pay gross margins are positively related to the ratio of private third-party to private-pay prescription volume within the pharmacy.

METHODOLOGY

A market survey of 1,653,593 prescriptions filled in 650 Georgia pharmacies during a representative one-month period was obtained from Pharmaceutical Data Services, Inc. Each record identified the dispensing pharmacy by type (i.e., chain or independent) and contained the price; the acquisition cost; and a payment indicator identifying private pay, Medicaid, or private third-party coverage. Records of 65 pharmacies were removed from the data set due to unreported prices. The prescription data of the remaining 585 pharmacies were aggregated at the individual store level into the data elements described below and summarized in Tables 32.1 and 32.2:

1. Number of private-pay prescriptions dispensed;
2. Ratio of Medicaid to private-pay prescription volume;
3. Ratio of private third-party to private-pay prescription volume;

TABLE 32.1. Data Summary (Chain Stores; n = 434)

Variable	Mean	Standard Deviation	Minimum	Maximum
Average private-pay gross margin	$3.42	1.10	1.34	8.37
Average private-pay prescription acquisition cost	$12.29	1.60	7.40	27.04
Number of private-pay prescriptions	2,194	953	751	9,504
Number of Medicaid prescriptions	198	240	0	2,944
Number of private third-party prescriptions	327	293	14	2,369
Ratio of Medicaid to private-pay prescription volume	*0.09	0.10	0	0.73
Ratio of private third-party to private-pay prescription volume	*0.15	0.13	0.009	1.14

*Ratio was calculated for each store; therefore, mean of ratios differs from ratio of means.

TABLE 32.2. Data Summary (Independent Stores; n = 551)

Variable	Mean	Standard Deviation	Minimum	Maximum
Average private-pay gross margin	$4.39	1.19	1.22	7.98
Average private-pay prescription acquisition cost	$12.47	1.91	8.29	17.94
Number of private-pay prescriptions	1,950	994	607	6,226
Number of Medicaid prescriptions	493	494	0	3,060
Number of private third-party prescriptions	186	188	0	1,047
Ratio of Medicaid to private-pay prescription volume	*0.30	0.32	0	2.98
Ratio of private third-party to private-pay prescription volume	*0.09	0.08	0	0.49

*Ratio was calculated for each store; therefore, mean of ratios differs from ratio of means.

4. Average acquisition cost of a private-pay prescription (based upon store-reported average wholesale prices); and
5. Average private-pay gross margin (calculated as reimbursement price less acquisition cost).

Multiple regression analysis was employed to test the linear relationship between average private-pay gross margin and the third-party to private-pay volume ratio. The average private-pay prescription acquisition cost was included to control for gross margin variance resulting from percentage markup pricing and interstore differences in drug mix. Because chains and independents differ in their strategic pricing postures and because they also differ in third-party program patronage, separate analyses were conducted for each store type. The regression statistics of the linear model are reported in Tables 32.3 and 32.4.

RESULTS

Tables 32.1 and 32.2 identify Medicaid as the predominant third-party patronizing independents, whereasenrollees of private third-party plans appear to patronize chains more heavily. The average ratio of Medicaid to private-pay prescription volume in independent stores (0.30) was significantly higher ($Z = 5.76$) than in chains (0.09). In contrast, chains' average ratio of private third-party to private-pay prescription volume (0.15) was significantly greater ($Z = 5.55$) than independents' (0.09). The average private-pay gross margin was higher ($Z = 8.79$) for independents ($4.39) than for chains ($3.42), although no significant difference was observed ($Z = 1.03$) between chains' and independents' average private-pay ingredient cost ($12.29 for chains versus $12.47 for independents).

Multiple regression analysis identified the private third-party to private-pay volume ratio as a statistically significant predictor of chains' private-pay gross margins (Table 32.3). A positive relationship was observed, indicating that higher private-pay markups are associated with chain stores exhibiting higher private third-party presence. The Medicaid to private-pay volume ratio was not significant in chains. In the contrasting regression of independents' gross margins, significance was observed for the ratio of Medicaid to private-pay volume, but not with respect to the private third-party ratio (Table 32.4).

The coefficient associated with private-pay acquisition cost was greater for independents (0.35) than for chains (0.11). The private third-party to private-pay volume ratio was the greatest contributor to explanation of

TABLE 32.3. Least-Squares Regression Summary (Chain Stores)

Dependent Variable: Average Private-Pay Gross Margin

Source	DF	Sum of Squares	Mean Square		R^2	F-Value	Prob. > F
Model	3	108.46	36.15		0.207	37.43	0.0001
Error	430	415.31	0.97	adj.	0.202		
C Total	433	523.77					

Variable	DF	Parameter Estimate	Standard Error	t	Prob. > t
Intercept	1	1,566	0.391	3.999	0.0001
Private-Pay Volume Ratio					
Medicaid	1	0.003	0.503	0.006	0.9949
Private Third Party	1	3.288	0.381	8.624	0.0001
Average Ingredient Cost (Private Pay)	1	0.110	0.031	3.517	0.0005

TABLE 32.4. Least-Squares Regression Summary (Independent Stores)

Dependent Variable: Average Private-Pay Gross Margin

Source	DF	Sum of Squares	Mean Square	R^2	F-Value	Prob. > F
Model	3	60.33	20.11	0.283	19.31	0.0001
Error	147	153.11	1.04	adj. 0.268		
C Total	150	213.44				

Variable	DF	Parameter Estimate	Standard Error	t	Prob. > t
Intercept	1	−0.291	0.621	−0.469	0.6398
Private-Pay Volume Ratio					
Medicaid	1	1.031	0.275	3.750	0.0003
Private Third Party	1	−0.351	1.064	−0.330	0.7422
Average Ingredient Cost (Private Pay)	1	0.353	0.048	7.418	0.0001

variance in chains' private-pay gross margins. In the contrasting analysis of independent pharmacies, average private-pay acquisition cost provided the greatest explanatory power of the model covariates.

The average private-pay prescription acquisition cost was significant for both chains and independents (Tables 32.3 and 32.4). Increased private-pay gross margins were associated with stores dispensing prescriptions with greater ingredient costs. These findings possibly indicate that percentage markup was a more heavily weighted pricing component for independents. Supporting evidence for this argument was provided by the differential intercepts between store types. A significant intercept was observed for chain stores (1.57), but not for independents. A zero intercept is consistent with pharmacies that primarily employ percentage markup pricing since no charge would result for drug products with an acquisition cost of zero. By controlling for acquisition cost, the intercept represents the all-payer gross margin that private-paying patients would pay for a prescription under conditions of no third-party market pressure and no product cost. In contrast, the significance observed for both intercept and acquisition cost indicates that chains apparently employ both fee- and cost-based pricing.

For independent pharmacies, the model accounted for 28.3% of the variance in private-pay gross margins compared to 20.7% of chains' private-pay gross margins. Removal of insignificant predictors from each model yielded no appreciable change in regression coefficients or respective model R^2.

DISCUSSION

As expected, chains demonstrated lower gross margins than independents; this appeared consistent with the purported lower price image of the chain store. The cross-sectional analysis of both chain and independent retail pharmacies demonstrated that private-pay gross margins increased with the degree of third-party market presence (third-party to private-pay volume ratio), a pattern consistent with the all-payer concept of cost shifting. However, this relationship was significant only with respect to the predominant type of third party facing the pharmacy. Chain stores faced a third-party market consisting largely of private plans, whereas Medicaid was the predominant third-party type served by independents.

One possible explanation is that stores do not cost shift in response to specific third parties below a market share (or impact) threshold. Stores are not likely to risk alienating the larger private-pay consumer group when faced with small third-party volume of minimal impact. It is also plausible that cost-shift responses to small numbers of third-party prescriptions could occur, but when assessed across a large private-pay consumer group, are not identifiable above the inherently large baseline variance.

The regression results were used to estimate the cost-shift premium levied upon private-pay prescriptions within chain and independent pharmacies. The average chain pharmacy within the sample faced a private third-party to private-pay volume ratio of 0.15. Regression analysis of chain pharmacies associated a gross margin increase of $3.29 per unit rise in the private third-party to private-pay volume ratio (Table 32.3).

Employing Equation 5, the cost-shift premium levied on each private-pay prescription within chain stores was estimated as:

$$(0.15) \times (\$3.29) = \$0.49 \text{ per private-pay prescription} \qquad \text{(Eq. 6)}$$

The estimated cost shift borne by private-pay patrons of independent pharmacies was less than that faced by chain store customers and consisted of a shift in response to Medicaid, the predominate third-party patronizing independents. The average independent store sampled faced a Medicaid to private-pay ratio of 0.30, with an associated dollar/ratio-unit regression coefficient of $1.03. Applying Equation 5 to the results for independent stores, the average cost shift per private-pay prescription due to Medicaid was estimated as:

$$(0.30) \times (\$1.03) = \$0.31 \text{ per private-pay prescription} \qquad \text{(Eq. 7)}$$

A greater cost-shift estimate in chain stores than in independents was somewhat unexpected. However, generally exhibiting a lower-price image, chains should be farther below the profit-maximizing pricing structure possible under existing demand conditions. Accordingly, chains should possess more latitude in which to increase private-pay prices when normally small operating margins are further squeezed by third-party market pressure.

In contrast, the higher-priced stature of independents might already have placed them close to a profit-maximizing price. Additionally, chain stores faced a third-party market largely comprised of private plans, whereas Medicaid constituted the predominant third-party served by independent stores. Private plans may impose greater costs upon participating chain stores than Medicaid imposes upon participating independents, thus promoting a greater cost-shift response to private plans.

Much of the variance in private-pay gross margins remained unexplained by the all-payer model, indicating that to some degree, cost shifting may not be a rational process. However, the unexplained variance may also result from pharmacies' likely deviation from assumed homogeneity of cost and target revenue and from lower-than-reported acquisition costs.

CONCLUSIONS

The regression findings suggest that the prices charged to private-paying patients reflect an added component that is associated with the degree of third-party incursion into the market, as well as the type of third-party involved. The pattern of this association appears consistent with the concept of cost shifting, whereby this added pricing component represents a subsidy paid by the private-pay patient to compensate the store for costs involved in serving the third-party market segment. Quantitatively, the results suggest that the average private-pay patient in Georgia paid a cost-shift subsidy approximating $0.31 per prescription in independent stores and $0.49 per prescription in chains. A greater shift estimate was observed for a given level of private third-party presence over the same level of Medicaid presence, possibly indicating that pharmacies perceive private third parties to be a greater burden than Medicaid.

In view of the rather rigid assumptions of the all-payer model, the results must be viewed with caution. Confirmation of the reported cost-shifting estimates can only be provided by longitudinal studies of pharmacies' actual price responses to changes in third-party market share and reimbursement. Considering the differences in computational method, time, and geographic region, however, the regression results appear to support cost-shift estimates previously reported by Pathak and Stone.[11,12]

Third-party insurers of prescription drugs may have exploited their market power to set low reimbursement rates, leaving pharmacists no alternative but to compensate by charging higher private-pay prices. From a policy perspective, the cost shift resulting from government programs such as Medicaid represents a hidden tax subsidy that is inequitably levied upon uninsured prescription users.

Of greater import is a cost-shift response to private third parties that represents the subsidization of these plans' profits at the expense of non-subscribers. Private plans can maintain this advantageous market position under the well-meaning constraints of antitrust laws, which prohibit pharmacists from banding together to bargain from a position of equal power. As government programs further restrict reimbursement to contain costs, private plans can "ride the bandwagon," using government rates as an indicator of what pharmacies are willing to accept.

It is unlikely that government programs will curtail the present direction of cost-containment efforts. However, profit-oriented private third parties should not enjoy the same market consideration as indigent-targeted public plans. Legislative action may be needed to protect the provider and the private-paying patient from the monopsonistic effects of private third parties.

REFERENCES

1. Kushner D, Feierman R. At the mercy of third-party payors. Am Druggist 1988;197(5):89+.

2. Schondelmeyer SW. Trends with third parties and managed health care: a pharmacy perspective. In: The changing health care environment: its impact on pharmacy and the pharmaceutical industry. Proceedings of the Midwest Conference, 11-14 Nov. 1987;17-39.

3. Morgan JP. Watching the monitors: "paid" prescriptions, fiscal intermediaries and drug-utilization review. N Engl J Med 1977;296:251-6.

4. Gagnon JP. How did we get where we are today? Am Pharm 1980;NS20: 703-10.

5. Knapp DA. Paying for outpatient prescription drugs and related services in third-party programs. Med Care Rev 1971;28(8):826-59.

6. Jones CM. Third-party prescription trends: experience in a community pharmacy. Pharm Manage 1980;152(4):157-60.

7. Siecker BR. Professional income under different payment plans. Am Pharm 1981;NS21(Aug.):49-50.

8. Anon. Pharmacists' administrative costs on 3rd-party Rx's range from 19¢ to $1.86. Pharm Times 1979;45(9):32-3.

9. Starr C. Pharmacists learn to save their skins in a managed care world. Drug Topics 1988;132(18):83-4.

10. Glaser M. Cuts from AWP will sink independents, WIPA warns. Drug Topics 1989;133(2):48.

11. Pathak DS. Cost shifting and third-party prescription drug programs. Ohio Pharm 1982;(Feb.):54-7.

12. Stone JT. Third party induced cost shifting in community pharmacy practice [Dissertation]. Lafayette, IN: Purdue University, 1985.

Chapter 33

Pharmacy Participation in Third-Party Contracts: Decision Making Through Economic and Financial Analysis

Dennis W. Raisch
Lon N. Larson
J. Lyle Bootman

INTRODUCTION

Third-party business is becoming more important to the financial success of the retail pharmacy industry.[1-5] Third-party programs are seeking price discounts in return for designating pharmacies as preferred or exclusive. The authors acknowledge that emotional factors may play a part in the decision to participate in third-party contracts. However, a method to more objectively evaluate these contracts may assist managers in making these decisions. This chapter presents a framework for evaluating the potential financial impact of specific third-party contracts, allowing comparison of decision alternatives.

ECONOMIC PRINCIPLES RELATED TO THIRD-PARTY CONTRACTS

Before discussing the evaluation methodology in detail, a brief review of cost behavior, economies of scale, and changes in demand associated with a third-party contract is in order.

Previously published in *Journal of Pharmaceutical Marketing & Management*, Vol. 3(4), 1989.

Cost behavior refers to the sensitivity of cost to a change in the volume of output. Generally, fixed costs (e.g., depreciation, legal fees) do not vary with output, while variable expenses (e.g., bad debts, advertising, cost of goods) are affected by changes in output; semifixed costs (e.g., personnel) may act as fixed or variable expenses.[6]

The concept of marginal cost helps to elucidate how cost behavior is related to third-party contracts. Marginal cost is the additional cost associated with an additional unit of output, in this case the additional cost associated with dispensing one more prescription. The marginal costs of dispensing additional prescriptions associated with a third-party contract may be lower than average dispensing costs because fixed costs and indirect variable costs do not necessarily increase with additional prescriptions.[6] Given these cost behaviors, an increase in output may not be associated with a proportional change in cost.

This leads to the concept of economies of scale. Economies of scale occur when larger production volumes result in lower average costs. When economies of scale exist, the marginal cost and average cost curves shift downward due to improved productivity. Reeder has found economies of scale present in retail pharmacies.[7]

Shifts in demand should also be considered in evaluating the effects of third-party contracts. As third-party contracts lower out-of-pocket expenses for the customer, demand for prescriptions increases. In some cases, the increased demand will offset reimbursement that is less than usual and customary charges. An example of this is Title XIX (i.e., Medicaid), which effectively lowers price (i.e., out-of-pocket expense) from the usual charge to zero (or a nominal copayment) for beneficiaries. Given the cost behavior discussed earlier, retail pharmacy–as an industry–is better off with Title XIX than without it.

In preferred provider contracting, however, demand may not increase overall, but it may increase for the preferred pharmacies vis-à-vis their competitors. If the enrollee's cost sharing is unchanged, the overall demand for prescriptions is unchanged; yet, demand may change dramatically for individual pharmacies. If the contract results in additional new customers for the pharmacy, it can increase the demand for prescription services and nonprescription merchandise. For example, among enrollees of that third-party program, the preferences for the participating pharmacy increase when compared to the preferences for nonparticipating pharmacies. Likewise, nonparticipation can decrease demand.

These economic principles can help to explain how third-party contract participation can be advantageous to pharmacies, even though the dispensing fees may be somewhat lower than the calculated average dispensing cost. Not all third-party contracts are desirable, but careful analysis can help determine the viability of participation in a particular contract. The next section presents a method for analyzing and comparing contracts.

A METHOD FOR ANALYZING THIRD-PARTY CONTRACTS

Problems encountered in the health care field can sometimes be more fully understood through decision analysis. Decision analysis involves the enumeration of possible alternatives and the assignment of probabilities and utilities to each alternative.[8] Hypothetical administrative and clinical choices in hospital pharmacy have been examined through decision analysis techniques.[9]

A similar technique was applied to a health care management problem by Christianson.[10] In his article, a case study was presented in which three organizations were competing to serve as a comprehensive health care program for a community's indigent population. The process of rate determination by each organization was presented. Each organization's set of potential rates was evaluated based upon potential financial benefits and probability of winning the contract.

The method proposed in this chapter involves assessing financial gains obtained by participation in the contract at varying levels of prescription volume. The effect of participation has two parts: an estimation of potential profitability per prescription and a prescription volume estimate. The volume estimate is further broken down into two parts: a prescription volume and a probability value for that volume. These are multiplied together. The concept is expressed in the following equation:

Effect of Participation =   Potential Profitability Per Prescription
$\times$ (Prescription Volume $\times$ Probability)

Changes from the current situation are another aspect of third-party contracts. This problem involves current customers who are likely to become members of the third-party program under consideration. Therefore, prescriptions from these patients are lost or may be reimbursed at a lower rate if the pharmacy does participate in the contract. Estimation of the changes from the current situation includes three parts: the current profitability per prescription, a volume loss estimate, and the probability associated with that volume loss, as shown in the following equation:

Changes from the Current Situation =   Current Profit Per Prescription
$\times$ (Volume Lost $\times$ Probability)

This amount is lost whether or not the pharmacy participates in the contract because it represents a change from the current situation. However, participation in a contract can offset these losses by generating revenue.

The concept of opportunity cost should also be considered. Opportunity cost is the alternative that is foregone when a particular good or service is produced. In the case of third-party contracts, the opportunity cost represents the alternatives to participation, that is, the other ventures that can be pursued if the pharmacy does not participate. The question is whether the resources used to fulfill a third-party contract can be used in other ventures that may be more profitable, such as expanding private-pay clientele, long-term care, home health care, or new pharmacy-based health services. Thus, the three decision alternatives are:

1. Participation.
2. Nonparticipation with continued emphasis on prescription business.
3. Nonparticipation with diversification or divestiture from prescription business.

The methodology discussed in this paper emphasizes the analysis of the effects of participation in third-party contracts.

FACTORS TO CONSIDER WHEN EVALUATING THE EFFECT OF PARTICIPATION

Three sets of factors are important in evaluating the expected outcome of participation in a third-party contract: pharmacy factors, third-party factors and contract terms, and community factors. Each set affects the results of participation and changes from the current situation. These factors were tabulated through review of the pharmacy literature on third-party contracts.[11-15]

Important pharmacy factors are listed in Table 33.1. Factors primarily affecting the profitability of the contract and current profit per prescription are separated from those affecting volume estimates. For example, purchasing methods and marginal cost affect profitability, while location and previous third-party experiences help determine volume estimates and their associated probabilities. Capacity limits affect profitability. If prescription volume exceeds capacity limits, costs rise (increased costs are associated with increasing capacity), and profitability per prescription decreases. Previous third-party experience affects volume and probability estimates because experience determines which values are likely to be assigned.

TABLE 33.1. Pharmacy Factors to Consider in Evaluating Third-Party Contracts

Factors Affecting Profitability:

Marginal cost	Marginal revenue
Purchasing methods	Capacity limits
Other merchandise	Computerization
Current profit per prescription	Nonprescription sales

Factors Affecting Volume and Probability Estimates:

Location	Competitors
Third-party experience	

Third-party factors and contract terms are displayed in Table 33.2. Ingredient cost reimbursement rates and dispensing fees obviously affect profitability per prescription, whereas current enrollment, projected enrollment, reputation, and other insurance plan competitors affect volume and probability estimates. Payment timeliness (although difficult to determine prior to participation) affects profitability because interest income is lost when receivables remain unpaid.

Community factors to consider in evaluating third-party contracts primarily relate to volume and probability estimates. These factors indicate how many community members are likely to join the third-party insurance plan. Age, family size, and income can affect enrollment because particular health care programs may be more attractive to specific age groups. For example, health maintenance organizations often enroll a high percentage of young families. The types of insurance plans available in the community and through prominent local employers also affect potential enrollments. These factors are listed in Table 33.3.

USE OF THE METHODOLOGY TO COMPARE THIRD-PARTY CONTRACTS

The owner of Anytown Pharmacy recently received offers from three health maintenance organizations to participate in their prescription drug programs. Each contract was reviewed by a lawyer and found legally acceptable. Each has been evaluated and compared to the others using the following method.

The dispensing fee offered by Contract A is $2.50 per prescription. The ingredient cost reimbursement is based upon AWP (average wholesale

TABLE 33.2. Third-Party Factors and Contract Terms to Consider in Evaluating Third-Party Contracts

Factors Affecting Profitability:

Dispensing fee	Payment timeliness
Ingredient cost	Formulary
reimbursement	Claim forms
Generic drug policy	Copayments
Quantity restrictions	% Rejections

Factors Affecting Volume and Probability Estimates:

Exclusivity	Reputation
Projected enrollment	Location
Current enrollment	Competitors
Satisfaction of clients	Participation of local employers

TABLE 33.3. Community Factors to Consider in Evaluating Third-Party Contracts

- Average age
- Family size
- Income
- Local employers
- Medical insurance plans available

price). The owner analyzed the expected outcome of the contract using the following data, incorporating the average prescription costs from the previous month:

POTENTIAL PROFITABILITY ANALYSIS
(Contract A)

Reimbursement:	
Dispensing fee	$ 2.50
AWP	10.00
Total reimbursement	$12.50
Total cost per prescription:	
Actual ingredient cost	$ 8.50
(85% of $10.00 AWP)	

Marginal cost of dispensing (includes all costs) (based upon 3000 RXs/month)	$ 1.50
Total cost	$10.00

Marginal profit per third-party prescription (Contract A) ($12.50-$10.00) $ 2.50

Similar analyses were conducted for Contracts B and C, resulting in estimated net profits per prescription of $2.00 and $3.50, respectively. Other factors listed in Tables 33.1 and 33.2 are considered in the estimates of total cost and reimbursement, but are not discussed individually in this paper to maintain simplicity.

Volume estimates associated with participation were made for each contract based upon the factors listed in Tables 33.1, 33.2, and 33.3. The results are shown in Table 33.4. For example, the pharmacy owner has estimated that 50 prescriptions per month will be filled under contract A. Because the owners is sure that this number of prescriptions will be filled under the contract, the assigned probability for this volume is 1.00. Similar estimates for minimum prescription volume were made for the other two contracts.

To provide a sensitivity analysis for each contract, several probabilities were selected (0.6, 0.4, 0.2). Estimates of potential prescription volumes were then made for each contract at each probability level. In making these estimates, the factors in Tables 33.1, 33.2, and 33.3 are considered. Alternatively, prescription volumes could be held constant for each contract and probability values estimated for the volumes in each contract. This would result in similar conclusions. In any case, when comparing third-party contracts, the pharmacy manager would want to hold probability values or volumes constant.

The effect of participation is then the calculated prescription volume associated with each contract. For the volume associated with a probability of 1.00, the effect is simply the marginal profit per prescription times the number of prescriptions. Because each higher prescription volume is based on the assumption that the previous volume is attained, a cumulative effect is calculated as follows:

FACTOR	EXAMPLE (Contract A at 100 Rxs/Month)
number of additional prescriptions	50

× probability	× 0.6
× marginal profit	×$2.50

The chance nodes of the decision tree associated with each contract are presented in Figure 33.1. The cumulative effects between contracts can be compared at each probability or at the end of the decision tree. The analysis in Table 33.4 discloses the effect of participation and implicitly compares it with nonparticipation. The profits of participation are foregone under nonparticipation.

The results shown in Table 33.4 (and Figure 33.1) indicate that Contract A is the most desirable in terms of overall potential profitability (cumulative effect), followed by Contract C. The least desirable is Contract B. However, all three contracts are profitable; this is the case as long as the

TABLE 33.4. Volume and Probability Analysis for Participation (Per Month)

	Marginal Profit/R_x	Total Contract Volume	Extra R_xs	Prob.	Cumulative Effect
Contract A	$2.50	50	--	1.00	125
	"	100	50	.60	200
	"	150	50	.40	250
	"	200	50	.20	275
Contract B	$2.00	25	--	1.00	50
	"	50	25	.60	80
	"	100	50	.40	120
	"	125	25	.20	130
Contract C	$3.50	20	--	1.00	70
	"	50	30	.60	133
	"	75	25	.40	168
	"	100	25	.20	186

Prob. = Probability assigned to the volume of prescriptions or additional volume gained or lost.

The cumulative effect values are affected by the probabilities assigned to them and therefore are weighted values associated with the probability that the volumes will be achieved.

Actual revenue is the dollar amount associated with the prescription volume (Marginal profit x Volume).

FIGURE 33.1. Profitability Analysis Associated with the Various Contracts

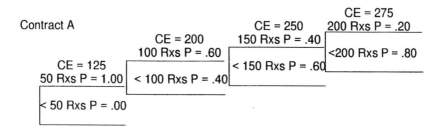

Contract A

CE = 125
50 Rxs P = 1.00

< 50 Rxs P = .00

CE = 200
100 Rxs P = .60

< 100 Rxs P = .40

CE = 250
150 Rxs P = .40

< 150 Rxs P = .60

CE = 275
200 Rxs P = .20

<200 Rxs P = .80

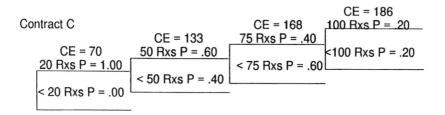

Contract B

CE = 50
25 Rxs P = 1.00

<25 Rxs P = .00

CE = 80
50 Rxs P = .60

< 50 Rxs P = .40

CE = 120
100 Rxs P = .40

<100 Rxs P = .60

CE = 130
125 Rxs P = .20

<125 Rxs P = .80

Contract C

CE = 70
20 Rxs P = 1.00

< 20 Rxs P = .00

CE = 133
50 Rxs P = .60

< 50 Rxs P = .40

CE = 168
75 Rxs P = .40

< 75 Rxs P = .60

CE = 186
100 Rxs P = .20

<100 Rxs P = .20

P = Probability that the prescription volume will occur

CE = Cumulative effect

At each intersection it is assumed that the previous probabilities have been attained.

marginal revenue associated with a contract's prescription exceeds its marginal cost.

Another concept displayed in Table 33.4 (and Figure 33.1) is that comparisons between contracts may vary based upon the prescription volume. For example, at a prescription volume of 50, Contract A yields an effect of 125 and Contract C yields 133. This makes Contract C the more desirable contract, especially if the pharmacy's optimal volume for additional prescriptions is 50.

The change from the current situation of each contract is shown in Table 33.5. Here, a probability of 1.00 is assigned to the prescription volume that the pharmacy owner expects to lose from current customers who enroll with the third party. The pharmacy owner noted that the marginal profit per prescription (i.e., marginal revenue minus marginal cost) for private pay patients is about $4.00. The owner has estimated that the current customers who will eventually be covered under Contract A account for 50 prescriptions per month and those under Contract B, 25 prescriptions per month. No current customers will be covered under Contract C. Third-party and community factors (Tables 33.2 and 33.3, respectively) are considered when making these estimates.

When the results in Tables 33.4 and 33.5 are compared, Contracts A and B may be less profitable than the precontract situation. Such is not the case with Contract C, which involves no current customers. The ultimate profitability of Contracts A and B depends upon the increased volume of prescriptions counteracting reduced profit margins.

STRATEGIC IMPLICATIONS

In assessing third-party contracts, a pharmacy is faced with three decision alternatives: (1) participation; (2) nonparticipation with continued emphasis on prescription business; and (3) nonparticipation with diversification or divestiture from prescription business.

A participation strategy relies on economies of scale or increased demand for prescription services and nonprescription merchandise to offset any price discount. A pharmacy may choose not to participate and may then devote the affected resources to another venture. If the rate of return associated with the new venture is estimated to exceed that of participation, then diversification is the preferable alternative.

The resources made available through nonparticipation may be used in other aspects of the prescription business or in other lines of business. As examples of the former, prescription-related services (e.g., blood-level

TABLE 33.5. Changes from the Current Situation (Per Month)

	Marginal Profit/R_x	Volume Lost	Probability	Losses from Current Situation
Contract A	$4.00	50	1.00	200
Contract B	$4.00	25	1.00	100
Contract C		0		0

monitoring) may be implemented or promotion may be increased to attract new market segments. Finally, the pharmacy can expend the resources in new endeavors. It can diversify, with or without divesting from the prescription business. Diversification may be into other health lines (e.g., home health, long-term care) or into retail lines of business that are not health related.

SUMMARY

As prescription revenue is increasingly affected by third-party programs, the pharmacy manager must be aware of the factors and implications of the decision to participate. This chapter has presented a framework in which some of the variables can be quantified. As with any decision-making tool, however, managerial judgment must be used.

REFERENCES

1. Anon., "State Executives Publish Survey of Third-Party Prescription Plans," *American Pharmacy*, n.s. no. 7, 24 (1984): 8-9.

2. Anderson, L. J., "Adapting to the New World of Pharmacy Economics," *American Pharmacy*, n.s. no. 7, 24 (1984): 33-36.

3. Schondelmeyer, S. W., "HMOs and PPOs: Strategy for Success Through Pharmacy Networks," *American Pharmacy*, n.s. no. 1, 26 (1986): 44-55.

4. Anon., "Executive Summary–APhA Commission on Third Party Programs," *American Pharmacy*, n.s. no. 4, 26 (1986): 49-58.

5. Ehrlich, F. J., "Learning to Live with Third Party," *Drug Topics*, 17 February 1986, pp. 38-40.

6. Larson, L. N., "Selective Contracting with Third-Party Programs," *Drug Topics*, 3 November 1986, pp. 35-39.

7. Reeder, C. E., "Returns to Scale in Retail Community Pharmacy Prescription Department Operations," *Journal of Pharmaceutical Marketing and Management*, no. 4, 1(1987): 115-125.

8. Weinstein, M. C., and H. V. Fineberg. *Clinical Decision Analysis*. Philadelphia: W. B. Saunders Company, 1980.

9. Einarson, T. R., W. F. McGhan, and J. L. Bootman, "Decision Analysis Applied to Pharmacy Practice," *American Journal of Hospital Pharmacy*, 42 (Feb. 1985): 364-371.

10. Christianson, J. B., "Competitive Bidding: The Challenge for Health Care Managers," *Health Care Management Review*, no. 2, 10(1985): 39-53.

11. Fink, J. L. III, "Evaluating Third-Party Prescription Program Contracts," *Pharmacy Management*, no. 3, 151 (1979): 114-119.

12. Boisseree, V., "Contracting for Pharmaceutical Services Part II," *California Pharmacist*, 33 (Feb. 1985): 28-35.

13. Glaser, M., "Independents Can Compete for Third-Party Business," *Drug Topics*, 18 November 1985, pp. 20-22.

14. Greifer, M., "What Are the Top 4 Problems Related to 3rd-Party Prescriptions?" *Pharmacy Times*, (Oct. 1984): 26-40.

15. Schondelmeyer, S. W., "Third Party Payment Policies: Design and Impact," *American Pharmacy*, n.s. no. 8, 26(1986): 41+.

Index

Page numbers followed by the letter "t" indicate tables; those followed by the letter "f" indicate figures.

MORE BOOKS FROM
HAWORTH PHARMACEUTICAL PRODUCTS

TAKE 20% OFF EACH BOOK!
Special Sale!